Review of ENT

Review of ENT

Sanjay Agarwal

Senior ENT Consultant
Surgeon and Teaching Faculty
New Delhi, India

Review of ENT

Preface

This is the second MCQ-based *Review of ENT* being written by me. In this book, I have used all the experiences of the previous book and the extra experiences that I have gathered since then.

This book is written by the most experienced ENT faculty which has been teaching students preparing for the various PG entrance examinations and MCI screening examination.

The need to write a new book arose because the pattern of PG entrance examination has changed completely. Now it is the **NEET** examination. In the **NEET** examination, the pattern of questions has changed, important topics have changed and, most importantly, **picture-based questions** are included. Only a very experienced faculty and the author can realize the subtle changes that the new pattern of examination needs. This new book is written keeping all this in mind. It caters to all the requirements of the new examination pattern.

Another hallmark of this book is the selection of only a few and relevant questions with absolutely correct answers from the most respected reference books. ENT is a short subject and so the books containing too many MCQs are NOT necessarily good (they can be counterproductive). I have also included **some picture-based questions** in this book. In short, this book has all that takes to crack ENT MCQs in any examination.

I feel that this book is an 'absolute must' for anyone who wishes to write any PG entrance examination.

Sanjay Agarwal

Acknowledgments

This book has come out of me and I am the sum of all the experiences throughout my life and all the people I have met in my life. Therefore, I thank and dedicate this book to every person I have ever met.

I would like to thank all my teachers and gurus for imparting on me all the knowledge that I have. It is their teaching and guidance that have made me capable of writing this book. I thank them from the bottom of my heart.

My special thanks to my parents **Shri SN Agarwal** and **Smt Savitri Agarwal**, whose blessings and motivation were a constant source of inspiration throughout my life.

This book would not have seen the light of the day without the support, inspiration and help of my wife **Dr Uma Agarwal** and my son **Pratik**. I appreciate the hardship they bear while I travel to different cities and countries to teach.

Finally, I must thank all my students, who are the real and true sources of inspiration behind this book. It is for them that I have written this book.

Contents

Part 4—Larynx

Annexures

ANNEXURE 1

MOST COMMON PATHOGENS IN ENT DISEASES

Diseases	Pathogens
• Perichondritis	Pseudomonas
• Furunculosis of ear	Staphylococcus aureus
• Malignant otitis externa	Pseudomonas
• Mastoiditis	Group A β-hemolytic streptococcus (GABHS)
• Acute suppurative otitis media (ASOM)	1. Streptococcus pneumonia (pneumococcus) 2. Haemophilus influenzae, and 3. Moraxella catarrhalis
• Glue ear/SOM	No pathogen
• Chronic suppurative otitis media (CSOM)	Pseudomonas
• Otosclerosis	Measles virus is believed to have some role in initiation of this condition.
• Ramsay hunt syndrome	Herpes zoster
• Otomycosis	Aspergillus niger
• Tonsillitis	Group A β-hemolytic streptococcus (GABHS) is the most common bacteria
• Quincy	Group A β-hemolytic streptococcus (GABHS)
• Ludwig's angina	Mixed pathogens
• Prevertebral space abscess	Tuberculosis
• Acute epiglottitis	Children—Haemophilus influenzae Adults—Streptococcus
• CROUP	Parainfluenza virus
• Nasopharyngeal carcinoma	Epstein-Barr virus (EBV)
• Laryngeal papilloma/JORRP	Human papilloma virus 6, 11
• Vincent's angina	1. Borrelia vincenti, and 2. Fusiformis
• Fungal rhinosinusitis	Aspergillus fumigates
• Acute bacterial sinusitis	1. Streptococcus pneumonia (pneumococcus) 2. Haemophilus influenzae, and 3. Moraxella catarrhalis
• Chronic bacterial sinusitis	Staphylococcus aureus
• Atrophic rhinitis	Klebsiella ozaenae
• Rhinoscleroma	Klebsiella rhinoscleromatis/Frisch bacillus
• Rhinosporidiosis	Rhinosporidium seeberi
• Maggots/myiasis	Larvae of chrysomya

ANNEXURE 2

IMPORTANT SIGNS IN ENT

Signs	Diseases
• Tragal sign	Furunculosis of ear
• Milian's ear sign	Erysipelas can spread to pinna whereas cellulitis cannot
• Laugier's sign	Collection of blood behind tympanic membrane. Usually longitudinal fractures of temporal bone
• Light house sign/pulsatile discharge	• Acute mastoiditis, and • Suppurative stage of ASOM
• Delta sign • Griesinger's sign • Crow beck sign • Tobey-Ayer/queckenstedt sign	Lateral sinus thrombophlebitis
• Aquino sign • Rising sun sign • Brown's sign • Phelp's sign	Glomus tumour (usually glomus tympanicum) Usually glomus jugulare
• Lyre sign	Chemodectoma
• Schwartz sign	Otosclerosis
• Hennebert's sign/false positive fistula test	1. Meniere's disease 2. Congenital syphilis 3. Hypermobile footplate 4. Adhesion in the medial surface of footplate
• Histelberger's sign	Acoustic neuroma/vestibular schwannoma
• Tea pot sign	CSF rhinorrhea
• Woods sign	Palpable jugulodigastric lymph nodes
• Antral sign/Holman miller sign • Hondusa sign	Juvenile angiofibroma
• Furstenberg sign	Encephalocoele
• Trotter's sign	Nasopharyngeal carcinoma
• Omega sign	Laryngomalacia
• Thumb sign	Acute epiglottitis
• Bryce sign	Laryngocoele
• Bocca sign	Post-cricoid growth
• Chevalier jackson sign	Foreign body/growth in pyriform fossa
• Steeple sign/pencil tip sign	CROUP
• Tea pot sign	CSF Rhinorrhea involving the sphenoid sinus
• Dodd's sign/crescent sign	Antrochoanal polyp
• Stankiewick's sign	Used during FESS surgery
• Tear drop sign/hanging drop sign	Blow out fracture
• Uvula pointing sign	Rhinoscleroma involving the pharynx
• Loss of scallops • Egg shell crackling sign	Mucocele of frontal sinus

ANNEXURE 3

TREATMENT OF CHOICE

Diseases	Treatment of choice
Furunculosis of ear	Ichthammol glycerin a hygroscopic solution
Malignant otitis externa	• **Ciprofloxacin** in doses of 1.5 g–2.5 g /day in divided doses can be administered for a period of 2 weeks. • Carbenicillin, piperacillin, ticarcillin can be used. • **Hyperbaric oxygen therapy may be useful in some patients** • **Surgical debridement is required in cases having necrosis or sequestrum**
ASOM	1st line- antibiotics and nasal decongestions 2nd line- Myringotomy
Glue ear	Myringotomy + grommet insertion +/– adenoidectomy
Safe CSOM	Myringoplasty/Tympanoplasty
Unsafe CSOM	Modified radical mastoidectomy (MRM)
Cholesteatoma	Modified radical mastoidectomy (MRM)
Bell's palsy	• 1st line-Steroids • 2nd line-surgical decompression of facial nerve
Otosclerosis	Active stage-sodium fluride Passive stage-Stapedectomy/Stapedotomy
Glomus tumour	Embolisation followed by surgical excision
Acoustic neuroma	Surgical excision and Gamma knife radiosurgery
BPPV	Epley's manoeuvre
Laryngomalacia	Reassurance Aryepiglottoplasty in severe cases
Thyroglossal cyst	Sistrunk's operation
Ranula	Marsupialization
Obstructive sleep apnea synd	• ***Weight loss*** • ***Oral devices*** • ***C-PAP machine*** *(Continuous positive airway pressure)* • ***Bi-PAP machine*** *(Bi-level positive airway pressure)* • ***Mandibular repositioning splints (MRS)*** • ***Surgeries***
Zenker's diverticulum	• ***Endoscopic stippling is the best option for small pouch*** • ***Dohlman's operation is an option***
Juvenile angiofibroma	• ***Radiotherapy*** • ***Chemotherapy*** • ***Embolisation*** • ***Hormonal therapy*** • ***Surgeries*** 1. *Per-oral approach* 2. *Transpalatal approach* 3. *Endoscopic intranasal approach (FESS)* 4. *Mid facial degloving approach* 5. *Lateral rhinotomy approach* ***Moure's incision*** ***Weber ferguson incision*** 6. *Infratemporal approach*
Nasopharyngeal carcinoma	• ***Radiotherapy-treatment of choice*** • ***Surgery*** • ***Photodynamic therapy***

(Contd...)

(Contd...)

Acute epiglottitis	• ***Higher generation cephalosporins*** • ***Supportive management***
CROUP	• ***Steroids*** • ***Epinephrine inhalation*** • ***Antibiotics (ampicillin)***
Reinke's edema	• ***Reduction glottoplasty***
Vocal cord nodule	• ***Voice rest*** • ***Microlaryngeal surgery*** • ***Botox injections***
Vocal cord polyp	• ***Microlaryngeal surgery*** • ***Pulse dye laser*** • ***Stop anticoagulants***
Puberphonia	• ***Counselling*** • ***Gutzmann's technique*** • ***Isshiki's thyroplasty type III***
Androphonia	• ***Counselling*** • ***Isshiki's thyroplasty type IV***
Spasmodic dysphonia	• ***Botox injections***
Adductor palsy	• ***Speech therapy*** • ***Medialization of vocal cord*** – ***Thyroplasty type I*** – ***Injection of Teflon paste/collagen/fat etc.*** • ***Arthrodesis of cricoarytenoid joint*** • ***Nerve or muscle pedicle grafting (Tucker's surgery)*** • ***Permanent Tracheostomy/Total Laryngectomy-****for aspiration.*
Abductor palsy of vocal cord	***Voice improvement*** • ***Thyroplasty Type I*** ***Relieve stridor*** • ***Tracheostomy*** • ***Thyroplasty Type II*** • ***Arytenoidectomy(woodman's surgery)*** • ***Cordectomy-usually by CO_2 laser excision*** • ***Dennis and Kashima's procedure*** • ***Nerve grafting*** • ***Muscle pedicle grafting (Tucker's)*** ***Relieve aspiration*** • ***Tracheostomy*** • ***Permanent Trachoestomy/Total Laryngectomy-****this is the* ***gold standard treatment*** *for aspiration.* • ***Epiglottopexy*** • *Vocal cord placation*
Laryngeal papilloma (JORRP)	• ***Microdebridement + intralesional cidofovir/Acyclovir*** • ***CO_2 laser*** • ***Photodynamic therapy***
Laryngeal CA	T1, T2 glottic-Transoral laser microsurgery (TLM) Radiotherapy is the 2nd option T1, T2 supraglottis- Horizontal partial laryngectomy is the best option Transoral laser microsurgery with regular follow-up Radiotherapy is the 2nd option T3- Radiotherapy plus chemotherapy (chemoradiation) Conservative/total laryngectomy & radiotherapy Bilateral neck dissection is combined T4- Radiotherapy plus chemotherapy (chemoradiation) Total laryngectomy followed by radiotherapy Salvage surgery and combined chemoradiotherapy Bilateral neck dissection done wherever possible

(Contd...)

(Contd...)

Verrucous carcinoma of larynx	Total laryngectomy Conservative laryngectomy
Epistaxis	**Pinch the nose for at least 10 min**. **Septal cautery** **1. Silver nitrate (Chemical cautery)**, or **2. Bipolar diathermy (Electrical cautery)** **Nasal packing**. **Artery ligation.**
Epistaxis in *Hereditary hemorrhagic telangiectasia*	Laser photocoagulation Septal dermoplasty
Vasomotor rhinitis	Vidian neurectomy
Mucormycosis	Steroids + antifungal + FESS
Turbinate hypertrophy	**Co-blation turbinectomy/radiofrequency turbinectomy** **Argon plasma turbinectomy.**
Atrophic rhinitis	**Alkaline nasal douching** *Sodium bicarbonate* *Sodium biborate and* *Sodium chloride* **25% glucose mixed in glycerin** There are **sprays of estrogen** Injections from **placental extract**. **Kemicetine solution** 1. Chloramphenicol 2. Oestradiol 3. Vitamin D_2 4. Propylene glycol • **Systemic use of streptomycin** • **Potassium iodide** Surgeries • **Young's and modified young's operation.** • **Lautenslager's surgery**
Maggots	• **10% diluted chloroform, or** • **Turpentine oil**
Maxillary sinusitis	• Antral wash • Inf. Antrostomy • Caldwell luc's Sx • FESS
Frontal sinusitis	• Trephining • Osteoplastic flap • Lynch-Howarth Sx • Rhinofrontal sinuseptotomy or Lothrop Sx • FESS
Ethmoidal sinusitis	• Lynch-Howarth Sx • Intranasal ethmoidectomy • Transantral ethmoidectomy or Jansen-Horgan Sx • FESS
Sphenoidal sinusitis	• Jansen-Horgan • FESS
Rhinosporidiosis	• Cautery excision + • Dapsone
Rhinoscleroma	• Cautery excision + • Streptomycin • For prophylaxis; Rifampcin can be given
Blow out fracture	• Caldwell luc surgery
CSF rhinorrhea	• Conservative management with head up position
Ringertz tumour	• Excision with wide margin
Sinonasal carcinoma	• Maxillectomy followed by radiotherapy

ANNEXURE 4

SPECIAL FEATURES

Diseases	Special features
Furunculosis	• Tragal sign
Acute mastoiditis	• Pinna pushed anteroinferiorly • Ironed out mastoid • Light house sign
ASOM	• Bulging TM • Fluid level seen • Cart wheel appearance • Light house sign • Reservoir sign
Glue ear/SOM	• Retracted TM • Foreshortened handle of ,malleus • Prominent lateral processs
Lateral sinus thrombophlebitis	• Tobey-Ayer sign/Queckenstedt sign • Griesinger sign • Crowe beck sign • Delta sign
Gradenigo's syndrome	• Discharge • Diplopia • Deep seated pain (retro-orbital pain)
Ear tuberculosis	• Multiple perforations • Painless • Pale granulations
Otosclerosis	• Schwartz sign • Paracusis willisi • Carhart's notch
Glomus tumour	• Rising sun sign • Brown's sign • Aquino sign • Phelp's sign
Meniere's disease	• Hennebert's sign (false positive fistula sign) • Tullio's phenomenon • Monaural diplacusis
BPPV	• Dix hallpike maneuver
Superior canal dehiscent syndrome	• Third window effect
Acoustic neuroma	• Loss of corneal reflex (most common manifestation) • Histelberger's sign
Laryngomalacia	• Omega shaped epiglottis
Acute epiglottitis	• Tripod position • Cherry red epiglottis • Thumb sign
CROUP	• Steeple sign (pencil tip sign)
Tuberculosis of larynx	• Turban epiglottis • Mouse nibbled/bitten appearance • Cobble stone appearance
Phonasthenia	• Posterior triangular glottis • Spindle/elliptical shaped glottis • Key hole glottis

(Contd...)

(Contd...)

Reinke's oedema	• Water balloon glottis (vocal cords)
Vocal cord nodule	• Hour glass glottis
Deviated nasal septum (DNS)	• Anterior ethmoidal syndrome, sometimes wrongly called- Sluder's syndrome
Ethmoidal polyps	• Bunch of grapes
Rhinophyma	• Potato nose
Rhinoscleroma	• Woody nose
Rhinosporidiosis	• Strawberry polyp
Wegener's granulomatosis	• Strawberry gingival
Adenoid facies	– ***Elongated face with dull expressions*** – ***Open mouth*** – ***Crowed upper teeth*** – ***High arched palate*** – ***Pinched nose***

PART 1

Ear

CHAPTERS

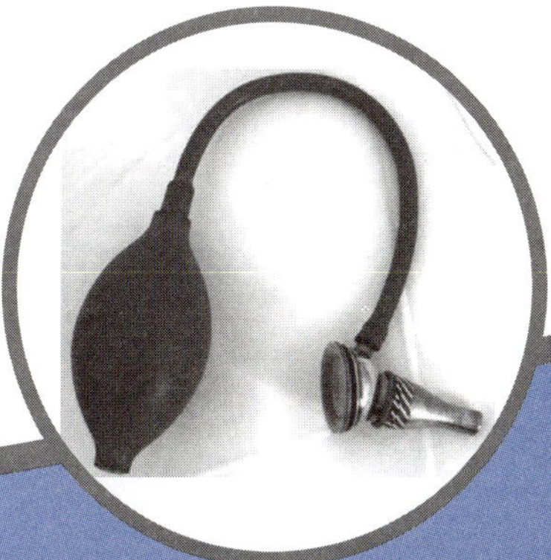

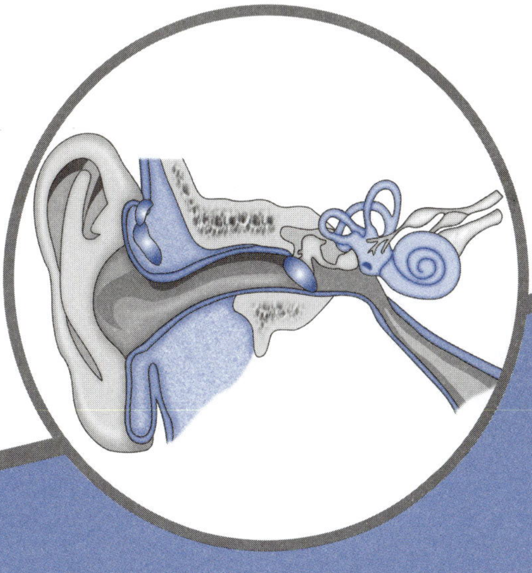

CHAPTER

1 Embryology and Congenital Anomalies of Ear

In the embryology of ENT, most important points are related to pharyngeal arches, pharyngeal clefts and pharyngeal pouches. Here are the most important facts that a PG aspirant needs to know.

The pharyngeal arches are mesodermal in origin and are **SIX** in number. They are numbered I to VI, starting from top going downward. Outside the arch is a layer of ectoderm forming clefts also called groove and inside the arch is a layer of endoderm which form pouches.

Given below are the important structures that develop from these arches, clefts and pouches. Also given are the common anomalies related to them.

IMPORTANT STRUCTURES FROM 1ST PHARYNGEAL ARCH

- Malleus and incus (THE FIRST TWO OSSICLES. They develop from ***Meckel's cartilage***.)
- Mandible and maxilla
- Muscles of mastication

Nerve supply of 1st arch is **mandibular branch** of trigeminal nerve.

MCQ

Structures that develop from Meckel's cartilage are:

a. *Malleus and incus from dorsal part*
b. *Anterior ligament of the malleus*
c. *Sphenomandibular ligament, and*
d. *Part of mandible*

IMPORTANT STRUCTURES FROM 2ND PHARYNGEAL ARCH

- Stapes **(except the inner surface of foot plate; the inner surface of stapes footplate develops from OTIC CAPSULE)**
- Upper ½ of body of hyoid (superior cornu) and styloid process.
- Muscles of facial expression.

Nerve of 2nd arch is facial nerve

MCQ

As noted above, the 1st ossicle (malleus) and 2nd ossicle (incus) develop from the 1st pharyngeal arch and therefore is supplied by the same artery. The 3rd ossicle (stapes) develops from the 2nd pharyngeal arch and is supplied by a different artery.
This lead to formation of end arteries at the incudostapedial joint (IS joint). Thus, IS joint becomes the MOST AVASCULAR AREA IN THE MIDDLE EAR. Therefore, this area is prone to necrosis.

IMPORTANT STRUCTURES FROM 3RD PHARYNGEAL ARCH

Rest of hyoid (lower ½ of body of lower or greater cornu)

Stylopharyngeus muscle

Nerve of 3rd arch is glossopharyngeal Nerve. Hence, stylopharyngeal muscle is the only pharyngeal which is supplied by glossopharyngeal nerve.

MCQ

Pinna develops due to fusion of Hillock's of His; which are partly from 1st arch and partly from 2nd arch but mainly from the 1st pharyngeal arch.

IMPORTANT STRUCTURES FROM 4TH PHARYNGEAL ARCH AND 6TH PHARYNGEAL ARCH

- Laryngeal cartilages **except epiglottis; which develops from hypobranchial eminence.**
- Laryngeal muscles.

MCQ

Epiglottis does NOT develop from pharyngeal arch. Epiglottis develops from HYPOBRANCHIAL EMINENCE.

The nerve of the 4th arch is **superior laryngeal nerve.**

The nerve of the 6th arch is **recurrent laryngeal nerve.**

Both these nerves are branches from **vagus nerve.**

MCQ

All the muscles of larynx develop from 6th pharyngeal arch except cricothyroid muscle.
Therefore, all the muscles of larynx are supplied by recurrent laryngeal nerve except cricothyroid muscle, which is supplied by superior laryngeal nerve

IMPORTANT STRUCTURES FROM PHARYNGEAL POUCHES

- First pouch develops **middle ear, Eustachian tube and the tubotympanic recess.**
- Second pouch develops **the bed of the tonsil.**
- The ventral wing of 3rd pouch develops **thymus.**
- The dorsal wing of 3rd pouch develops **inferior parathyroid glands.**
- The dorsal wing of 4th pouch develops **superior parathyroid glands.**
- The ventral wing of 4th pouch (some books say 5th pouch) develops **parafollicular cells that secret calcitonin.**

IMPORTANT STRUCTURES FROM PHARYNGEAL CLEFTS

- The 1st pharyngeal clefts develops into external auditory canal rest of the clefts do not develop into any significant structures. However, they can give rise to various anomalies like **branchial sinus, fistulas and cysts.**

ANOMALIES OF PHARYNGEAL ARCHES, POUCHES AND CLEFTS

1. **Canal atresia is a hypoplasia of external auditory canal.** It may be associated with the hypoplasia of middle ear and inner ear. In few cases, it may be associated with facial nerve anomalies and/or pinna anomalies like **microtia, i.e. small pinna.**

   It is more common in males and is usually unilateral.

   Management

   In all these patients, HRCT of the ear should be done.

   If the problem is unilateral patient may hear normally from the other ear and so may require NO treatment. However, in case of bilateral atresia, surgical correction may be required along with **bone anchored hearing aid (BAHA) implant.** In patients with microtia; cosmetic surgery of the pinna may be required.

   In case the above-mentioned surgeries are required, they should be done after the completion of the external ear growth which is **4–5 years of age.**

MCQ

External ear correction surgeries, if required, should be done after the age of 5 years.

2. **Pharyngeal/branchial sinus, fistulas and cysts.**

   Various sinuses, fistulas and clefts are possible. Of these, the 2ND **PHARYNGEAL ARCH ANOMALIES ARE THE MOST COMMON.**

MCQ

The 2nd arch anomalies are the most common anomalies.

3. **Stahl's bar (abnormal folds):** It is an abnormal fold or third crust in the pinna.
4. **Lop ear:** In this, the upper lobe of the ear folds over or flops over.
5. **Bat ear (prominent ear):** In this, the main defect is the **absence of the anti-helix with deep conchal cave.**
6. **Congenital perilymphatic fistula:** In this, there is a fistula connecting middle ear with inner ear. The presentation of this condition may be similar to Meniere's disease. The child presents with fluctuating sensorineural hearing loss with vertigo. Surgical correction may be required.
7. **Inner ear anomalies like:**
   a. **Michel's aplasia:** There is complete absence of the inner ear. Therefore, **cochlear implant is NOT possible. There is no cochlea.**
   b. **Mondini's dysplasia:** Only 1.5 turns of the cochlea are present instead of 2.5 turns. Base is present and the apex is absent.
   c. **Scheibe dysplasia:** Also called **cochleosaccular dysplasia** because there is absence of membranous saccule and cochlea. Rest is normal. This is the **most common inner ear deformity.**

Part of ear	Age of development
• External ear	Is incomplete at birth. It completes at 4-5 years of age
• Middle ear	It attains the adult size before birth
• Inner ear	Completes at 25 weeks of intrauterine life (IUL)

QUESTIONS

1. **Spiral ganglion and organ of Corti are fully developed in a fetus by?**
   a. 20 weeks b. 25 weeks
   c. 30 weeks d. 35 weeks
2. **Fetus starts hearing by what time in intrauterine life (IUL):**
   a. 15 weeks b. 20 weeks
   c. 25 weeks d. 30 weeks
3. **Commonest genetic defect of inner ear is:**
   a. Michel aplasia
   b. Mondini aplasia
   c. Alexander aplasia
   d. Scheibe aplasia
4. **Which of these may be a Korner's septum?**
   a. Petrosquamous suture
   b. Petromastoid suture
   c. Tympanopetrous suture
   d. Tympanomastoid suture
5. **Which of the following statement about development of external is true?**
   a. Pinna develops from second branchial arch
   b. External auditory canal develops from first branchial pouch
   c. Collaural fistula is second branchial cleft anomaly
   d. Second arch anomalies are the most common arch anomalies
6. **A child is born with bilateral canal atresia. You have planned to do canaloplasty (repair of canal). What is the right time of the surgery:**
   a. 6 months b. As soon as possible
   c. 5-7 years d. Puberty
7. **Most common cause of congenital hearing loss:**
   a. Ankylosis of stapes alone
   b. Aplasia of long process of incus and congenital anomalies of ossicular chain
   c. Congenital aplasia or severe dysplasia of oval and round window
   d. Persistence of stapedial artery
8. **Which is the most common type of congenital ossicular dysfunction?**
   a. Isolated stapes defect
   b. Stapes defect with fixation of foot plate and lenticular process involvement
   c. Defective lenticular process of incus
   d. None of the above

ANSWERS AND EXPLANATIONS

1. **b. 25 weeks**
   Spiral ganglion is ganglion of cochlear branch of vestibulocochlear nerve.
   Although the development of spiral ganglion starts at 4 weeks of intrauterine life (IUL), it completes at around 25 weeks IUL.
   The ganglion of vestibular nerve is **Scarpa's ganglion.**
   Both these ganglions are bipolar.
2. **b. 20 weeks**
   The inner ear or labyrinth has two coverings:
   - ***Bony labyrinth (otic capsule).***
   - ***Membranous labyrinth (saccus endolymphaticus)***

   Bony labyrinth completes its growth by 16 weeks IUL and membranous labyrinth completes its growth by 20 weeks IUL.
   It is clear that labyrinth is complete by 20 weeks IUL and henceforth the embryo can hear.
   Other facts about auditory pathway development:

Gestational age	Auditory structure development
6 weeks	Cochlear ganglion cell move toward brainstem
7 weeks	Appearance of cochlear nerve
23 weeks	Inner ear developed
30 weeks	Auditory pathway complete

3. **d. Scheibe aplasia**
   - **Scheibe dysplasia**—also called **cochleosaccular dysplasia.**

   In Scheibe aplasia, there is absence of membranous saccule and cochlea.

Rest of the labyrinth is normal.

- This is the **most common inner ear deformity.**
- Michel aplasia has complete absence of labyrinth
- Mondini aplasia has only $1^1/_2$ turns
- Alexander aplasia is reverse of Mondini aplasia. In this, base is absent and the apex of cochlea is normal.

4. **a. Petrosquamous suture**
Korner's septum is a bony covering that may be present lateral to the mastoid antrum. It appears like a bony septum. This is formed as a result of ***persisting petrosquamous suture.***
The important of this septum is that it gives a false sense of having entered the mastoid antrum during mastoidectomy.

5. **d. Second arch anomalies are the most common arch anomalies.**
   - Pinna develops from the six ***Hillocks of His.*** Hillocks of His develop from the combination of first and second branchial arches. This means that pinna develops from first and second branchial arches.
     However, if we have to select between first and second branchial arch, then ***first arch is the better answer.***
   - External auditory canal develops from ***first branchial cleft (groove)*** and NOT the first pouch.
   - First pouch develops into middle ear and Eustachian tube.
   - Collaural fistula is the ***first branchial cleft/groove anomaly.***
   - ***Second arch anomalies are the most common arch anomalies.***

6. **c. 5-7 years**
It is common knowledge that the repair of bone should be done after the completion of the growth of that bone. For the same reason, septoplasty is done after the age of 16-17 years.
The external canal is incomplete at the time of birth. It completes its growth by 4-5 years. Therefore, correction of the canal should be done after 5 years of age.
If the child is unable to hear for 5 years, the child may become ***deaf-mute child.***
To prevent this, the child is fitted with special hearing aid called ***bone anchored hearing aid (BAHA).***
When the child attains 5 years of age, the hearing aid is removed and repair of the canal is done.

Structures of Ear and their Time of Completion

Structures	Completion
• External ear	4-5 years
• Middle ear	Complete at birth
• Ossicles	Complete at birth
• Mastoid process	Appears at second year Completes at 12 years
• Labyrinth	Complete at birth

7. **b. Aplasia of long process of incus and congenital anomalies of ossicular chain**

8. **b. Stapes defect with fixation of foot plate and lenticular process involvement**
Congenital anomalies of ossicular chain in the middle ear are not very common.
Various classifications of the congenital ossicular anomalies are present.
One such classification is by Clemens'.
Important points are given below:

Class	Anomaly	Incident
1	Isolated congenital stapes ankylosis/fixation	30.6%
2	Stapes ankylosis with another ossicular chain anomaly	38.2%
3	Congenital anomaly of ossicular chain but mobile footplate	21.6%
4	Congenital aplasia of oval or round window	9.7%

From the above table, we can see that the most common anomaly is:

- ***Stapes footplate ankylosis with other anomaly of ossicle like:***
  - *Aplasia of long process*
  - *Aplasia of lenticular process*
  - *Aplasia of malleus*
  - *Fixation of malleus/incus, etc.*

CHAPTER

2 Anatomy and Physiology of Ear

Most books divide the ear into three parts:

- External ear
- Middle ear and
- Inner ear

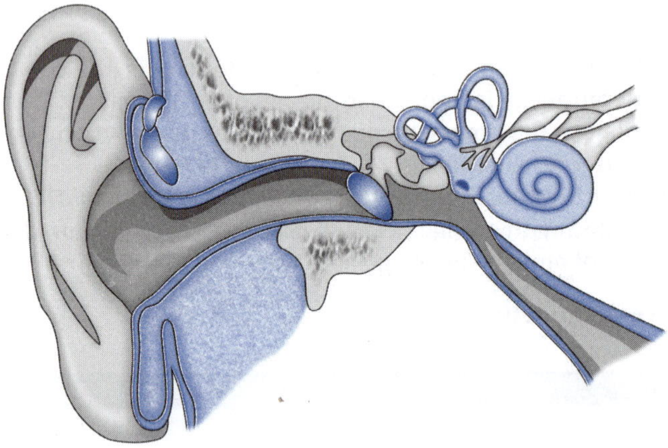

From functional point of view, it is always better to divide the ear into four parts. They are:

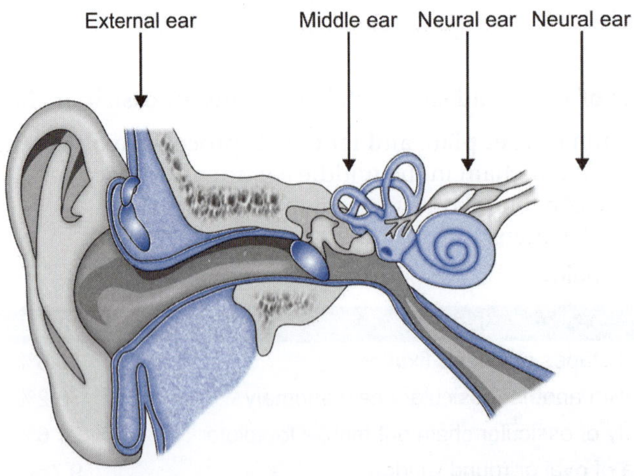

EXTERNAL EAR

External ear has two parts. They are:

a. Pinna and
b. External auditory canal

IMPORTANT POINTS FROM ANATOMY OF EXTERNAL AUDITORY CANAL

- Almost the entire pinna is made of cartilage, EXCEPT
  1. Lobule and
  2. **Insicura terminalis**

Insicura terminalis used during **endaural incision** in case of ear surgery

Approaches during ear surgeries	
Postaural approach	• Incision is behind the pinna • This is the most common approach during ear surgeries • Cosmetically it is the most acceptable approach
Transmeatal approach/Intrameatal approach	• Second most common approach
Endaural approach	• This incision passes through insicura terminalis

- The skin on the pinna is:
  1. ***tightly attached on the lateral surface of the pinna, and***
  2. ***loosely attached on its medial surface***
  3. Because of this the ***cellulites cannot spread through the lateral surface of the pinna whereas erysipelas can spread into the ear through the lateral surface of the pinna.*** This is called **MILIAN'S EAR SIGN**.
- External auditory canal is 24-25 mm long and the outer 1/3 is cartilaginous, whereas the inner 2/3 is bony.
- The cartilage part of canal is directed ***inwards, forwards and downwards.***
- Therefore, to straighten the external canal, the pinna should be pulled.

Outward, Backward and Upward Directions

- The narrowest part or isthmus is approximately 6 mm before tympanic membrane.
- Foreign body of external audtitory canal is removed by syringing. The direction of jet should be in the postero-superior.
- In the external canal, there are 2-3 *foramen of santorini* on anterior wall.
- In a child < 4-5 years old, external canal has a **fossa of Huschka**.
- **Fossa of Huschka** is formed due to incomplete formation of canal.

IMPORTANT POINTS IN THE ANATOMY OF THE TYMPANIC MEMBRANE

- It is oval in shape and is ***pearly white*** to grey white in color.
- The thickness of tympanic membrane is 0.1 mm.
- The most mobile part of the tympanic membrane is **on both the sides of the handle of malleus.**

Note

The most mobile part is neither the central part nor the peripheral part.
The correct answer is paramedian part, i.e. on either side of the handle of malleus.
When this is not given in the choices, peripheral part is the acceptable answer.

- The landmark of tympanic membrane may be any of the following:
  1. Umbo
  2. Handle of malleus
  3. Cone of light
  4. Lateral process of malleus

Note: The best answer for landmark of tympanic membrane is ***lateral process of malleus,*** whereas the best answer for *reliable landmark is* ***Handle of Malleus.***

Nerve Supply of External Ear

Pinna/auricle	External auditory meatus	Tympanic membrane
• Auriculotemporal nerve—most of lateral surface • Greater auricular nerve (C2, 3)—lobule • Lesser occipital nerve (C2, 3)—upper part of medial surface • Arnold—concha area • Facial nerve upper concha	1. Anterior wall • Auriculotemporal nerve 2. Posterior wall and floor • Arnold nerve (vagus) 3. Posterosuperior wall • Branch from facial nerve • Note: when acoustic neuroma involves VII nerve, posterosuperior wall has hypoesthesia. This is **Hitzelberger's sign**	1. Outer surface • Anterior part by auriculotemporal nerve • Posterior part by Arnold nerve a branch of vagus 2. Inner surface • Tympanic plexus (IX)

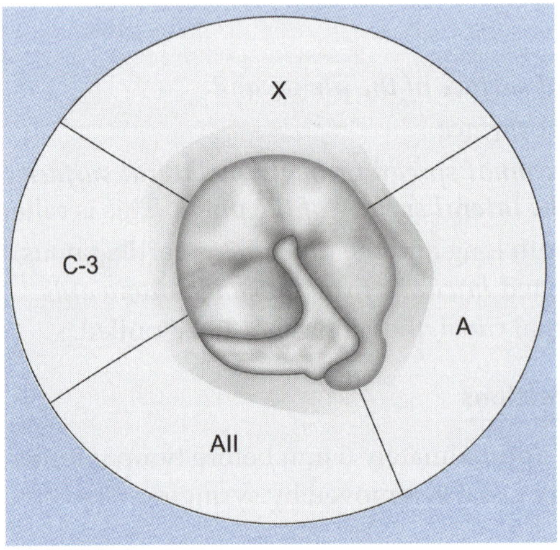

Nerve of external ear

Blood Supply of External Ear

External auditory meatus	Tympanic membrane
• Branches from external carotid artery	• Maxillary artery • Stylomastoid branch of post auricular artery • Branch from middle meningeal artery

IMPORTANT POINTS FROM ANATOMY OF MIDDLE EAR

The shape of middle ear is biconcave and is compared to a match box.

It is divided into three compartments and has six boundaries and the main contents are:

- Three ossicles
- Two nerves (facial nerve with branches and tympanic plexus), and
- Two muscles (tensor tympani and stapedius)

The three compartments are:

- *Epitympanum/Attic*
- *Mesotympanum*
- *Hypotympanum*

The narrowest part of middle ear is ***mesotympanum*** *and is 2 mm in width/depth.*

Attic of middle ear has four important structures. They are:

1. Head of malleus
2. *Body of incus*
3. ***Ligaments for suspension of ligaments and***
4. ***Corda tympani nerve, which passes between the first two ossicles.***

BOUNDARIES OF MIDDLE EAR

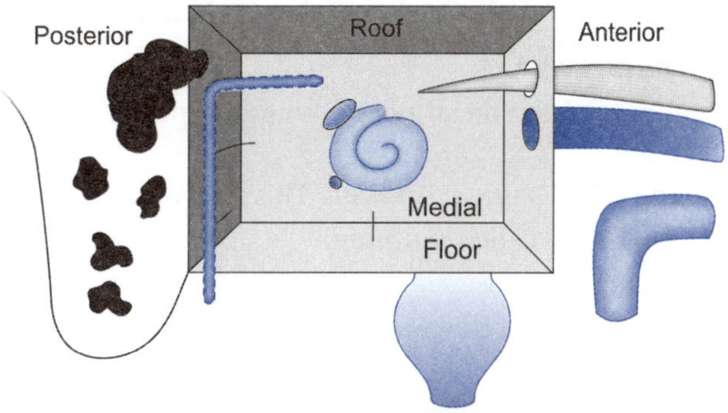

The outer boundary or lateral boundary of the middle ear is formed mainly by the tympanic membrane.
The lateral wall of attic is formed by:

- **A bony speculum called scutum.** When scutum is not given in the choices, the accepted second best answer is
- **Pars flaccida/Shrapnell's membrane.**

Between pars flaccid and the neck of malleus is a space called **Prussak's space.**

Prussak's space

The three boundaries of Prussak's space are:
1. Pars flaccida/Shrapnell's membrane
2. Neck of malleus, and
3. Lateral malleolar ligament

Prussak's space is the most common site of formation of primary acquired cholesteatoma.

Anterior wall of middle ear separates the middle ear from internal carotid artery.
The most important structure on the anterior wall are:

- the Eustachian tube and,
- canal of the tensor tympani muscle

Medial wall of the middle ear is formed by the bony labyrinth
Medial wall of the middle ear has a bulge called ***promontory***
Promontory is formed by ***basal coil of cochlea***
Behind the promontory are two windows:

1. ***Oval window***—it is covered by the foot plate of stapes
2. ***Round window***—it is covered by ***secondary tympanic membrane***

Oval window and round window should be at opposite phase of each other for proper hearing.
This means that the phase difference between the two windows should be 180 degrees.

The round window is useful in the following procedures:

1. MicroWicks/microtubules are placed at the round window during intratympanic gentamycin instillation, and
2. During the procedure of cochlear implant, the electrodes of cochlear implant are inserted through the round window into the scala tympani of cochlea.

Just anterior to the oval window is ***fissula ante fenestram.***

This is the most common site of ***otosclerosis.***

Medial wall has a bony projection called ***processus cochleariformis.***

Processus cochleariformis
• *the tendon of tensor tympani muscle winds around it and changes direction* • *processus cochleariformis acts as a pulley for this tendon* • *processus cochleariformis acts as a surgical landmark for the first genu of facial nerve*

The medial wall and the posterior wall have a canal called the ***fallopian canal.***

Through this canal of runs the ***facial nerve.***

Medial wall has the horizontal part of the facial nerve, whereas, posterior wall has the vertical part of facial nerve.

The posterior wall has an opening called *aditus ad antrum*. This is a connection between the antrum and the attic.

Posterior wall also has a bony projection called ***pyramid.***

Stapedius muscle originates from the pyramid.

In addition to all these, the posterior wall of the middle ear also has the following ridges and sinuses:

Ridges on the posterior wall of middle ear	Sinuses on the posterior wall of middle ear
1. Pyramidal eminence	1. Facial recess
2. Suprapyramidal eminence	2. Sinus tympani
3. Chordal ridge	3. Posterior tympanic recess
4. Ponticulus	4. Lateral tympanic recess

Among the above mentioned ridges and sinuses/recesses, the two important ones are:

Facial recess	Sinus tympani
The boundaries of facial recess are: 1. Facial nerve or facial ridge 2. Corda tympani nerve or annulus of tympanic membrane, and 3. Fossa incudis or short process of incus	The two boundaries are: 1. Ponticulus and 2. Subiculum Note: Sinus tympani is one of the most difficult areas of middle ear form where disease/cholesteatoma can be removed
Note: Facial recess is one of the entry sites to the middle ear during ear surgeries. This surgical approach is called "posterior tympanotomy/ facial recess approach". This surgery is used during cochlear implant	

OSSICLES OF THE MIDDLE EAR

Middle ear has three ossicles. They are connected to each other through synovial joints to form an ossicular chain. The main role of the ossicular chain is to **amplify the sound.**

The amount of **amplification done by the ossicular is about 1.3-1.7 times.**

However, total amplification done by the middle ear is **17 to 22 times.**

Joints between ossicles	Name of joint	Type of joint
Between head of malleus and body of incus	Incudomalleolar joint	Saddle joint (synovial joint)
Between incus and stapes	Incudostapedial joint	Ball and socket joint (synovial)

Important points about ossicles and joints
Ossicles ossify at 4th month of intra uterine life
Ossicular chain amplifies the sound 1.3-1.7 times
The incudostapedial joint (I-S joint) has end arteries. Therefore, it is the most avascular area of the middle ear. Hence, it is the most commonly damaged/necrosed area of the middle by the cholesteatoma
When ossicles are damaged but tympanic membrane is intact, the hearing loss is very high. The hearing loss in this case is 55-60 dB
The damage of ossicles is classified by Austin and Kartush. This classification is given below:

Depending on the types of ossicular defects, the following classification is used:

	Austin and Kartush classification
Group O	All ossicles intact M+I+S+ (all ossicles present)
Group A	Malleus and stapes present M+S+ (incus absent)
Group B	Malleus present stapes absent M+S– (incus and stapes absent)
Group C	Malleus absent stapes present M–S+ (incus and malleus absent)
Group D	Malleus absent stapes absent M–S– (all ossicles absent)
Group E	Intact chain but malleus head fixed (all present but malleus head fixed)
Group F	Intact chain but stapes fixed (all present but footplate fixed)

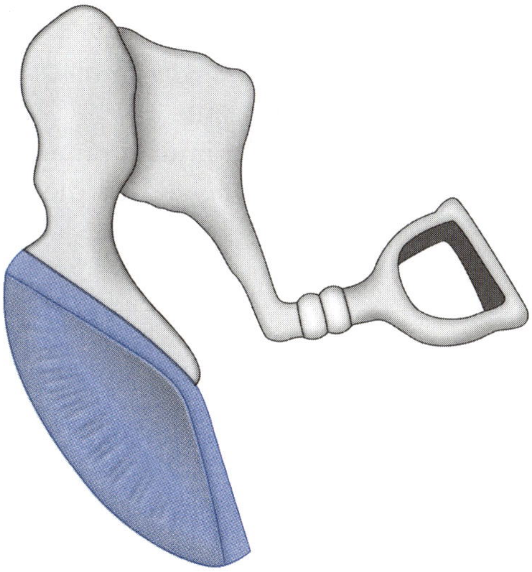

Tympanic membrane with ossicular chain
You are expected to identify the three ossicles

MUSCLES OF MIDDLE EAR

Two important muscles of middle ear are:

1. *Tensor tympani and*
2. *Stapedius.*

Tensor tympani is supplied by:

Nerve to medial pterygoid (a branch of mandibular division of trigeminal nerve).

Important points about the two main muscles of middle ear

Tensor tympani	Stapedius
Comes from the canal of tensor tympani muscle, on the anterior muscle	Comes from the pyramid, on the posterior wall
The tendon curves around the processus *cochleariformis* and is inserted on the manubrium of malleus	Is inserted onto the neck on stapes
Supplied by mandibular nerve (*nerve to medial pterygoid*)	Supplied by nerve to stapedius, a branch of facial nerve
Contraction of this muscle tenses the membrane, which causes dampening of sound	Contraction causes dampening of sound Is an important component of stapedial reflex

STAPEDIAL REFLEX/ACOUSTIC REFLEX

Normal stapedial reflex needs the following structures:

- ***Vestibulocochlear nerve*** – is **afferent nerve of the reflex**
- ***Facial nerve*** – is **efferent nerve of the reflex**
- *Stapedius muscle, and*
- *Ossicular chain*

  Therefore, defect to any of these may result in the absence of the reflex.

  This reflex is present/normal in **cochlear disease** and is absent in **retro cochlear disease.**

  This reflex is produced when the sound is ***70dB -80dB above the threshold*** of the person.

  In a normal person the reflex is produced between ***70-100dB sound level.***

  Absence of this reflex results in *"**Hyperacussis**".*

NERVES OF THE MIDDLE EAR

Middle ear is mainly supplied by *tympanic plexus which is formed by the combination of*

- **Jacobsen's nerve (a branch of glossopharyngeal nerve) and**
- **Coraticotympanic nerve (carrying sympathetic fibers for middle ear and *parotid gland*).**

Facial nerve passes through the middle ear but does not supply the middle ear.

EUSTACHIAN TUBE

Eustachian tube is 36 mm long.

It is directed ***downwards, anteriorly and medially.***

The angulation of the tube is approx. **45 degrees** in adults and almost ½ of this in children.

The tube has two parts:

1. Outer 1/3 is bony and inner 2/3 is cartilaginous
2. Isthmus is at junction of bone of cartilage

   The cartilage part of the Eustachian tube opens on the lateral wall of the nasopharynx.

   In the nasopharynx, it forms a bulge called **torus tubaris.**

Torus tubaris mainly formed because of:

1. **Cartilage of the Eustachian tube**
2. **Tensor veli palatini muscle, and**
3. **Salpingopharyngeus muscle**

This nasopharyngeal end of the Eustachian tube is **1.25 cm below and behind the inferior turbinate.** This is also called the landmark of the tube.

Small part of the tube is covered with fat. This fat is called **Ostmann's pad of fat.**

The nasopharyngeal end has some **lymphoid tissue around it.** This lymphoid tissue around the Eustachian tube is part of the **Waldeyer's ring and is called "Tubal Tonsils of Gerlach".**

Just behind this area in the nasopharynx is the **Fossa of Rosenmuller.**

Fossa of Rosenmuller is the most common site of nasopharyngeal carcinoma.

Eustachian tube has three functions. They are:

- Maintains air pressure of middle ear.
- Drainage of secretions from the middle ear.
- Protection of middle ear from infection of nasopharynx.

In the resting state, the Eustachian tube remains in a closed position.

The opening of Eustachian tube is caused by the contraction of:

- ***Tensor veli palatini muscle (more important), and***
- ***Levator palati muscle***

If the tube remains in an open position, this condition is called ***patulous eustachian tube.***

The most common complaint of ***patulous tube is "autophony"***

Causes of patulous eustachian tube

- *Idiopathic*
- *Loss of Ostmann's pad of fat*
- *Old age*
- *Pregnancy*
- *Dehydration*
- *Connective tissue disorders and disorders of the cartilage e.g multiple sclerosis.*

Some of the important tests done for eustachian tube disorders are:

- **Tympanometry (the best test for eustachian tube)**
- **Politzerization test (politzerization is more important for opening/treating the tube)**
- **Toynbee's test**
- **Sonotubometry**

BLOOD SUPPLY OF MIDDLE EAR

The main arterial supply:

- *Anterior tympanic branch of maxillary artery*
- *Stylomastoid branch of posterior auricular artery.*

MASTOID BONE AND MASTOID CAVITY

Mastoid lies behind the ear and is connected with the epitympanum through aditus ad antrum

Mastoid antrum is almost **completely developed at birth but the mastoid process is absent at birth.**

The mastoid process appears at **2nd year and completes at 12 years.**

Pneumatization of mastoid completes at 4-5 years of age.

As a result, the mastoid antrum is only **2 mm deep in a newborn child** whereas it is **12-15 mm deep in adults.**

Because of the same reason, facial nerve is more commonly damaged in children as compared to adults during postaural approach (Wilde's incision).

In order to avoid the damage of facial, this incision is given at a much lower level in children as compared to adults.

In some individuals, there is **persisting petrosquamous suture.** This persisting petrosquamous suture form a **"Korner's septum".**

The surgical/anatomical landmark of the mastoid antrum is **MacEwen's triangle/Suprameatal triangle.**

Boundaries of MacEwen's/Suprameatal triangle

1. Posterosuperior meatal wall/Spine of Henle
2. Superior temporal line, and
3. A tangent drawn between the above two

When mastoid antrum is exposed during surgery, the follow may be seen:

Mastoid antrum has these	
Solid angle	Angle formed by the three semicircular canals
Citelli's angle/Sinodural angle	Angle formed by sinus plate and dural plate
Trautman's triangle	Triangle formed by: 1. Sinus plate 2. Dural plate, and 3. Bony labyrinth or solid angle Note: Trautman's triangle and sinodural angle are the same area. Through this area disease/cholesteatoma can spread intracranially
Donaldson's line	It is an imaginary line that passes from lateral semicircular canal and bisects posterior canal perpendicularly. This line is used during endolymphatic sac decompression done for Menniere's disease.

FACIAL NERVE

Facial nerve is the most important nerve in ENT because it passes through the middle ear and inner ear.

Facial nerve is a mixed cranial nerve

Facial nerve has four components. They are:

Component of facial nerve	Comes from	Types of fibres	Supply
Special visceral efferent	Motor nucleus in lower pons	Motor fibres	Muscles of face and ear
General visceral efferent	Superior salivary nucleus	Preganglionic parasympathetic	• Lacrimal gland • Submandibular gland • Sublingual gland • Minor glands
Special visceral afferent	Nucleus of tractus solitarius	Taste fibres	Anterior 2/3 tongue
Somatic afferent fibres		General sensory fibres	Skin of posterosuperior canal

The sensory root of the facial nerve is ***Nervus Intermedius or Nerve of Wirsberg***.

This root joins the main trunk at the lateral end of internal acoustic meatus.

The course of the facial nerve is divided into various parts:

Part of facial nerve	Important points	Branches
Intracranial part	It is 24 mm long This part has no perineurium It is commonly affected by C-P angle tumours	Has no branch
Meatal part	It is 5-12 mm long It runs in anterosuperior part of meatus This part is very close to VIII nerve	Has no branch
Labyrinthine part	This is the *narrowest and smallest (3-5mm) part of facial nerve* This part is also called *Fisch physiological bottle neck* This part is most commonly damaged in Bell's Palsy	This gives rise to • *Greater superior petrosal nerve (GSPN).* • *GSPN is the 1st branch of facial nerve* • *It arises from geniculate ganglion* • *This part is involved in Ramsay Hunt Syndrome*
Horizontal/tympanic part	This part is on the medial wall of medial ear. *Dehiscence is commonly seen in this part*	No branch here

(Contd...)

(Contd...)

Part of facial nerve	Important points	Branches
Vertical/mastoid part	This is on the posterior wall of ear This part is *commonly damaged during ear surgeries* This form boundary of facial recess	• *This part has three branches* • *Nerve to stapedius* • *Auricular branch* • *Corda tympani*
Extrauricular part	Outside the ear and *stylomastoid foramen* *Has only motor fibres* *Passes through parotid gland*	All the motor branches for the face

Labyrinthine part of the facial nerve is the ***narrowest part of facial nerve*** and Hence is called **Fisch physiological bottle neck**.

BRANCHES OF FACIAL NERVE IN THE EAR

- **Greater superior petrosal nerve**—This is the first branch of facial nerve.
  It arises from the geniculate ganglion in the labyrinthine part of facial nerve.
  It joins with deep petrosal nerve to form ***vidian nerve/nerve of pterygoid canal***
  This carries secretomotor fibres for *lacrimal gland.*
  Hence, trauma to the facial nerve **proximal to geniculate ganglion (i.e, labyrinthine part) may cause dryness of eye.**
- **Nerve to stapedius**–2nd branch of facial nerve. It participates in *stapedial reflex.*
- **Corda tympani nerve**–4th branch of facial nerve.
  This forms boundary of facial recess.
  It travels between the ***malleus and*** incus and also through the ***fibrous layer and mucosal layer of tympanic membrane***
  It comes out of the ear through the ***Canal of Hugieur***.
  Corda tympani nerve:
  - *Carries the taste from the anterior 2/3 of the tongue*
  - *Secretomotor fibres* to the submandibular gland, and
  - *Secretomotor fibres* to the sublingual gland.

Duct of submandibular gland is called **wharton's duct**.

Duct of parotid gland is called **Stensen's duct**

Stensen's duct opens opposite crown of upper 2nd molar.

Calculus in most commonly seen in Wharton's duct

When the facial nerve passes through the temporal bone, it is covered a bony canal called ***the fallopian canal.*** Since the nerve is covered by the protective fallopian canal, it cannot be seen during ear surgeries. Therefore, we need few surgical landmarks during surgeries.

Important Landmarks of Facial Nerve in Middle are:

Landmarks of facial nerve	Landmark for which part of the nerve
• COG/jog	For 1st genu
• Processus cochleariformis	For 1st genu
• Pyramid	For 2nd genu
• Short process of incus	For vertical part
• Bulge of lateral semicircular canal	For vertical part
• Digastric ridge	For lower part of vertical nerve

Whereas facial nerve landmark during parotid surgery are:
- Tragal Pointer
- Styloid Process

INNER EAR

Otic capsule is a ***cancellous bone*** and develops from 14 ossifying centre.
It starts to fuse at around 16 weeks of intrauterine life and completes the fusion at 20th wk of IUL.

	Labyrinth has three parts	
1. Cochlea Has 2½ turns. Has three compartments: • Scala vestibule • Scala media/cochlear duct • Scala tympani	2. Vestibule Vestibule has two parts: • Saccule • Utricle	3. Semicircular canals SCC has three canals: • Superior canal • Posterior canal • Lateral/horizontal canal

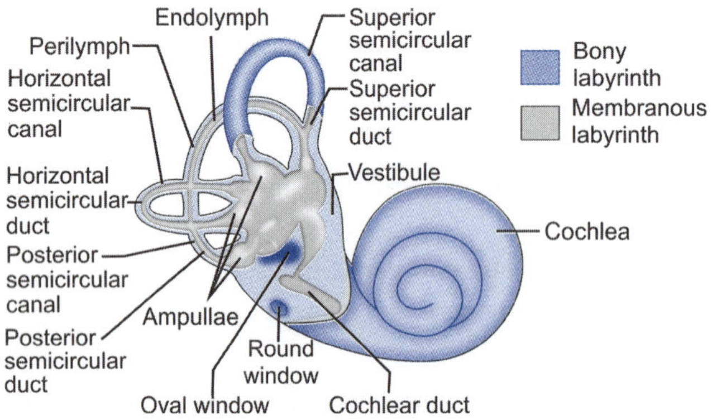

Diagram of labyrinth

Labyrinth has Two Types of Fluid

- **Endolymph—*present in the membranous labyrinth.*** Therefore this part is called ***endolymphatic sac.*** Sometimes the quantity of endolymph increases to distent the endolymphatic sac to cause ***hydrops.*** This happens in a disease called **Meniere's disease.**
- **Perilymph—*present between the bony and membranous labyrinth.***

Differences between perilymph and endolymph are given below:

Endolymph	Perilymph
• Present in membranous sac • Has more potassium ions • The electrical potential is +80-100 mV • Formed from perilymph • Absorbed in endolymphatic sac	• Present between perilymph and endolymph • Has more sodium ions • The potential is 0 mV • Formed from CSF • Gets converted into endolymph

CSF from ***subarachnoid space*** enters into scala tympani of cochlea through a duct called **the cochlear aqueduct.**

Stria vascularis and **dark cells** then convert perilymph into endolymph.

The endolymph in turn is drained, through endolymphatic duct, into the ***dural duplication in the posterior cranial fossa*** *so as* to form CSF again.

Hence, a cycle is created.

Therefore, the infection from the meninges may travel into the inner ear causing *labyrinthitis via* the **cochlear aqueduct** and

The pathogens from the labyrinth may cause meningitis via **endolymphatic duct.**

COCHLEA

Cochlea is for hearing. It has 2.5 turns.

The length of uncoiled cochlea is **35 mm.**

This turn of the cochlea takes place around a central axis called **modiolus.**

The main function of cochlea is to **convert mechanical energy of sound to action potential.**

This process is called **transduction.**

Transduction is done by the sensory organ of hearing called *organ of Corti.*

The base of cochlea preserves sound of high frequency whereas the apex preserves sound of low frequency.

This is explained by ***place theory*** also called ***Bekesy's travelling wave theory.***

Sensory organ of hearing is called *organ of Corti.*

Transduction takes place due to hyperpolarization of hair cells. Hyperpolarization of hair cells takes place due to entry of **potassium ions** into the hair cells which takes place through the **voltage gated ion channels.**

Hyperpolarization of hair cells cause releases neurotransmitter called **"glutamate"** into the postsynaptic part of cochlear nerve.

Perception of sound
Vibration of sound reaches the hair cells ↓
Opening of voltage-gated ion channels ↓
Hyperpolarization of hair cell due to entry of K^+ ions ↓
Release of neurotransmitter glutamate ↓
Action potential in the VIII nerve

Organ of Corti is present on the basilar membrane inside the scala media.

It has two types of cells:

a. Hair cells and

b. Supporting cells.

Names of supporting cells are:

- Hansen
- Claudius
- Deiters

Hair cells are of 2 types:

Outer hair cells	Inner hair cells
3,500 in number	12,000-13,000 in number
Arranged in single row	Arranged in multiple rows
Flask-shaped	Cylindrical-shaped
Synapses with afferent fibres	Synapses with mainly efferent fibres
Not so	Easily damaged by loud noise and drugs causing ototoxicity
The function is transduction of sound	It enhances the function of inner hair cell It also acts as mechanical amplifier of inner hair cells
Not so	Responsible for production of: • Cochlear microphonics (CM), and • Otoacoustic emission (OAE)

AUDITORY PATHWAY

The cochlear division of vestibulocochlear nerve supplies the hair cells of cochlea.
The ganglion of cochlear nerve is called ***spiral ganglion*** which has ***bipolar cells.***

Cochlea and the Rest of Auditory Pathway with their Functions

Pathway	Function
Cochlea ↓	Frequency and intensity determination
Cochlear nucleus ↓	First site for neural procession
Trapezoid body with superior olivary nucleus ↓	For localization of sound
Lateral lemniscus ↓	Not known, probably Resolution and organization of sound
Inferior colliculus ↓	Analyze sound stimuli
Medial geniculate ganglion ↓	Sound consciousness
Auditory cortex • Superior temporal gyrus (Brodmann's area 41) • Wernicke's area 22	Identify pattern of sound, like pitch and rhythm Differentiate between noise and music

VESTIBULE

Function of vestibule to balance the body.
Saccule and utricle are for ***linear acceleration.***
Semicircular canals are for ***angular accelerarion.***
And there are **five openings** of semicircular canals on the posterior wall of utricle.
The joining of the ***nonampullatory end of posterior canal and superior canal is called*** **"Crus commune".**
The sensory organ of saccule and utricle is called **macula** and the sensory organ of semicircular canals is called **cristae ampullaris.**

Both macula and crista ampullaris have type I and type II cells. The main difference is:

- Macula has calcium bodies called **otoliths/otoconia**
- Crista ampullaris has a **gelatinous membrane called *cupula***

Note: When this **otoconia (calcium bodies) dislodges from macula of utricle and settles in the posterior semicircular canal, the condition is called benign paroxysmal positional vertigo (BPPV).**

VESTIBULOCOCHLEAR NERVE

The ganglion of Vestibular nerve is called ***Scarpa's ganglion. It is present in the lateral part of internal acoustic meatus.***
It has ***bipolar cells,*** and connects macula and crista with vestibular nucleus.

Arterial Supply

Labyrinth is supplied by *labyrinthine artery.*
Labyrinthine artery is branch of ***anterior inferior cerebral artery (AICA).***
In some individuals (20%), it arises directly from ***basilar artery.***

Vestibulocochlear Nerve (VIII Cranial Nerve)

This is the nerve that supplies the hair cells of the cochlea and vestibule.
It comes out of the brainstem in the pons area and then travels through the C-P angle and then enters the internal auditory meatus (IAM) along with VII nerve, before it reaches the hair cell in the labyrinth.

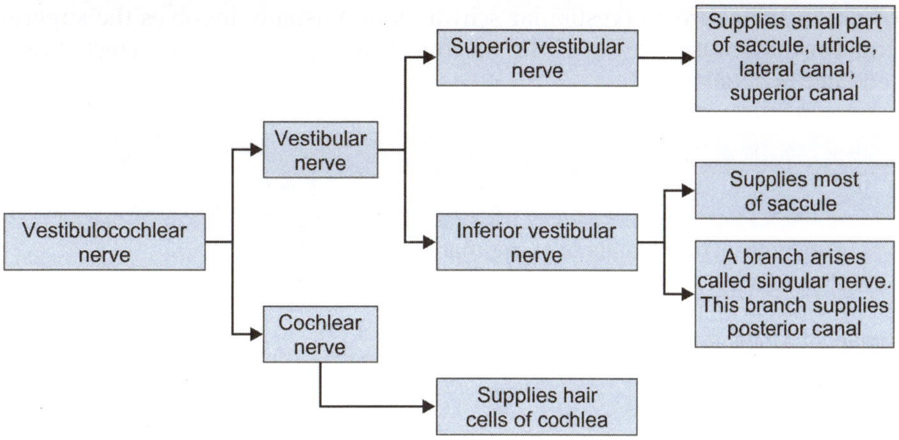

Internal Auditory Meatus

As has been discussed already, the three main branches of VIII nerve and the VII nerve pass through the internal auditory meatus (IAM).

IAM is at the medial most end of the temporal bone. It is a cone-shaped canal.

The **length of IAM is 10 mm or 1 cm.**

The width varies from **2 mm to 8 m** (because it is cone-shaped).

IAM has a **horizontal bony crest** called **falciform crest.** This crest divides the meatus into superior part and inferior part.

There is also a **vertical bar** that divides the meatus into anterior part and posterior part. This vertical bar is called **Bill's bar.**

This creates four regions in the meatus and through each region, a nerve passes. This is given below:

Part of IAM	Nerve passing through part
1. Anterosuperiorly	Facial nerve
2. Posterosuperiorly	Superior vestibular nerve NOTE: Superior part has superior nerve *Acoustic neuroma usually involves this area*
3. Anteroinferiorly	Cochlear nerve
4. Posteroinferiorly	Inferior vestibular nerve NOTE: Inferior part has inferior nerve

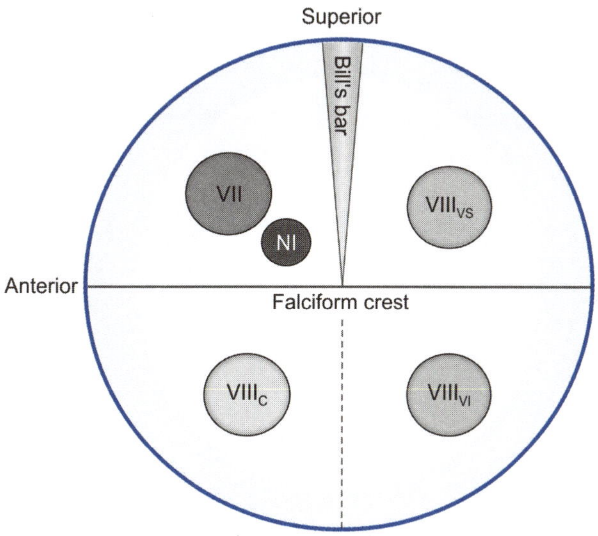

As mentioned above, acoustic neuroma (vestibular schwannoma) usually involves the superior vestibular nerve in the IAM. This tumour may cause erosion of the meatus. This erosion may be detected on a scan and help in diagnosis (discussed later in details).

Last minute revision

- Foramen of Santorini are present on the anterior of external auditory canal
- They can cause parotitis
- Tympanic membrane is pearly white in colour
- Umbo is the landmark of tympanic membrane

The boundaries of facial recess are:

1. Facial nerve or facial ridge
2. Corda tympani nerve or annulus of tympanic membrane, and
3. Fossa incudis or short process of incus
    - Incudostapedial joint is a type of ball and socket joint
    - Ossicular chain damage with intact TM causes highest hearing loss
    - Tensor vali palatini muscle helps in opening the eustachian tube
    - This muscle is supplied by nerve to medial pterygoid a branch of mandibular nerve
    - Tympanometry is the best test for eustachian tube
    - Korner's septum is petrosquamous suture
    - Ist branch of facial nerve is greater petrosal nerve
    - Labyrinthine part of facial nerve is the narrowest and smallest part
    - Vertical bar in the internal meatus is Bill's bar
    - Labyrinthine artery is the branch of AICA

QUESTIONS

1. **Which of the following conditions causes the maximum hearing loss?**
   a. Ossicular disruption with intact tympanic membrane
   b. Disruption of malleus and incus as well tympanic membrane
   c. Partial fixation of the stapes footplate
   d. Otitis media with effusion
2. **Nerve supply of tragus is:**
   a. Auriculotemporal nerve
   b. Greater auricular nerve
   c. Lesser occipital nerve
   d. Arnold nerve
3. **Vestibular labyrinth attaches with cochlea by which structure:**
   a. Ductus reunion
   b. Endolymphatic duct
   c. Saccule
   d. Utricle
4. **The cough response caused while cleaning the ear canal is mediated by stimulation of which of these:**
   a. The V cranial nerve
   b. Innervation of external ear canal by C1 and C2
   c. The X cranial nerve
   d. Branches of the VII cranial nerve
5. **Stapes footplate covers which of these:**
   a. Round window.
   b. Oval window.
   c. Inferior sinus tympani.
   d. Pyramid
6. **Eustachian tube open into**
   a. Anterior wall of the middle ear
   b. Posterior wall of the middle ear
   c. Medial wall of the middle ear
   d. Internal ear
7. **All are components of epitympanum EXCEPT**
   a. Body of incus
   b. Head of the mallus
   c. Chorda tympani
   d. Footplate of stapes
8. **First branch of the facial nerve is:**
   a. Greater petrosal nerve
   b. Lesser petrosal nerve
   c. Chorda-tympani nerve
   d. Nerve to the stapedius
9. **The effective diameter of the tympanic membrane is**
   a. 25 mm^2 b. 30 mm^2
   c. 40 mm^2 d. 45 mm^2
10. **Stapedius muscle is supplied by:**
   a. 5th nerve
   b. 6th nerve
   c. 7th nerve
   d. 8th nerve
11. **Perilymph contains:**
   a. Na+ b. K^+
   c. Mg++ d. CI
12. **Tegmen tympani separates middle ear from the middle cranial fossa containing temporal lobe of brain by:**
   a. Medial wall of middle ear
   b. Lateral wall of middle ear
   c. Roof of middle ear
   d. Anterior wall of middle ear
13. **True about Eustachian tube is:**
   a. Lateral one-third is bony
   b. Lateral two-third is bony
   c. Lateral one-third is fibrocartilaginous
   d. Lateral two-third is fibrocartilaginous
14. **Secondary tympanic membrane is present over:**
   a. Round window
   b. Oval window
   c. Lateral wall of middle ear
   d. Scala media
15. **Hyperacusis in Bell's palsy is due to the paralysis of the following muscle:**
   a. Tensor tympani b. Levator veli palatini
   c. Tensor veli palatini d. Stapedius
16. **What is attenuation reflex?**
   a. Stapedial reflex
   b. Tensor tympani reflex
   c. Stapedial reflex + tensor tympani reflex
   d. none of these
17. **First branch of the facial nerve is:**
   a. Greater petrosal nerve
   b. Lesser petrosal nerve
   c. Chorda-tympani nerve
   d. Nerve to the stapedius
18. **Function of stapedial reflex is:**
   a. Protection against loud sounds
   b. Increase movement of ossicular chain
   c. It may be absent in normal individuals
   d. Mediated by 9th nerve
19. **All are boundaries of facial recess except:**
   a. Facial ridge/vertical part of facial nerve
   b. Chorda tympani nerve
   c. Short process of incus
   d. Horizontal part of facial nerve
20. **All are true of facial recess except:**
   a. Supra pyramidal recess
   b. Medially has chorda tympani and laterally facial nerve
   c. Important in cochlear implant
   d. Middle ear can be approached through it
21. **While doing posterior tympanotomy through the facial recess there is chance of injury to all except:**
   a. Horizontal part of facial nerve
   b. Vertical part of facial nerve
   c. Chorda tympani nerve
   d. Dislodgement of short process of incus from fossa incudis
22. **Pain of which of these areas cannot be referred to the ear:**
   a. Pharynx b. Tongue
   c. TM joint d. Vestibule of nose

23. **Endo-cochlear potential is:**
   a. +45 b. -45
   c. -60 d. +85
24. **Blood supply of facial nerve is:**
   a. Ascending palatine artery
   b. Facial artery
   c. Ascending pharyngeal artery
   d. Stylomastoid artery
25. **All of these are surgical landmark of facial nerve except:**
   a. Below the processus cochleariformis
   b. Above and posterior to the oval window
   c. Medial to short process of incus
   d. Behind the pyramid
26. **According to the WHO definition of hearing loss, what is the value to classify as profound hearing loss?**
   a. 61-71 dB
   b. >81 dB
   c. >91 dB
   d. >101 dB

IMAGE BASED QUESTIONS

27. **In the below diagram, the ossicle marked anvil is also called:**

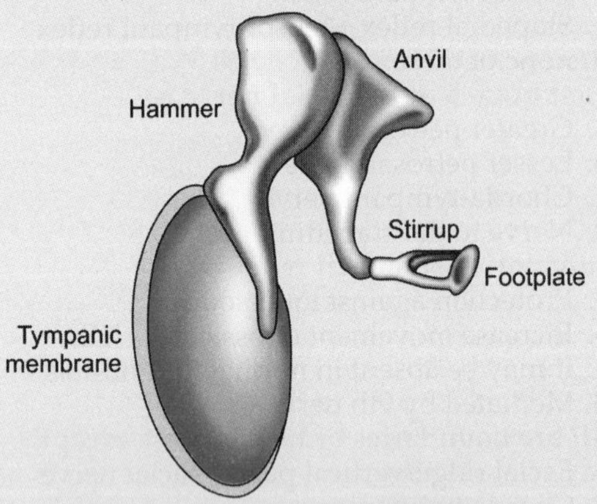

   a. Malleus b. Incus
   c. Stapes d. None
28. **The below picture is a picture of which bone:**

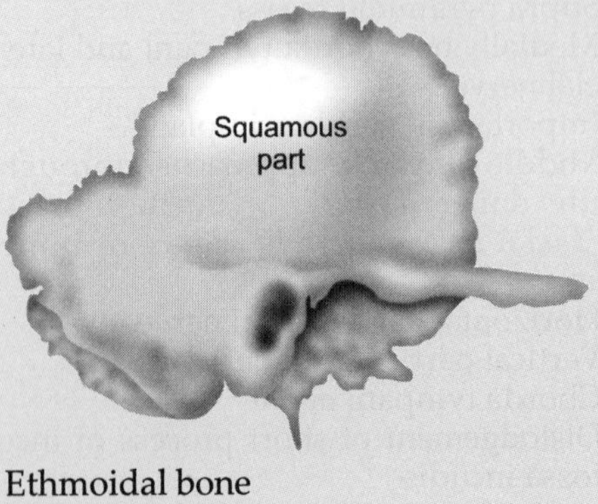

   a. Ethmoidal bone
   b. Temporal bone
   c. Sphenoidal bone
   d. Maxillary bone
29. **This is a diagram of tympanic membrane. Which side membrane is it?**

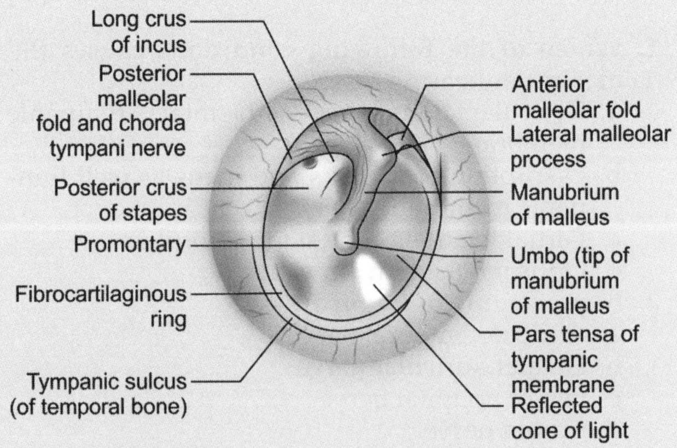

   a. Right side b. Left side
   c. Can be any side
   d. Complete information is not given
30. **This is a picture of crista ampullaris. What is the structure with arrow pointed at called?**

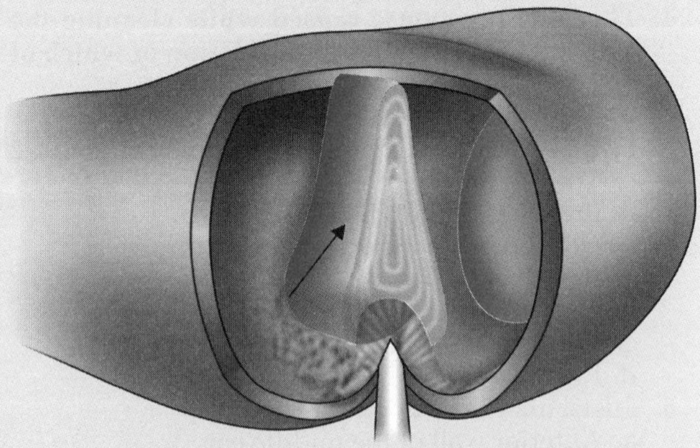

   a. Cupula b. Otolithic membrane
   c. Cristae d. None of the above
31. **Look at this picture. All are true of this picture *except*:**

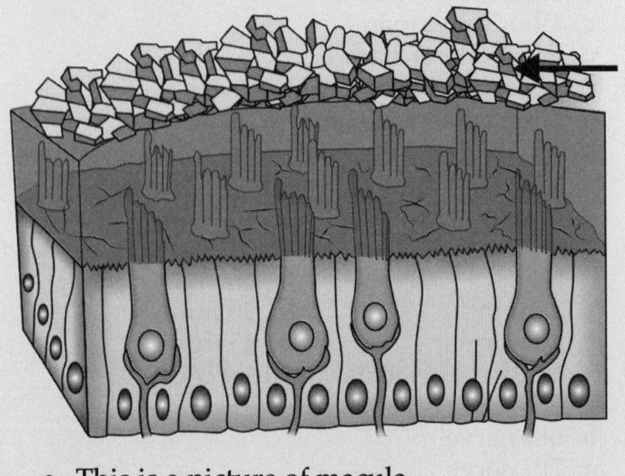

   a. This is a picture of macula
   b. This is a picture of crista ampullaris
   c. The arrow marked structure is called Otolith
   d. This is present in saccule and utricle

ANSWERS AND EXPLANATIONS

1. **a. Ossicular disruption with intact tympanic membrane**
Ossicular disruption with intact tympanic membrane will cause about 54 dB hearing loss.
The only other condition that can cause more than this conductive hearing loss is complete closure of oval window (this causes about 60 dB hearing loss).

2. **a. Auriculotemporal nerve**

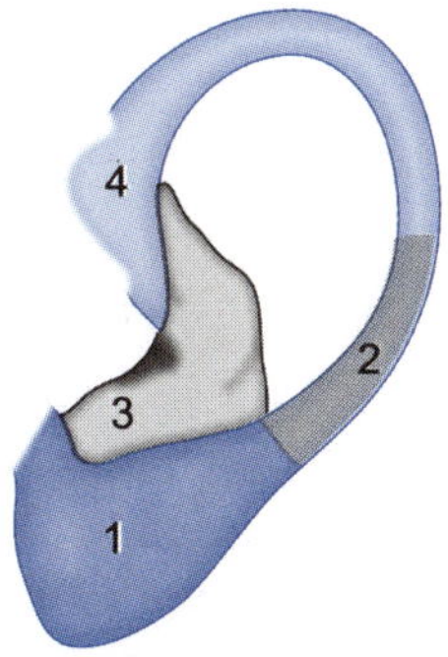

Key:
1. Greater auricular nerve
2. Lesser occipital nerve
3. Auricular branch of vagus nerve
4. Auriculotemporal nerve

From the diagram shown above, we understand that auricle is supplied by four nerves. These nerves are:
1. **Auriculotemporal nerve**. This supplies the anterior part of the auricle including ***tragus.***
2. **Greater auricular nerve**. This supplies the lower part of auricle including the lobule (medial and lateral surface).
3. **Lesser occipital nerve**. This supplies the descending helix and upper part of medial surface.
4. **Arnold nerve**. This supplies the concha area near the canal.

3. **a. Ductus reunion**

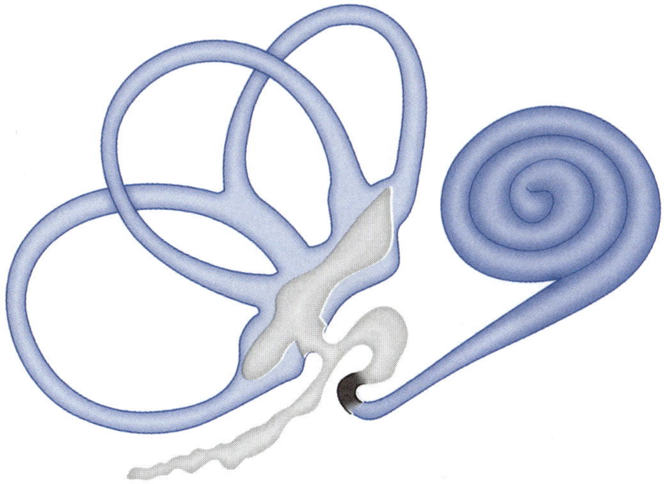

Shaded area is the ductus reunion

Developmentally cochlea and saccule together and utricle and semicircular canals develop separately. The saccule along with utricle and semicircular canals become the vestibule.
The connection between the cochlea and saccule becomes the ***ductus reunion.***
Endolymph flows from cochlea to saccule through this ductus reunion.

4. **c. The X cranial nerve**
External ear has mainly four nerves supplying it. These nerves are:

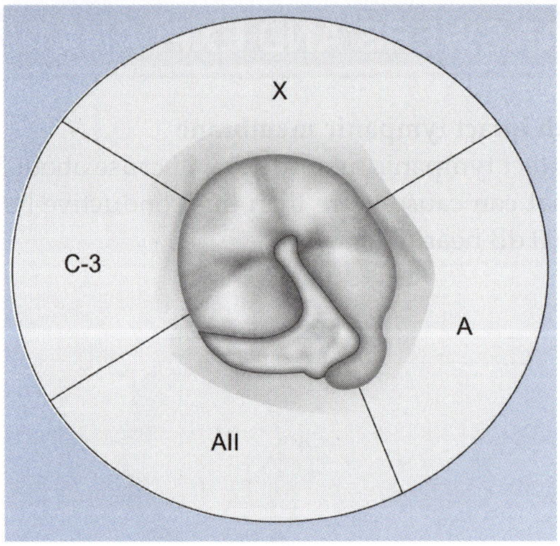

We can see from the above diagram that vagus is one of them.
The vagus nerve (X) nerve sends a branch to the external auditory canal.
The name of this branch is ***Arnold's Nerve or Alderman's Nerve***.
Vagus (X) nerve also supplies the larynx through two branches. These are
Superior laryngeal nerve, and
Recurrent laryngeal nerve.
We now understand that both ear and larynx have a common nerve, this nerve is vagus.
Hence, while cleaning the external auditory canal this nerve, i.e. vagus, gets stimulated causing coughing.

5. **b. Oval window.**
Oval window is a window on the bony labyrinth and so is part of the bony labyrinth. The inner surface of the foot plate also develops from bony labyrinth (common development).
Stapes footplate covers the oval window and this is responsible for transmission of vibrating sound energy from middle ear to inner ear.
The round window, on the other hand, is covered by secondary tympanic membrane.
These two coverings (stapes foot plate and secondary tympanic membrane) must be at opposite phase of each other for proper hearing.
Otosclerosis, which is a disease of ***fissula ante fenestram,*** spreads from ***fissula ante fenestram*** onto the oval window and so involves footplate (on the oval window).
When footplate gets involved, the ossicular chain is unable to vibrate properly.
This is the ***cause of conductive hearing loss in otosclerosis.***

6. **a. Anterior wall of the middle ear**
Eusachian tube which is approximately 36 mm in adults is partly cartilaginous and partly bony. The bony part which is the outer 1/3 opens into the anterior wall of the middle ear and the medial cartilaginous part opens into the nasopharynx. Thus it connects the nasopharynx to the middle ear.
The main function of the Eustachian tube are :
- Balance the middle ear air pressure
- Drains the secretions of the middle ear, and
- Protection of middle ear from nasopharyngeal infections.

Therefore, any problem/blockade of the Eustachian tube leads to problems of the middle ear like:
- Retraction of the tympanic membrane
- ASOM and glue ear
- CSOM etc.

Besides the eustachian tube, the anterior wall of the middle ear also has the canal of tensor tympani muscle.

7. **d. Footplate of stapes**
Epitympanum also called the attic is the upper 1/3 of the middle ear.
Most of the structures of the middle ear are present in the mesotympanum.
Hardly anything is present in the hypotympanum.

Few important structures present in the attic are:
- **Incudomalleolar joint.** This is the joint between the head of the malleus and the body oincus. Rest of the ossicular structures are present in the mesotympanum.
- **Chorda tympani nerve.** This nerve arises from facial nerve on the posterior wall of the middle and then passes between the head of malleus and body of incus in the epitympanum, before exiting from the middle ear through ***canal of hugieur***.
- **Few ligaments** for suspension of the ossicles.

8. **a. Greater petrosal nerve**

Greater petrosal nerve also called Greater superficial petrosal nerve is the first branch of the facial nerve and arises from the ***geniculate ganglion*** of facial nerve which is situated just proximal to the first genu in the ***labyrinthine part of facial nerve***.

This branch carries
- Secretomotor fibres for the lacrimal gland and minor glands of nose, nasopharynx, palate and paranasal sinuses.
- Taste fibres for the palate (NOT CONFIRMED YET)

The second branch of the facial nerve is the nerve to the stapedius and then arises the corda tympani nerve.
Lesser petrosal nerve is not a branch of facial nerve.
Instead it is a branch from tympanic plexus and carries parasympathetic fibres for the parotid gland.

Route of parasympathetic of lacrimal gland

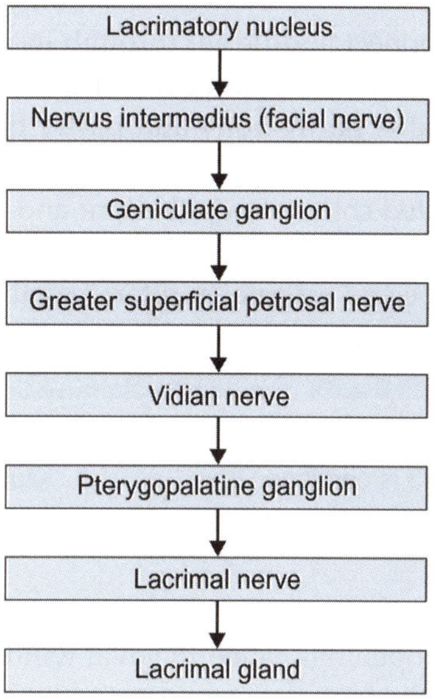

9. **d. 45 mm^2**

The greatest lengh of tympanic membrane is 9-10 mm and the breadth is 8mm.
The total area of tympanic membrane is 80-90mm^2.
Since pars flaccida does not vibrate, less than 2/3 of tympanic membrane is effective.
Hence the effective area of tympanic membrane is 45-55mm^3.

10. **c. 7th nerve**

Stapedius muscle is one of the two important muscles of middle ear. It originates from pyramid and inserts into the neck of stapes.
The function of stapedius muscle is to dampen loud sound.
It is supplied by a branch from facial nerve called nerve to stapedius.

11. **a. Na+**

Perilymph is present between membranous labyrinth and bony labyrinth.
It resembles the extracellular fluid and mainly has Na+.
Whereas, endolymph is present within the membranous labyrinth.

It resembles intracellular fluid and hence mainly has K+.
Because to this difference (in the ionic contents of these inner ear fluids), the potential of the two fluids are also different.
The potential of endolymph is approximately 80-100 mV and the potential of perilymph is 0 mV.
However, the major content of both these fluids is protein.

12. **c. Roof of middle ear**
Tegmen tympani is the roof of ear and it separates the middle ear from middle cranial fossa.
This roof of the ear has a bulge called ***arcuate eminence.*** The arcuate eminence is formed due to ***superior semicircular canal.***
On this run two important nerves:
1. *Greater superficial petrosal nerve and*
2. *Lesser petrosal nerve*

The six wall of middle ear are:
- The medial wall separates middle ear from inner ear,
- The anterior wall from internal carotid artery,
- Posterior wall from mastoid antrum,
- Inferior wall from jugular vein and
- Lateral wall from external ear
- Roof from the midial cranial fossa.

13. **a. Lateral one-third is bony**
Eustachian tube is a tube which connect middle ear through its anterior wall to the nasopharynx.
In the nasopharynx it is about 1.25 cm behind and below the end of the inferior turbinate.
This tube is 35-36cm in length and is partly bony and partly fibro-cartilaginous. The outer 1/3 is bony and inner 2/3 cartilaginous.
It is lined by pseudostratified ciliated columnar epithelium and
NOTE: In case of external canal the reverse of this is true.
Difference between eustachian tube and external auditary canal

External canal	Eustachian tube
• Is 24 mm in length	• Is 36 mm in length
• The outer 1/3 is bony and inner 2/3 is cartilage	• Outer 2/3 is bony and inner 1/3 is cartilage
• Has shape of 'S'	• Is angled

14. **a. Round window**
Middle ear has two windows like openings called the oval window and the round window.
The oval window is covered with the foot plate of stapes and the round window is covered with a membrane called the secondary tympanic membrane.
The two windows should be at a phase difference to each other for effective hearing.

SURGICAL IMPORTANCE OF ROUND WINDOW

- Electrodes of cochlear implant are inserted into the cochlea through the round window.
- A cochleostome is made on the anterior lip of round window, through which the electrodes are passed.
- During intratympanic gentamycin (ITG) procedure, the ***microwicks are placed at the round window.***
- ***In type VI tympanoplasty, the graft is placed over the round window unlike type IV tympanoplasty in which graft is placed over the oval window.***

15. **d. Stapedius**
Bell's palsy is idiopathic palsy of the facial nerve.
Of the four muscles mentioned, stapedius is the only one supplied by a branch of facial nerve.
The stapedius muscle produces the ***stapedial reflex which dampen sounds which are very loud.***

Hyperacussis

When the stapedial reflex is NOT produced (is absent), the loud sound is NOT reduced in intensity.
Patient hears the loud sound louder. This is called ***hyperacussis.***
In other words, when the patient hears loud sound louder, due to absence of stapedial reflex, the condition is called hyperacussis.
For the normal stapedial reflex the four things that are needed are:

1. Normal ossicular chain
2. VIII cranial nerve which is the afferent nerve of the reflex
3. VII cranial nerve which is the efferent nerve of the reflex, and
4. Stapedius muscle which is supplied by the facial nerve.

Damage to any of these four structures can lead to loss of stapedial reflex and hyperacussis.

For further information on this topic, kindly read the next question.

16. **c. Stapedial reflex + tensor tympani reflex**

We already know that middle ear has two muscles. The two muscles are:

1. ***Tensor tympani and***
2. ***Stapedius***

Stapedius muscle	Tensor tympani muscle
• *It originates from pyramid on posterior wall* • *It inserts on the neck of stapes* • *It is supplied by branch of facial nerve* • *It produces stapedial reflex which dampens loud noise*	• *It originates from canal of tensor tympani on anterior wall* • *It inserts on the neck of malleus* • *It is supplied by nerve to medial pterygoid from trigeminal* • *It produces tensor tympanic reflex causing dampening of loud noise.*

Please notice that one is inserted to first ossicle (Malleus) and the other is inserted onto last ossicle (Stapes).
The basic fuction of both these muscles is the same i.e dampens the loud noise.
In cases of loud noise, both the muscles contract together and the ***ossicular chain becomes rigid leading to reduced vibration and therefore, attenuation of sound (this is similar to dampening of sound)***
It is clear that attenuation requires both the reflexes.

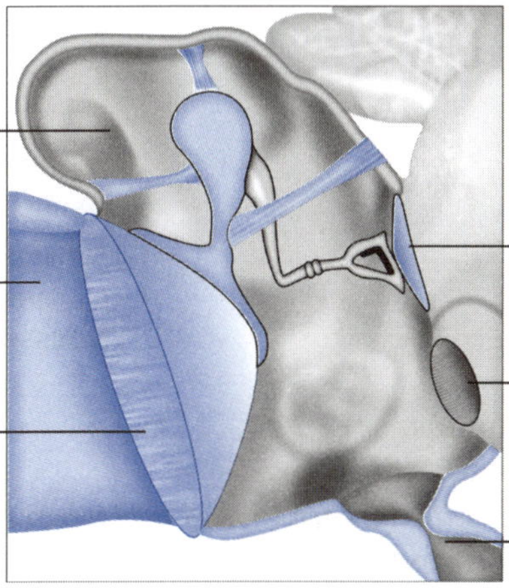

Both the middle muscles

Form the above mentioned facts it is clear that ***palsy of both the muscles of middle ear can cause hyperacussis.***
But of these only the stapedius is supplied by the facial nerve.
Hence, facial nerve palsy will not affect the tensor tympani muscle.

17. a. Greater petrosal nerve

Greater petrosal nerve also called Greater superficial petrosal nerve is the first branch of the facial nerve and arises from the geniculate ganglion of facial nerve which is situated just proximal to the first genu in the ***labyrinthine part of facial nerve***.

VII facial nerve

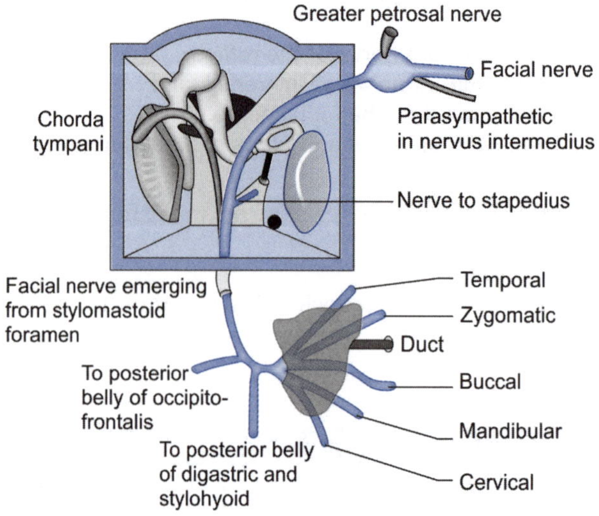

Origin of this nerve

This branch carries secretomotor fibres for the lacrimal gland and glands of nose, nasopharynx, palate and paranasal sinuses.

- The second branch of the facial nerve is the nerve to the stapedius after which arises the third branch, the corda tympani nerve.
- Lesser petrosal nerve is not a branch of facial nerve. It is a branch from ***tympanic plexus and carries fibres for the parotid gland***.

Braches of facial nerve in the temporal bone	
1. Greater petrosal nerve	• It is first branch of facial nerve • It arises from ***labyrinthine part*** of facial nerve.
2. Nerve to stapedius	• It is second branch of the facial nerve • It arises near 2nd genu in middle ear • It participates in stapedial reflex
3. Auricular branch	• It supplies sensory to postero-superior canal wall • This branch is responsible for ***Hiztelberger's sign.***
4. Corda tympani	• It arises near stylomastoid foramen • It passes between the first two ossicles in attic

18. a. Protection against loud sounds

Stapedial reflex is also called acoustic reflex.

Primary function of this reflex is to ***dampen loud sound when the sound exceeds 85 dB so as to protect the inner ear from noise-induced hearing loss (NIHL).***

This is achieved by the contraction of stapedius muscle and ***reducing the vibration of the ossicular chain.***

It is mediated by two cranial nerves i.e VII nerve (efferent nerve) and VIII nerve (afferent nerve). IX nerve is NOT used in this reflex.

19. d. Horizontal part of facial nerve

20. b. Medially has chorda tymapnia and laterally facial nerve

21. **a. Horizontal part of facial nerve**

There are four recesses on the posterior wall of middle ear. They are:

FOUR RECESSES
1. Facial recess 2. Sinus tympani
3. Posterior tympanic recess
4. Lateral tympanic recess

Out of these, facial recess and lateral tympanic recess are ***supratympanic recess.***
Facial recess is located lateral to facial ridge.
The boundaries of facial recess are:

1. Medial boundary	• Facial ridge with vertical part of facial nerve
2. Lateral boundary	Either • Chorda tympani nerve or • Annulus of tympanic membrane
3. Superior boundary	Either • Short process of incus or • Fossa incudis

- Horizontal part of facial nerve is on the medial wall of middle ear and so cannot be a boundary of facial recess.
- Facial recess is a route or approach for the middle ear. When middle ear is approached through the facial recess, it is called ***posterior tympanotomy.***
- The most commonly use of this approach is for ***cochlear implant.***
- During this approach the boundaries may be damaged, i.e.
  - Vertical part of facial nerve
  - Chorda tympani nerve
  - Dislocation of incus from fossa incudis

22. **d. Vestibule of nose**

Pain can be referred from a site to another site only if they have common nerve supply.

IMPORTANT NERVE SUPPLY OF EAR

Part of ear	Nerve supply
Pinna	• Auriculotemporal nerve (mandibular division of Trigeminal) • Greater auricular nerve • Lesser occipital nerve • Arnolds nerve (Vagus) • Facial nerve
Exernal auditory canal	• Auriculotemporal nerve (mandibular division of Trigeminal) • Arnold's nerve (Vagus) • Facial nerve
Middle ear	• Tympanic plexus (jacobsen's nerve from glossopharyngeal)

From the table given above we can see the important branches supplying ear are from four cranial nerves:

1. Mandibular division of Trigeminal nerve (V)
2. Facial nerve (VII)
3. Glossopharyngeal nerve (IX), and
4. Vagus nerve (V)

Therefore, any area having sensory supply from any of these nerves may cause referred pain inot the ear.
- Pharynx has supply from glossopharyngeal nerve and so can cause referred pain into the ear.
- Larynx has supply from vagus and so can cause referred pain
- TM joint has supply from auriculotemporal nerve (mandibular) and so can cause referred pain
- Posterior $^1/_3$ of tongue has supply from glossopharyngeal nerve
- Anterior $^2/_3$ of tongue has sensory from mandibular nerve (lingual nerve) and so can cause pain.
- Nasal vestibule has supply from maxillary division of trigeminal and so CANNOT cause referred pain into the ear.

23. **d. +85**

Endo-cochlear potential is the electrical potential of endolymph in the scala tympani of the cochlea. In other words, it is the potential of endolymph and therefore is also called endolymphatic potential (EP).
Different part of the cochlea has different potential and varies between +80 mV to +100 mV.
The potential of perilymph is 0 mV.
We are well aware of the fact that endolymph has mainly the K+ ion and perilymph has Na+ ion.

24. **d. Stylomastoid artery**

The temporal part of the facial nerve receives blood supply from three main sources:
1. **Labyrinthine artery** – A branch of anterior inferior cerebellar artery
2. **Superficial petrosal artery** – A branch of middle meningeal artery
3. **Stylomastoid artery** – A branch of occipital artery

25. **a. Below the processus cochleariformis**

During mastoid surgery, the trauma to facial nerve is common. In order to avoid the trauma, some landmarks are used.

Landmarks of facial nerve
• COG/jog • PROCESSUS COCHLEARIFORMIS • OVAL WINDOW • PYRAMID • SHORT PROCESS OF INCUS • BULGE OF LATERAL SEMICIRCULAR CANAL • DIAGASTRIC RIDGE

Facial nerve lies anterosuperior to procesus cochleariformis.

26. **b. >81 dB**

There are many classifications for hearing impairment. Of which the WHO classification is given below:

World Health Organization's Grades of Hearing Impairment (WHO, 2008)			
Grade of impairment*	Corresponding audiometric ISO value**	Performance	Recommendations
0 – No impairment	25 dB or better (better ear)	No or very slight hearing problems. Able to hear whispers.	
1 – Slight impairment	26-40 dB (better ear)	Able to hear and repeat words spoken in normal voice at 1 metre.	Counselling. Hearing aids may be needed.
2 – Moderate impairment	41-60 dB (better ear)	Able to hear and repeat words spoken in raised voice at 1 metre.	Hearing aids usually recommended.
3 – Severe impairment	61-80 dB (better ear)	Able to hear some words when shouted into better ear.	Hearing aids needed. If no hearing aids available, lip-reading and signing should be taught.
4 – Profound impairment including deafness	81 dB or greater (better ear)	Unable to hear and understand even a shouted voice.	Hearing aids may help understanding words. Additional rehabilitation needed. Lip-reading and sometimes signing essential.

However, the WHO classification is NOT used in practice. The more practical classification especially for interpretation of pure tone audiometry is given below:

0–25dB	Normal hearing
26-40dB	Mild hearing loss
41–55dB	Moderate hearing loss
56–70dB	Moderately severe hearing loss
71–90dB	Severe hearing loss
>91dB	Profound hearing loss

IMAGE BASED ANSWERS

27. **b. Incus**
    Hammer is malleus, Incus is anvil and stirrup is stapes.
28. **b. Temporal bone**
29. **a. right side**
    Look at the cone of light. The cone of light is always in the antero-inferior quadrant. Therefore, this is a right sided tympanic membrane.
30. **a. Cupula**
    The structure marked in this picture of crista ampullaris is a gelatinous material called cupula.
    - Otolithic membrane is seen in macula and not in crista ampullaris
31. **b. This is a picture of crista ampullaris**
    This is a picture of macula which is present in saccule and utricle and is responsible for linear acceleration.

CHAPTER

3 Diseases of the External Ear

The external ear comprises of three parts, they are:

1. Pinna
2. External auditory meatus, and
3. Outer surface of the tympanic membrane

In this chapter, we shall discuss:

1. Diseases of pinna

2. Diseases of outer surface of tympanic membrane

3. Diseases of external meatus

INFECTIOUS DISEASES OF EAR

1. Diseases of Pinna

A. Hematoma of pinna/**cauliflower ear/boxer's ear**

Hematoma of the pinna is usually caused due to trauma to ear and there is collection of blood in the sub-perichondrial space.

In this, the swelling is described as C**auliflower of ear.**

It is a highly necrotizing disease. The chances of necrosis increases in three situations as follows:

i. Seen in elderly patients
ii. Patient having diabetes
iii. Associated with severe pain

Treatment mainly involves incision and drainage with tight bandage. Antibiotics are also added.

B. Perichondritis/relapsing polychondritis

(Sometimes also called *seroma*)

It is usually ***pseudomonas*** infection of the perichondrium of pinna. Sometimes, it may be immunological in nature.

On the other hand, relapsing polychondritis is usually autoimmune in nature.

In perichondritis, only the pinna cartilage is involved and, in polychondritis, along with the pinna other cartilages are also involved.

Management:

Perichondritis—antibiotics are the main line of treatment. Sometimes drainage may be required.

Iontophoresis—is a process of delivery of antibiotics to local area without systemic absorption. This therapy is needed because the cartilage is devascularised.

In cases of recurrent polychondritis, **steroids** may be added.

The main line of treatment in both the conditions are incision and drainage along with tight bandage.

NOTE

Erysipelas—inflammation of overlying skin
Cellulitis—inflammation of the soft tissue
Perichondritis—inflammation of the cartilage

Milian's ear sign: Erysipelas from adjoining area can spread to pinna (cuticular affection), where as cellulitis cannot.

MCQ'S

Cauliflower ear—another name of hematoma of pinna
Pseudomonas—pathogen causing perichondritis
Iontophoresis—may be treatment option in perichondritis
Milian's ear sign—erysipelas can spread to pinna but cellulitis cannot—sometimes useful in differentiating the two conditions

2. **Diseases of outer surface of tympanic membrane:**

   A. **Bullous myringitis/bullous myringitis haemorrhagica**

   - Bullous myringitis is caused by **influenza virus**. In some cases, it may caused by ***Mycoplasma pneumonia.***
   - In this condition, there is a bullae/large swelling/vesicle on the tympanic membrane. It could be due to **blood** collection between the outer layer and middle layer of the tympanic membrane.
   - These large swellings filled with blood are called **haemorrhagic bleb/bullae.**
   - It presents as **sudden, severe and throbbing ear ache on one side with hearing impairment.**
   - It is usually a self relieving disease.

   B. **Granular myringitis**

   It has **granular tissue on the outer surface of the tympanic membrane, which may extend onto the canal wall.**

   - It presents as foul smelling ear discharge with irritation in the ear. Pain may be absent.
   - Histopathological examination may show oedematous granulation tissue with capillaries and chronic inflammatory cells.
   - On examination, the red granulation tissue may be seen which sometimes appear as **"red carpet"** on the membrane.
   - Topical antibiotics and steroids may treat the condition.

3. **Diseases of the ear canal**

   The external ear canal is exposed to outside and is, therefore, prone to diseases. Some of the important external canal diseases are:

A. **Furunculosis/localized otitis externa**
B. **Generalized/diffuse otitis externa**
C. **Benign necrotizing otitis externa**
D. **Malignant otitis externa**
E. **Otomycosis**
F. **Herpes zoster oticus/Ramsay Hunt syndrome**
G. **Primary auditory canal cholesteatoma.**
H. **Ear wax/foreign body**
I. **Keratin obturans**
J. **Exostosis of the ear**

A. Furunculosis or Localized Otitis Externa is Very Common

- It is usually caused by ***Staphylococcus aureus.***
- Severe pain in the canal is the predominant symptom.

  Important findings are:

- **Tragal sign** is +ve (patient has severe pain on pressing tragus) .
- Pinna pushed outward due to edema (this may confuse this condition and mastoiditis)
- Retroauricular sulcus is obliterated

Untreated cases may progress to form abscesses.

Treatment

These are the option:

1. Antibiotics and symptomatic treatment is required.
2. If pain is very severe, then, ear is packed with ***Ichthammol glycerine.***

Ichthammol glycerine helps in two ways:

- It is a hygroscopic solution and therefore absorbs moisture and thus edema subsides, thus relieving pain.
- It has specific antistaphylococcal action.

3. Aluminium acetate solution—this is hygroscopic as well as astringent

Carrier of staphylococcus in the nasal cavity may lead to recurrent disease. In such cases, the following therapy may be helpful.

1. Nasal mupirocin
2. Oral flucloxacillin for 14 days
3. Bacterial interference therapy—non-pathogenic stains of staphylococcus **(stain 502A)** is inoculated in the nasal cavity.

B. Diffuse Otitis Externa

Also called ***topical ear or Singapore ear.***

This condition is similar to localized otitis externa but is more widespread

C. Benign Necrotizing Otitis Externa

In this condition, there is necrosis of a localized area of the bone with secondary inflammation of the overlying soft tissue and skin

The necrosis leads to sequestrum formation and it involves only the superficial cortical layer of bone.

The condition is idiopathic.

Treatment

Surgical removal of the bony sequestrum is sufficient.

D. Malignant Otitis Externa

Malignant otitis externa is seen in **elderly diabetic patients**, and is caused by ***pseudomonas.***

In diabetics, host response is impaired due to the following reasons:

- **Impaired leukocyte mobility**
- **Microangiopathy**
- **Impaired phagocytosis**
- **The pH of ear cerumen is high. This reduces its antibacterial property**

In this condition, the discharge emanating from the external canal is scanty and foul smelling in nature. When the discharge is foul smelling, it indicates the onset of osteomyelitis. Ironically, the patient does not have fever or other constitutional symptoms.

Otoscopy: reveals **granulation** tissue at the bony cartilaginous junction.

Microabscesses may also be seen.

Common complications are:

- **Osteomyelitis**
- **Multiple cranial nerves palsy.**

The commonly involved nerves are **VII (most common)**, IX, X, XI and XII.

LEVENSON'S CRITERIA FOR DIAGNOSIS OF MALIGNANT OTITIS EXTERNA

- Refractory otitis externa
- Severe nocturnal otalgia
- Purulent otorrhoea
- **Granulation** tissue in the external canal
- Growth of Pseudomonas aeruginosa from external canal
- Presence of diabetes and other immunocompromised state

Investigations

Imaging algorithm in these patients are:

1. **TC99 scan** to seek evidence of bone involvement
2. If this is positive, CT scan and MRI scan is a must to rule out bone and soft tissue involvement
3. Serial Ga 67 scans to assess the efficacy of treatment modality.

Staging and Classification

Stage	Ga67	TC99	Extent of disease
I	+	--	Soft tissue (necrotizing otitis)
II	+	+	Ear and mastoid (skull base osteomyelitis)
III	+	+	Extensive skull base osteomyelitis

Treatment:

- **Ciprofloxacin** in doses of 1.5 g–2.5 g /day in divided doses can be administered for a period of 2 weeks.
- Carbenicillin, piperacillin, ticarcillin can be used
- **Hyperbaric oxygen therapy may be useful in some patients**
- **Surgical debridement is required in cases having necrosis or sequestrum.**

E. Fungal otitis externa—is also called *otomycosis*

The most common fungus causing otomycosis is ***Aspergillus Niger.***

The main complaints are itching and pain with reduced hearing.

On examination, one can see dark fungal spores in the canal. At times, it gives a look of **wet blotting paper.**

Ear cleaning with antifungal ear drops is usually sufficient.

F. Viral Otitis Externa/Ramsay Hunt Syndrome

A number of viruses are known to cause otitis externa.

The most prominent virus is **herpes otitis externa,** which is caused by *herpes zoster.*

Patient presents with sever pain with presence of ***vesicles in the canal.***

Sometimes this is associated with ***facial nerve palsy.*** When herpes otitis externa is associated facial nerve palsy, it is called **Ramsay Hunt syndrome.**

The characteristic or defining feature of ram say hunt syndrome is *facial nerve palsy.*

Treatment mainly involves acyclovir 800 mg 5 times a day and steroids. Acyclovir should be started only if the patient presents within 3 days (72 hours). If the patient presents after 3 days; only steroid is given.

G. Primary Auditory Canal Cholesteatoma

This is due to abnormal migration or invasion of canal squamous epithelium into the localized bone of the canal.

This may lead to keratin formation in the canal bone causing localized osteitis or erosion of the bone; sometimes forming sequestrum.

Hence, surgical debridement of the involved bone may be needed.

H. Ear Wax/Foreign Body

Ear wax is formed when the following combine and collect in the ear canal:

- **Keratin (desquamated skin)**
- **Cerumen-released from apocrine glands.** Hence, Apocrine glands are **ceruminous glands.**
- **Sebum-secreted from sebaceous glands, and**
- **Dust**

Major components of earwax are:

- **Long chain fatty acids (both saturated and unsaturated)**
- **Alcohol**
- **Squalene, and**
- **Cholesterol**

Treatment

Syringing is the common option used.

FOREIGN BODY IN EAR CANAL

The most common foreign body in the external ear is **cotton.** Sometimes, living things and insects like cockroach may also enter the canal.

Syringing is the most common procedure for removal of wax and foreign bodies.

However, syringing should be avoided in the following situations:

1. In case of **insect** in the canal. In such cases; few drops of **OIL** should be put in the canal before syringing.
2. When the foreign body organic like pulse, wheat, rice, etc. such a foreign body may absorb water and swell in size.
3. **Button battery** in the canal. It may leak on syringing.

I. Keratin Obturans

This is accumulation of large plug of desquamated keratin in the external canal; but, **NO bony erosion as seen in primary auditory canal cholesteatoma.**

The keratin in the canal skin gives "**onion skin appearance".** This also causes expansion of the canal lumen, but **NO canal erosion.**

J. Exostosis of the External Ear

Exostosis is a kind of benign growth in the external auditory meatus. It affects the periosteum of the canal bone. They may be multiple such growths in one ear.

Exostosis is more common in people who are exposed to cold water frequently; for example, **surfers in cold water.** For this reason, it is also called **"surfer's ear".**

Usually, **NO** treatment is required.

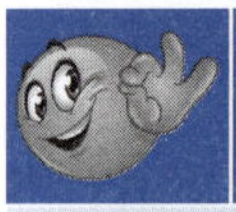

Last minute revision

- Hematoma of the pinna is also called cauliflower ear
- Exostosis is also called surfer's ear
- Tragal sign can be diagnostic of furunculosis
- Malignant otitis externa is common in elderly person with uncontrolled diabetes
- Pseudomonas is the most common pathogen
- Keratin obturans has onion skin appearance
- In case of insect in canal, oil should be put in the canal
- Button battery in the canal should be removed with forceps. Syringing should be avoided.
- Granulomatous myringitis has granulation on the tympanic membrane, giving it red carpet appearance, whereas malignant otitis externa has granulation at the junction of bone-cartilage in the external auditory meatus
- Ciprofloxacin is now the first line drug in malignant otitis externa

QUESTIONS

1. **Malignant otitis externa is seen in:**
   a. External ear malignancy
   b. Glomus tumor
   c. Pseudomonas infection in a diabetic patients
   d. Mycotic infection in a diabetic patient
2. **All of the following are true for Ramsay Hunt syndrome, except:**
   a. It has viral aetiology b. Involves VIIth nerve
   c. May involve VIIIth nerve
   d. Results of spontaneous recovery are poor
3. **Age for surgery of bilateral external canal atresia with microtia.**
   a. < 1 yr b. 5-7 yrs
   c. Puberty d. As soon as possible
4. **Dehiscence of anterior wall of the external auditory canal cause infection to the parotid gland known as:**
   a. Fissure of santorini b. Notch of Rivinus
   c. Petrous fissure
   d. Retropharyngeal fissure
5. **Organism causing otitis externa includes all *except*:**
   a. E. coli b. Candida albicans
   c. Strep pyogenes d. Staph aureus
6. **Keratosis obturans is:**
   a. Foreign body in external auditory canal
   b. Desquamated epithelial cell + cholesterol
   c. Cholesterol crystals surrounded by calcium
   d. Wax in external auditory canal
7. **A 60-year-old with complain of left ear discharge associated with mild pain for last 7 years. No complain of hearing loss on examination of ear tympanic membrane normal with discharge coming from posterior canal. Right ear canal and tympanic membrane normal. Diagnosis:**
   a. Keratosis obturans b. Left sided CSOM
   c. Left side chronic otitis externa
   d. Carcinoma external auditory canal
8. **All are true about malignant otitis externa except:**
   a. ESR is used for follow-up after treatment
   b. Granulation tissues are seen on superior wall of the external auditory canal
   c. Severe hearing loss is the chief presenting complaint
   d. Pseudomonas is the most common cause
9. **A 75 years diabetic patient with severe ear pain and granulation tissue in the external auditory canal with facial nerve involvement. The most likely diagnosis is:**
   a. Malignant otitis externa
   b. Carcinoma of external ear
   c. ASOM d. CSOM

ANSWERS AND EXPLANATIONS

1. **c. Pseudomonas infection in a diabetic patients**
   Malignant otitis externa is the most important infective disease of the external ear.
   It is caused by pseudomonas infection of the external canal.
   This is mainly seen in elderly diabetics (immunocompromised). The usual presentation is pain with otorrhea. In severe cases, there may be necrosis and so may have dark-coloured discharge from the ear.
   Because the patient is elderly and immunocompromised, the disease spreads very fast and therefore complications are very common.
   - It is NOT a malignancy
   - Glomus tumor is tumour of glomus bodies in the middle ear or jugular fossa
   - Mycotic infection in a diabetic is called ***otomycosis.***
2. **d. Results of spontaneous recovery are poor**
   Ramsay hunt syndrome is caused by varicella zoster virus infecting geniculate ganglion of facial nerve causing facial nerve palsy.
   Since the vestibulocochlear nerve is close to the facial nerve, it may be involved causing symptoms like hearing loss, tinnitus, vertigo and nausea.
   The recovery is excellent, especially, if treatment started within the first 72 hours. However, the outcome depends on the degree of damage.
   In case of degree 1 damage (***neuronopraxia***), the chance of complete recovery if 70–75%.
   Whereas, in case of degree 2 (***axonometesis***) damage, the chance of recovery is 50%.
3. **b. 5–7 yrs**
   Microtia is a congenital disease of where pinna is not developed properly.
   Microtia is divided into four grades.
   Microtia with bilateral canal atresia is grade II which is also the commonest type.
   External canal is incomplete when a child is born. It completes at 4–5 years of age.

Therefore, external ear surgeries should be done only after 4–5 years age.
Till the surgery is done, BAHA (a type of bone anchoring hearing aid) should be fitted on to the child so that the child can hear and can learn to speak.
NOTE: The same principle also applies to septoplasty.
Septoplasty should be done after 16 years of age because septum completes the growth at 16 years.

4. **a. Fissure of Santorini**
Fissure of santorini are fistulas or foramen, which are few in number and are present on the anterior wall of external auditory canal at the junction of bony canal and cartilaginous canal.
These are natural dehiscences on the anterior canal wall which may result in spread of infection from external auditory canal into the parotid and vice versa.

5. **a. E. coli**
Otitis externa is the inflammation of the external ear. It could be of the following types:
- Viral otitis externa. In this, the virus is usually ***herpes zoster*** and it spreads through the auricular branch of facial nerve in patients with ***Ram Say Hunt syndrome.***
- Fungal otitis externa also called ***otomycosis.*** Otomycosis is caused by ***Aspergillus niger and Candida albicans.***
- Bacterial otitis externa like furunculosis, malignant otitis externa, etc. the common pathogens are:
  - ***Pseudomonas***
  - ***Other Gram negative organisms***
  - ***Staphylococcus aureus***
  - ***Streptococci***

6. **b. Desquamated epithelial cell + cholesterol**
Keratosis obturans is collection of desquamated epithelial cell and cholesterol in the externa auditory canal.

Cause of Keratin Obturans

It is usually caused by abnormal migration of the canal epithelium. It may be seen in patients having ciliary defects like bronchitis and sinusitis.
Removal of the keratin plug is required.
This condition must be differentiated from ***primary auditory canal cholesteatoma.***
Primary auditory canal cholesteotoma is derived from defective epithelium migration due to defective bone (osteitis or osteomyelitis) of the canal.

Differential Diagnosis of a Plug in the Canal

- Wax. This is mixture of keratin, dust and canal secretions.
- Foreign body
- Keratin obturans
- Benign necrotizing otitis externa
- Canal cholesteatoma (***primary auditory canal cholesteatoma).***
- Osteoradionecrosis of external canal
- Tumors, etc.

7. **c. Left side chronic otitis externa**
A 60 years old person with chronic history (7 yrs) of mild pain and ear discharge is most likely having chronic otitis externa.
- Keratosis obturans has a keratin plug in the canal. Discharge is uncommon.
- In CSOM, hearing loss is very common and pain is uncommon. CSOM is very easy to diagnose clinically.
- Carcinoma cannot have such a long history of 7 years. By this much time, it would have caused massive destruction.

8. **c. Severe hearing loss is the chief presenting complaint**
We all know that malignant otitis externa is ***pseudomonas infection of the external auditory canal seen in diabetics.***
Since it is a disease of the external ear, it will cause ***conductive hearing loss.***
- ***Conductive hearing loss can never of severe or profound.***
- ***Severe and profound hearing loss which has hearing threshold >70 dB, is only possible in sensorineural hearing loss.***
- *Rest of the given options are true for malignant otitis externa.*

9. **a. Malignant otitis externa**
The above-mentioned case is a classical presentation of malignant otitis externa with facial nerve involvement.
Facial nerve is the most commonly involved nerve in malignant otitis externa.

CHAPTER

4 Inflammatory Diseases of the Middle Ear

INTRODUCTION

The four important inflammatory diseases of the middle that will be discussed are:

1. Acute suppurative otitis media/acute otitis media/ASOM/AOM
2. Otitis media with effusion/serous otitis media/non-suppurative otitis media/glue ear
3. Chronic otitis media
4. Tuberculosis of the middle ear

1. Acute Otitis Media/ASOM

ASOM is infection and inflammation of the mucosal lining of middle ear and mastoid.

It is caused by the following organisms:

- ***Streptococcus pneumonia or pneumococcus***
- ***Haemophillus influenzae***
- ***Moraxella catarrhalis.***

NOTE

The most common pathogen causing ASOM is Streptococcus pneumonia or pneumococcus.
Although some books claim that H.influenza is the most common pathogen.
Pneumococcus is the most acceptable answer.

In HIV-positive patients,it is caused Staphylococcus aureus.

AETIOLOGY OF ASOM

1. The most common cause that leads to ASOM is **viral infection** of the nasopharynx and eustachian tube. It is more common in children because eustachian tube of a child compared to adult is:
   - *shorter,*
   - *wider, and*
   - *straighter*
2. It may be seen in patients with some syndromes. Two common syndromes having ASOM are:
   a. Down's syndrome and
   b. Turner's syndrome.

ASOM has four stages. These stages are:

1. Stage of tubal occlusion
2. Stage of presuppuration
3. Stage of suppuration
4. Either stage of resolution or stage of complication

The findings are as given below:

- ***Bulging tympanic membrane***
- ***Change in color (red, congested)***
- ***Cart wheal appearance due to dilated blood vessel,***

- *Fluid level of middle ear in seen*
- *Reduced mobility of tympanic membrane. Mobility of membrane is checked by Siegel's speculum*
- *Foreshortened handle of malleus*
- *Pulsatile discharge seen as light house sign, and*
- *Reservoir sign is seen*

Uses of Siegel's speculum:

- Check the mobility of membrane
- Instillation of powered medication in ear
- Magnification
- Elicit signs like **fistula sign and Brown's sign**.
- During a tuning fork test called **Gelle's test.**

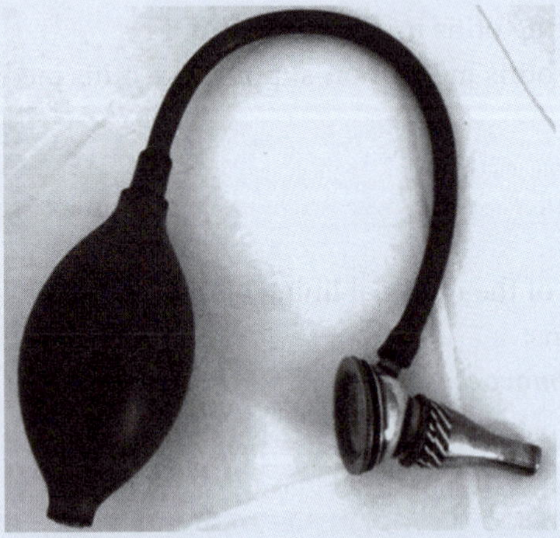

Siegel's speculum

Investigation

Tympanometry is the investigation of choice. It usually shows "Type B" tympanogram.

Treatment

Eighty five to ninety five percent of ASOM heals spontaneously and so NO treatment is required in these patients.
Where medicines are needed; **antibiotics with nasal decongestions** are useful.
However, the treatment of choice in ASOM is **myringotomy**.
Myringotomy is usually done in *Posteroinferior quadrant* of tympanic membrane

2. Otitis Media with Effusion/Glue Ear

Also called *serous otitis media*/adhesive otitis media
Serous otitis media is chronic accumulation of mucus in the middle ear and mastoid air cell.
Chronic serous otitis media is the collection of mucus for more than 12 weeks.
The mucus is ***sterile fluid*** and so does not have infection.
Glue ear is the ***commonest cause of hearing loss in children.***

Findings in Glue Ear

- *Retracted tympanic membrane*
- *Prominence of lateral process of malleus*
- *Pale / yellow look / bluish look of tympanic membrane with* ***dull look***
- *Fluid level is seen along with* ***air bubble****.*
- *Reduced mobility of tympanic membrane*
- *Foreshortened handle of malleus.*

Whereas ASOM has bulging tympanic membrane; glue ear has retracted tympanic membrane.
When tympanic membrane is retracted, it is also called "atelectasis"
The retraction of the tympanic membrane is due to negative pressure in the middle ear.
As the disease progresses, the pressure becomes more and more negative. The retraction also keeps on increasing.
The retraction of the membrane is graded between "Grade I to Grade IV"
This grading was done by a person called SADE

SADE'S grading of tympanic membrane
Grade I - tympanic membrane is retracted but does not touch incus or stapes
Grade II- tympanic membrane touching either incus or stapes, but not touching promontory
Grade III-tympanic membrane touching the promontory but is not adherent onto it
Grade IV-tympanic membrane is adherent onto the promontory

Treatment of choice of Glue ear is **myringotomy with grommet insertion with adenoidectomy.**
Grommet is usually inserted in the *anteroinferior quadrant*

3. Chronic Suppurative Otitis Media/CSOM

CSOM is defined as inflammation of middle ear cleft (middle ear cleft includes 1. Middle ear 2. Mastoid and 3. Eustachian tube) with perforation and discharge, for more than 3 months.

The **most common pathogen is *Pseudomonas***

CSOM can be divided into different types in two different ways:

1. Two types-

1. Safe type (Tubo-tympanic type)	2. Unsafe type (Atticoantral type)

2. Four types-

1. Inactive mucosal COM	2. Active mucosal COM	3. Inactive squamous COM (retraction pockets)	4. Active squamous COM. (cholesteatoma)

1. Differences between sand and unsafe are given below:

Safe or tubo-tympanic type	Unsafe or attico-antral type
Mucosal disease	Bony disease
More discharge	Little / scanty discharge
Interrupted or discontinuous discharge	Continuous and foul swellingdischarge
Central perforation	Attic or marginal perforation
Pale ear polyp	Fleshing / red ear polyp
No granulation	Granulation is fleshy colored
No cholesteatoma	Cholesteatoma seen
Less complication	More complications

2. Relevant differences between inactive mucosal, active mucosal, inactive squamous and active squamous are below:

Inactive mucosal COM	Active mucosal COM	Inactive squamous COM (retraction pockets)	Active squamous COM (Cholesteatoma)
Has TM perforation without discharge	Has TM perforation with active discharge	Has retraction pockets with keratin debris	Has cholesteatoma in the middle ear
Rx is myringoplasty or type I tympanoplasty	Antibiotics followed by myringoplasty	Regular cleaning of retraction pocket. Severe cases MRM	MRM is the treatment of choice

RETRACTION POCKETS (INACTIVE SQUAMOUS COM)

Retraction pockets are different from retracted tympanic membrane that was discussed in glue ear. Retraction of tympanic membrane is also called **"atelectesis".**

Differences between Retraction Pockets and Retracted Tympanic Membrane

Retracted TM (Atelectasis)	Retraction pockets
Diffuse retraction towards promontory	Focal retraction towards attic
Usually seen in glue ear (already discussed)	If allowed to expand; will lead to primary acquired cholesteatoma formation
Graded into four stages by Sade	Graded into four stages by Tos (grading is given below)
Regular cleaning of retraction pocket. Severe cases MRM	MRM is the treatment of choice

Tos's staging of retraction pocket
Stage I- Retracted but NOT adherent onto malleus
Stage II- Retracted and adherent onto neck of malleus
Stage III- Causes partial erosion of bony attic wall
Stage IV- Causes full erosion of bony attic wall

Kindly note the difference between Sade's staging used during glue ear and Tos's staging used for retraction pocket which may form cholesteatoma, if allowed to progress

CHOLESTEATOMA/KERATOMA/EPIDERMOSIS

It is sac of keratinized or desquamated squamous epithelium in the middle ear.

It comprises of two things:

1. **The matrix**- keratinizing squamous epithelium, and
2. **Keratin debris**- the central mass

The commonest site of cholesteatoma is **Prussak's space.**

It is also frequently seen in the *posterosuperior quadrant of middle ear.*

Cholesteatoma can be divided into two types:

1. Congenital cholesteatoma, and
2. Acquired cholesteatoma

Theories of Cholesteatoma Formations

1. Congenital cholesteatoma: Develops from ***residual cell; rest cell or nest cell.***

Derlaki and Clemis laid down four criteria for congenital chloesteatoma and **levenson** added the fifth criteria. These criteria are given below:

Derlaki and Clemis criteria
1. White mass present medial or deep to intact tympanic membrane
2. Normal pars tensa and pars flaccida
3. No previous history of otorrhea (ear discharge) or tympanic membrane perforation, and
4. No past history of ear procedure or ear surgery
5TH CRITERIA ADDED BY LEVENSON
5. Recurrent attacks of otitis media does not rule out congenital cholesteatoma

The three common sites of congenital cholesteatoma in order of preference are:

1. Anterior part of middle ear
2. Petrous bone/petrous apex, and
3. C-P angle

2. Primary acquired cholesteatoma:

Theories of primary acquired Cholesteatoma

1. Invagination or negative pressure theory also called Wittmaack's theory- is the most acceptable theory. This can also form secondary cholesteatoma.
2. Basal cell hyperplasia or Ruede's theory, and
3. Metaplasia or Sade's theory

According to the invagination theory; the primary acquired cholesteatoma is usually formed due to *retraction pocket formed, which is due to negative pressure in the middle ear.*

Primary Acquired

Primary acquired cholesteatomas arise as the result of tympanic membrane retraction. The classic primary acquired cholesteatoma develops from progressively deeper medial retraction of the pars flaccida into the epitympanum. As this process continues, the lateral wall of the epitympanum (called the scutum) is slowly eroded, producing a defect in the lateral wall of the epitympanum that slowly expands. The tympanic membrane continues retracting medially until it passes over the heads of the ossicles and into the posterior epitympanum. Ossicular destruction is common. If the cholesteatoma pokes posteriorly into the aditus ad antrum and the mastoid itself, erosion of the tegmen mastoideum, with exposure of the dura and/or erosion of the lateral semicircular canal with deafness and vertigo, may result.

A second type of primary acquired cholesteatomas arises when the posterior quadrant of the tympanic membrane is retracted into the posterior middle ear. The drum initially adheres to the long process of the incus. As retraction continues medially and posteriorly, squamous epithelium envelops the superstructure of the stapes and retracts into the sinus tympani. Primary cholesteatomas arising from the posterior tympanic membrane are likely to produce facial nerve exposure (and occasionally paralysis) and destruction of the stapedial superstructure. Surgical removal from the sinus tympani may be extremely challenging.

3. Secondary acquired cholesteatoma:

Theories of secondary acquired cholesteatoma

1. Retraction pockets.
2. Migration theory also called Habermann's theory,
In this case *Trail sign* may be seen- in this sign keratin is present in the ear canal, which can be followed through the perforation, into the middle ear.
3. Metaplasia theory
4. Inoculation of squamous tissue during ear procedures.

NOTE:

Levenson's criteria is used for malignant otitis externa and congenital cholesteatoma

Metaplasia may explain both primary acquired cholesteatoma as well as secondary acquired cholesteatoma

Tuberculosis of Ear

Tuberculosis into the middle ear usually spreads through the following routes:

1. **Eustachian tube- Most common route**
2. **Bloodstream from distant sites**

3. **Direct spread from adjoining area, and**
4. **From mother during birth**

When to suspect tuberculosis of ear-

- ***The triad of the following should raise the suspicion of ear tuberculosis***
- ***Delayed presentation of chronic otitis media***
- ***Not responding to medication***
- ***Having regional lymphadenopathy***

Diagnostic features of ear tuberculosis are:

- **Multiple perforations on tympanic membrane**
- **It is a painless disease**
- **Ear discharge is serous or watery and NOT purulent**
- **Pale granulations seen in the middle ear.**

Common complications of ear tuberculosis are:

- Facial nerve palsy
- Profound hearing loss

Diseases of ear having granulations	Types of granulation
Malignant otitis externa	Red granulation in the external canal, at the bone-cartilage junction
Granular myringitis	Red granulation on the tympanic membrane. This gives "red carpet" appearance on the membrane
Unsafe CSOM	Red granulation in the middle ear
Tuberculosis of ear	Pale coloured granulation in middle ear

Last minute revision

- *Streptococcus pneumoniae and Haemophilus influenzae are common pathogens in ASOM*
- *Glue ear usually has no pathogen*
- *CSOM is usually caused by pseudomonas*
- *Light house sign is seen in two diseases*

1. ASOM

2. Mastoiditis

- *Sade graded tympanic membrane retraction seen in serous otitis media. In grade II retraction, tympanic membrane touches the Incus*
- *Tos graded retraction pocket which may lead to primary acquired cholesteatoma*
- *First line management of ASOM is nasal decongestions and antibiotics*
- *Glue ear requires myringotomy with grommet insertion and adenoidectomy*
- *Grommet insertion is preferred in the antero-inferior quadrant of tympanic membrane*
- *In adults with unilateral glue ear; nasopharyngoscopy should be done*
- *Most common site of acquired cholesteatoma is Prussak's space. If this is not given in the choices then, postero-superior quadrant is an acceptable answer*
- *Most important feature of ear tuberculosis is multiple perforations*
- *Ear tuberculosis is painless whereas laryngeal tuberculosis is painful.*

QUESTIONS

1. **Acute otitis media in children is most commonly due to:**
   a. Moraxella catarrhalis
   b. H. influenzae
   c. Streptococcus pneumoniae
   d. Staphylococcus aureus
2. **A 7-year child presenting with acute otitis media does not respond to ampicillin. The examination reveals is full and bulging tympanic membrane. The treatment of choice is:**
   a. Systemic steroid
   b. Ciprofloxacin
   c. Myringotomy
   d. Cortical mastoidectomy
3. **Unilateral secretory otitis media in an adult is associated with:**
   a. Mastoiditis
   b. CSOM
   c. Carcinoma nasopharynx
   d. Foreign body
4. **True statement about ASOM is:**
   a. Most frequently it resolves without sequelae
   b. Commonly follows painful parotitis
   c. Radical mastoidectomy is required for treatment
   d. Most common organism is pseudomonas
5. **The fluid level and air bubble level in otoscopy indicates:**
   a. CSOM b. ASOM
   c. Middle ear effusion d. Otosclerosis
6. **Dangerous ear is associated with:**
   a. Central perforation
   b. Attico antral perforation
   c. Subtotal perforation
   d. Tuberculous perforation
7. **Cholesteatoma is usually present at:**
   a. Anteroinferior quadrant of tympanic membrane
   b. Posteroinferior quadrant of tympanic membrane
   c. Attic region d. Central part
8. **The posterosuperior retraction pocket, if allowed to progress, will lead to:**
   a. Sensori-neural hearing loss
   b. Secondary cholesteatoma
   c. Tympanosclerosis
   d. Primary cholesteatoma
9. **In which of the following condition there will be watery discharge from the ear:**
   a. ASOM
   b. Endolymphatic sac decompression
   c. CSF otorrhea
   d. Parotid fistula

IMAGE BASED QUESTIONS

10. **This is an otoscopic finding of tympanic membrane of a patient presenting with hearing loss. Which of these is true?**

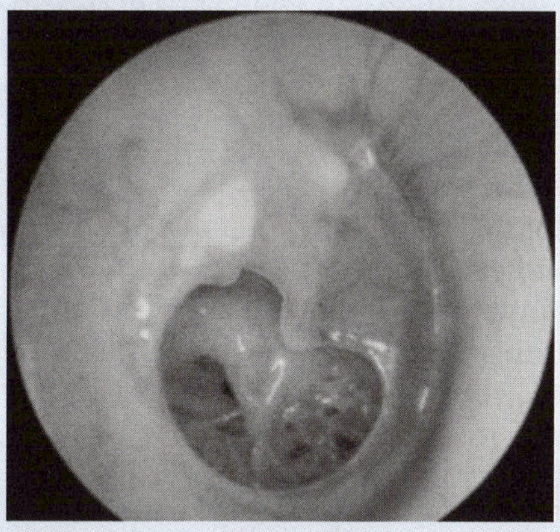

   a. This is a case of central perforation of tympanic membrane
   b. Myringoplasty is contraindicated in this patient
   c. Trauma to the ear is the probable cause of this condition
   d. All are true
11. **A 30 years old lady has a history of ear discharge off and on for the past few months. On otoscopic examination, the following is the finding:**

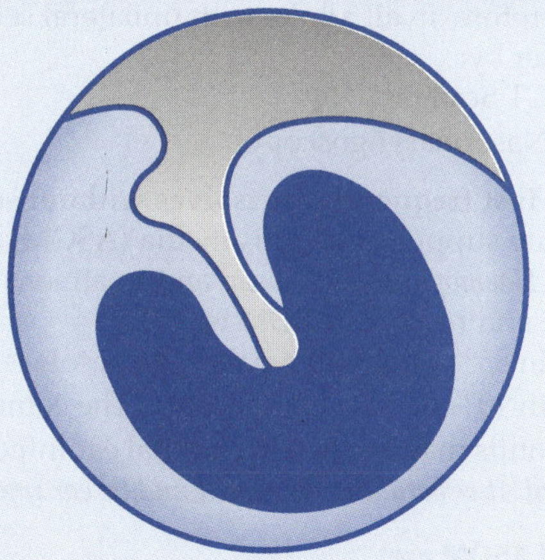

Which of these is correct?
   a. This is a case of unsafe CSOM
   b. The finding is showing a marginal perforation
   c. Myringoplasty is the best treatment option
   d. All are true

ANSWERS AND EXPLANATIONS

1. **b. H. influenzae**
   This question is controversial.
   Lot of books say that *Streptococcus pneumoniae* is the most common organism causing ASOM in infants and children.
   However, according to Scott Brown's book, ***H. Influenza is the most common organism.***
   The three important pathogens in ASOM are:
   1. Streptococcus pneumoniae
   2. H. infleunzae, and
   3. Moraxella catarrhalis

2. **c. Myringotomy**
   A child with full and bulging TM is ***a case of acute suppurative otitis media (ASOM).***
   Treatment options in ASOM are:
   1. Antibiotics with nasal decongestant is the initial treatment.
   2. If this fails to relieve then ***myringotomy is second line of treatment.***
   3. ***Myringotomy is also the treatment of choice.***

   NOTE: *In SOM/glue ear, the treatment of choice is myringotomy+grommet insertion+/- adenoidectomy.*

3. **c. Carcinoma nasopharynx**
   Secretory otitis media (SOM) is a disease of middle ear which is usually caused due to blockade of eustachian tube.
   Causes of eustachian tube blockade could be many. Important causes of eustachian tube blockade are:
   1. **Adenoid hypertrophy:** This is more common in children.
   2. **Nasopharyngeal carcinoma:** This is more common in adults.

   SOM is more common in children and is bilateral.
   However, it may also be seen in adults but is usually bilateral (like in children).
   If SOM is seen in adults and is unilateral then it should raise the suspension of nasopharyngeal carcinoma.
   This is because the most common site of nasopharyngeal carcinoma is ***fossa of Rosenmuller, which is just behind the eustachian tube.***
   Hence, CA of this area may block the tube leading to unilateral secretory otitis media in adults.
   Therefore, in all adults with unilateral secretory otitis media, nasopharyngeal carcinoma should be ruled out either by:
   - CT Scan or
   - Nasopharyngoscopy.

4. **a. Most frequently it resolves without sequelae**
   Acute suppurative otitis media (ASOM) is caused most commonly by *Streptococcus pneumoniae* (some books say *Haemophilus influenza)* and treatment of choice is myringotomy.
   The end result os ASOM is:
   1. In 85%–90% of the patients it resolves without sequelae.
   2. In 10%–15%, it complicates. The common complications of ASOM are glue ear and CSOM.

   Parotitis may be seen in external ear infections because of ***foramen of Santorini*** *which are present in the external canal. It is very uncommon in middle ear infections like ASOM.*

Stages of ASOM are:

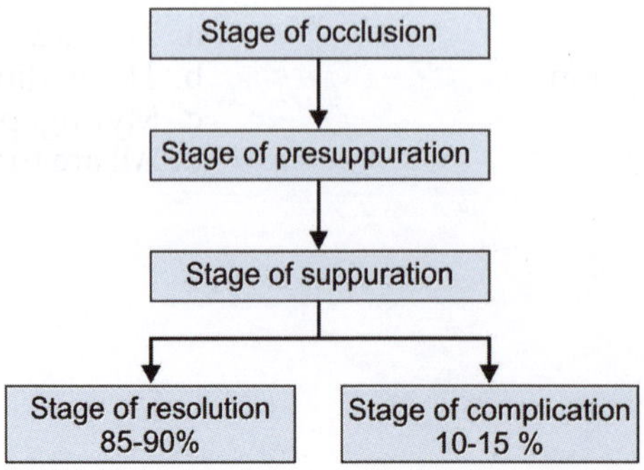

PART 1: EAR

Resolution is seen in about 85-90% of these patients and complications in only 10-15%.
Hence, most commonly *i.e* 85-90% of patients, it heals without sequelae.

5. **c. Middle ear effusion**

Middle ear cavity is lined with ciliated columnar epithelium with secretory glands in it.
These glands have secretion in the middle ear cavity. The secretion of the middle ear drain into the nasopharynx through the eustachian tube.
Any abnormality causing the blockade of the eustachian tube may cause stasis of the secretion in the middle ear, leading to diseases like:

1. ASOM. This has fluid collection but NO air bubbles.
2. Glue ear/ SOM. This has fluid collection with air bubbles. The presence of fluid with air bubbles is a characteristic otoscopic finding of middle ear effusion or glue ear.

Some of the Other Findings of Otoscopy are:

1. Retracted and bluish/straw coloured tympanic membrane with reduced mobility and foreshortened
2. Handle of malleus in glue ear.
3. Fluid may also be seen in ASOM, but in this air bubbles are absent.
4. In otosclerosis, Schwartze sign is seen on otoscopy.
5. In CSOM, tympanic membrane perforation is seen on otoscopy.

Differences in the Otoscopic Findings of ASOM and Glue Ear

ASOM	Glue ear
• Bulging tympanic membrane	• Retracted tympanic membrane
• Red and congested membrane with cart wheel	• Blue to yellow membrane
• Fluid level is seen	• Fluid level with air bubbles seen

6. **b. Attico antral perforation**

Several types of perforations may be seen in patients having ear diseases. Some of the common types of perforations in the tympanic membrane are:

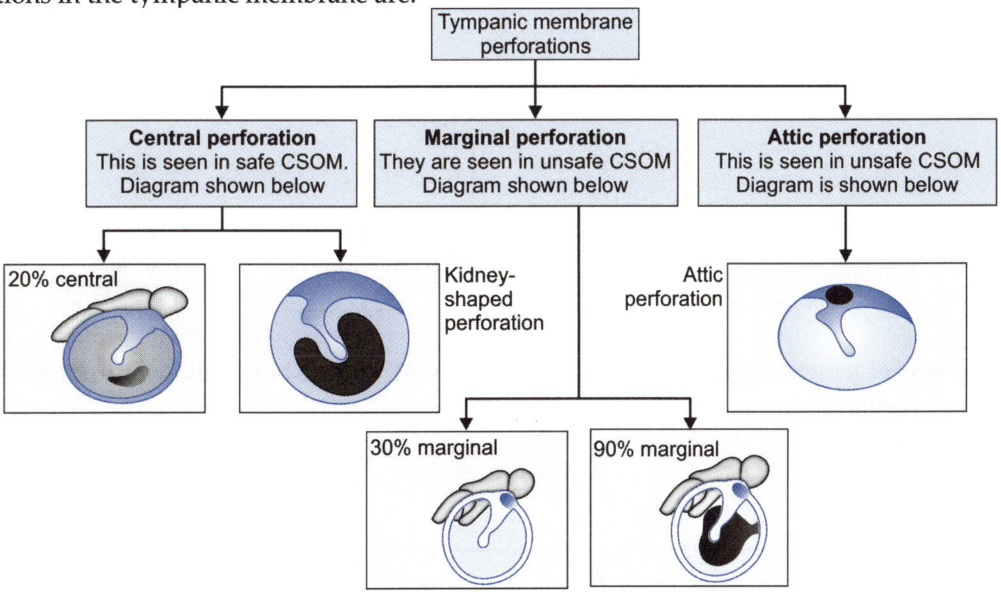

Important Points about Tympanic Membrane Perforations

1. Safe CSOM has:
   a. *Central perforation*
   b. *Kidney-shaped perforation*
   c. *Subtotal perforation*

2. Unsafe CSOM has:
   a. ***Marginal perforation***
   b. ***Total perforation***
   c. ***Attic perforation (Attico-antral)***
3. Tuberculosis of ear has:
   a. ***Multiple perforation***
4. Traumatic perforation has:
   a. ***Rugged margin with blood stains on it***
   b. ***They do not require repair/surgery***

We can see that damgerous ear (unsafe CSOM) can have attico antral perforation.

7. **c. Attic region**

The commonest site of cholesteatoma is the ***Prussak's space*** which is in the attic (epitympanum) of middle ear.

Prussak's Space

This space is bounded medially by:

1. ***The neck of malleus (medially)***
2. ***Laterally by the pars flaccida of tympanic membrane and***
3. ***Superiorly by the lateral malleolar fold.***

Therefore, when Prussak's space is not given in the choices then attic is the acceptable answer.
The most common site of cholesteatoma in the mesotympanum is posterosuperior quadrant of tympanic membrane which becomes the ***second most common site*** over all.
NOTE:- Posterosuperior guadrant is nearly as common a site of cholesteatoma as Prussak space.

Pathophysiology

1. Prussack space is in the attic which has pars flaccid as on of the boundary.
   Pars flaccida is a loose part of the membrane. therefore ***retraction pockets are formed easily here.*** *This in turn leads to formation of cholesteatoma.*
2. Posterosuperior quadrant of the tympanic membrane is ***the most vascular part of the membrane.***
   Therefore inflammation of this part is common and recurrent. This leads to thinning and loosening of the membrane. Therefore retraction pocket and cholesteatoma is easily formed.

8. **d. primary cholesteatoma**

Chronic otitis media are of four types. These types are:

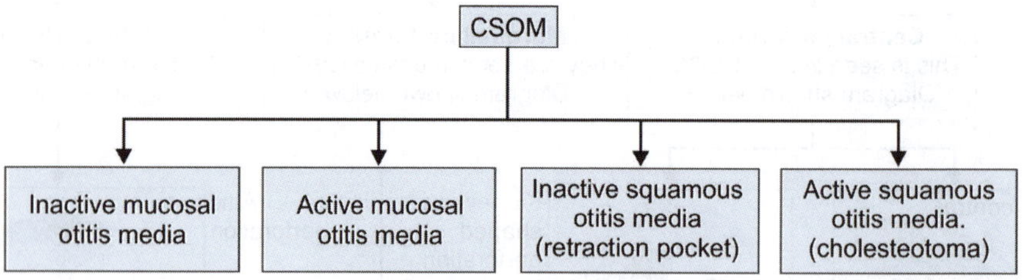

If retraction pocket (inactive squamous otitis media) is NOT treated but is allowed to progress, one of the following may result:

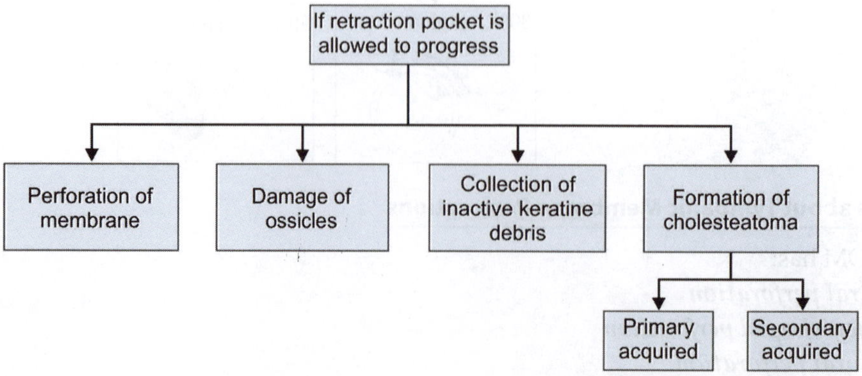

Cholesteatoma are of three types

1. *Congenital cholesteatoma*
2. *Primary acquired cholesteatoma and*
3. *Secondary acquired cholesteatoma*

NOTE: Tertiary cholesteatoma is NOT a type of cholesteatoma.

Common Complications of the Different Types of Chronic Otitis Media (Com)

Types of chronic otitis media	Complications
Inactive otitis media	• Normal healing • Tympanosclerosis • Becomes active otitis media
Active otitis media	• Normal healing • Tympanosclerosis
Inactive squamous media (retraction pocket)	As mentioned above, besides other complications it may form: • ***Primary cholesteatoma or*** • ***Secondary cholesteatoma***
Active squamous media (cholesteatoma)	Besides may other complications, it may form: • ***Sensorineural hearing loss***

As noticed above:

If a posterosuperior retraction pocket is allowed to progress
↓
Forms of primary acquired cholesteatoma
↓
If this is not treated
↓
Leads to sensorineural hearing loss

As we notice, retraction pocket (inactive squamous COM) may ultimately lead to sensorineural hearing loss. Tympanosclerosis on the other hand is the end stage healing of inactive mucosal COM and active mucosal COM. NOTE: If primary acquired cholestotoma is NOT given in choices then secondary cholesteatoma is an acceptable answer.

9. **a. ASOM**

ASOM is an acute inflammatory disease of the middle ear. In the suppurative stage of this disease, there is discharge from the middle ear. This discharge is from the glands of the middle and is therefore mucoid in nature and watery.

In come cases this mucoid discharge is infected with bacteria and the discharge becomes ***muco-purulent.***

- In endolymphatic sac surgery, the discharge is the endolymph and is watery.
- In CSF otorrhea, the discharge is CSF and is therefore watery.
- In parotid fistula, the discharge is from parotis and is watery in nature.

IMAGE BASED ANSWERS

10. **a. This is a case of central perforation of tympanic membrane**

The picture is that of central perforation which is usually seen in tubotympanic disease and is NOT caused by trauma.

In such cases, *myringoplasty* is the treatment of choice.

- ***Traumatic perforations have rugged and have blood stained margins.***

11. **c. Myringoplasty is the best treatment option**

Discharge from ear which is off and on for few months is a feature of **Safe CSOM band not Unsafe CSOM.**

The picture shows a ***central perforation because the annulus is NOT involved.***

The treatment of choice in Safe CSOM with central perforation is *Myringoplasty*.

CHAPTER

5 Complications/Sequel of CSOM

All types of CSOM may cause complications. Complications are most commonly seen in active squamous COM or cholesteatoma. In lot of patients, the membranes heal on their own.

HEALED TYMPANIC MEMBRANE IN CHRONIC OTITIS MEDIA

Sometimes the condition heals normally.

Other times, the healing of the membrane is not normal and may lead to **thin membrane/dimeric membrane.** This is due to the following reasons:

1. Loss of lamina propria of the membrane
2. Atrophy/failure of complete healing

As a result of this, the membrane has only two layers instead of three layers.

The tympanic membrane becomes thin it may:

- Get retracted due to negative pressure
- Flap in and out with change of ear pressure during swallowing.
- Patient may hear a click sound caused due to flapping membrane during swallowing.

Complications can be Divided into Two Main Types. They are:

Extracranial/Intratemporal complications	Intracranial complications
Tympanosclerosis	Meningitis
Ossicular damage	Lateral sinus thrombophlebitis
Mastoiditis	Subdural abscess
Labyrinthine fistula	Extradural abscess
Labyrinthitis	Cerebral abscess
Petrositis	Otitis hydrocephalus
Gradenigo's syndrome	
Facial nerve palsy	

The important features of these complications are given below:

Tympanosclerosis

Tympanosclerosis is hyalinization of tympanic membrane and middle ear followed by calcification, ossification and hyalinization.

It is usually the ***end stage of healing of mucosal chronic otitis media.***

The most important feature of this condition is that the tympanic membrane begins to look **"chalky white"** in color.

Different Conditions Resulting in Different Color of RHE Tympanic Membrane

Diseases	Color of tympanic membrane
Normal ear	Pearly white/grayish white
ASOM	Red and congested
Glue ear/SOM	Blue/yellow/straw colored
Otospongiosis	Flamingo pink
Tympanosclerosis	Chalky white

Acute or Coalescent Mastoiditis

Acute mastoiditis is seen when the infection from the middle ear cavity reaches into the mastoid cavity causing inflammation of the mucosal lining of the mastoid cavity.

It is more common in children and is caused by **B- hemolytic Streptococcus.**

In this the finding are as given below:

- Mastoid tenderness may be seen in late stages. At early stage tenderness may be present at *cymba concha.*
- Light house sign may be seen (this is also a feature of ASOM).
- **Reservoir sign** may be seen
- Pinna is pushed downward and forward.
- Retroauricular sulcus deepens/enhance **BUT** later on it may obliterate.
- **Ironed out mastoid is an important feature.**

Conditions having reservoir sign
1. ASOM
2. Acute mastoiditis

X-ray shows **clouding/sclerosed** mastoid air cells (normally it is ***honeycomb appearance***)

Investigation of choice is CT scan.

Most patients can be treated by antibiotics and symptomatic.

Cortical mastoidectomy or complete mastoidectomy is the treatment of choice.

Differentiating Furunculosis from Mastoiditis

Furunculosis	Acute mastoiditis
Caused by Staphylococcus	**Caused by GABHS**
Seen in any age	Seen in children
Inflammation in the external canal	Inflammation over the mastoid area
Tragal sign is positive	Tragal sign is negative
No tenderness at mastoid tip	Tenderness either at mastoid tip or at cymba concha
Obliteration of retroaural sulcus	Prominence of retroauricular sulcus which later on may obliterate
Mastoid is NOT ironed out	Mastoid may be ironed out
X-ray of mastoid is normal	Clouded mastoid on X-ray

Masked Mastoiditis

Masked matoiditis is subclinical types of mastoiditis. This is usually seen in patients of mastoiditis who have received partial treatment and therefore the symptoms disappear but damage/erosion inside the mastoid continues slowly.

Treatment is similar to coalescent mastoiditis.

Complication of Mastoiditis

A complicated mastoid may lead to formation of abscess in the following areas:

- **Retro-auricular /Postauricular**—when the abscess is behind pinna.
- **Zygomatic abscess**—when the abscess at the root of zygoma
- **Luc's abscess**—when the abscess in the superior canal wall causing *sagging of the canal wall.*
- **Bezold's abscess**—when the abscess is in the sheath of *sternocleidomastoid muscle.* This may sometimes lead to **torticollis/wry neck.**
- **Citelli's abscess**—when the abscess is in the sheath of post belly of *digastric.*

CT scan is the investigation of choice.

Treatment of choice is *cortical mastoidectomy + Incision and drainage of the abscess*

The commonest abscess is post auricular abscess and second most common abscess is Bezold's abscess

Common Infective Diseases of Ear and their Pathogens

Diseases	Pathogens
Perichondritis of pinna	Pseudomonas
Furunculosis/folliculitis	Staphylococcus
Malignant otitis externa	Pseudomonas
Bullous myringitis	Influenza virus
ASOM	Streptococcus pneumoniae and Haemophilus influenzae
Glue ear	No pathogen/has sterile fluid
CSOM	Pseudomonas
Acute mastoiditis	Group A beta hemolytic Streptococcus

Petrositis

Like mastoiditis; when infection from the middle ear spread to the petrous bone, it leads to petrositis.

- Petrositis (inflammation of petrous part of temporal bone) is usually a complication of CSOM. In these cases the infection reaches through two routes
  1. From behind and above the bony labyrinth- **posterosuperior tract**
  2. From hypotympanum near the eustachian tube and around the cochlea- **Anteroinferior tract**
- It may also be seen in cases with congenital cholesteatoma of the petrous bone.

  Petrositis may present with ***persistant pulsatile discharge.***

In some patients of petrositis, the infection may reach the petrous apex and involve V and VI cranial nerves leading to **Gradenigo's syndrome.**

Important Points about Gradenigo's Syndrome are

- It is usually seen in case of petrous apex abscess
- In this two cranial nerves are involved. These nerves are Vth and VIth nerves
- It has three features. They are:
  1. ***Ear discharge***
  2. ***Retro orbital pain and***
  3. ***Diplopia.***

Surgery of petrous bone is done in this case. The surgical approaches for petrous bone are given below:

- *Lempert's and Ramadier's*
- *Almoor's*
- *Eagleton's*
- *Thornvolt's*
- *Frenckner's*

Three important causes of pulsatile discharge from ear are
1. ASOM–called light house sign
2. Acut mastoiditis–called light house sign
*3. Petrositis–***causes persistent pulsatile discharge**

LABYRINTHINE FISTULA/CIRCUMSCRIBED LABYRINTHITIS

Labyrinthine fistula is the most common complication of CSOM
Labyrinthine fistula is most commonly seen in the bulge of **lateral semicircular canal.**
The main complain is vertigo.
In this **fistula test/sign will be present**.
Treatment is **immediate exploration of mastoid and closure of fistula**.

Important conditions with positive fistula test/sign
1. Labyrinthine fistula/Circumscribed labyrinthitis
2. Superior canal dehiscent syndrome/Minor's syndrome
3. After Tympanoplasty type V
4. After Stapedectomy and Stapedotomy

Labyrinthitis

Labyrinthitis is inflammation of the inner ear
It is of three main types:

1. Circumscribed labyrinthitis/labyrinthine fistula- Already discussed
2. Serous or toxic labyrinthitis, and
3. Suppurative labyrinthitis

The Important Differences between Serous Labyrinthitis and Suppurative Labyrinthitis are

Serous/toxic labyrinthitis	Suppurative labyrinthitis
Caused by "toxins" of bacteria in the middle ear. There are NO pathogens in the labyrinth. Only their toxins are present in the inner ear	There is bacterial infection of the labyrinth
There are NO polymorphonuclear leukocytes in the inner ear fluids	Polymorphonuclear leukocytes are present in the inner ear fluid
Symptoms of vertigo, nausea and sensorineural hearing loss are mild	Symptoms are severe. Sometimes leads to dead ear (permanent hearing loss)
Symptoms are reversible	Symptoms are irreversible
Antibiotic + steroids + symptomatic treatment	Antibiotic + steroids + symptomatic treatment

FACIAL NERVE PALSY

Since a large part of facial nerve runs through the middle ear, it may be involved in various middle ear infections. There are more than 80-90 causes of facial palsy. They can be divided into six broad categories. These categories are:

Facial nerve palsy causes
1. Idiopathic/Bell's palsy–The most common cause of facial palsy
2. Infections–Most commonly CSOM/Cholesteatoma, herpes zoster etc.

(Contd...)

(Contd...)

3. Tumors—Most commonly acoustic neuroma/parotid gland tumors
4. Trauma either accidental or iatrogenic
5. Systemic diseases like diabetes, sarcoidosis, etc.
6. Syndromes like Moebius syndrome, Melkersson-Rosenthal syndrome, etc.

Causes of recurrent facial nerve palsy
Bell's palsy
Diabetes
Melkersson-Rosenthal syndrome
Sarcoidosis

BELL'S PALSY/IDIOPATHIC FACIAL NERVE PALSY

Bell's palsy is the most common cause of facial palsy. It is lower neuron type of facial palsy.

The accepted minimum criteria for diagnosis of facial palsy are:

1. ***Sudden onset of the condition***
2. ***Palsy of all muscle groups on one side of the face***
3. ***No obvious ear diseases, cerebellopontine angle diseases and central diseases***

Most of the patients recover completely but complete recovery is NOT the rule. Poor outcome or prognosis is seen in the following conditions:

- ***Old age***
- ***Diabetes in the patient***
- ***Absence of stapedial reflex***
- ***Grade V palsy (complete palsy)***
- ***Involvement of the lacrimal fibres and taste fibres.***

	Classification/Grading of facial nerve damage
Grade I	This is also called neuropraxia. All nerve fibres are intact anatomically.
Grade II	This is also called axonotmesis. All the three layers are intact but nerve axons are damaged.
Grade III	It is also called neurometesis. Along with fibres, endoneurium is also damaged. In this condition, synkinesis may be seen.
Grade IV	It is called partial resection. In this perineurium gets damaged. Recovery is poor.
Grade V	Nerve is completely resected including epineurium. Almost no spontaneous recovery seen.

Management of Bell's Palsy

The management of Bell's palsy is controversial. However, the best way to proceed is as follows:

- If the patient reports in the **first 72 hours /3 days** of palsy—**start steroids (prednisone) and acyclovir (antiviral)**. Vitamin B2, B6 and B12 are optional. Steroid should be given for 10 days and then tapered off.
- If the patient reports **after 72 hours/3 days** of palsy—**start only steroids**. Vitamins are optional.
- In both the above situations; **physiotherapy and electrophysiotherapy (NOT electrophysiological tests)** may be helpful but they are not necessary.
- If the patient fails to respond to the above mentioned treatment for more than 2 weeks:
  1. The next line of **management** is to carry out **electrophysiological tests (NOT electrophysiotherapy)** and **topodiagnostic tests.** Based on the results of these investigations; ***surgical decompression of the facial nerve may or maynot be required.***
  2. However, the next line of **treatment is *surgical decompression of the facial nerve.***

     NOTE:- When surgical decompression of the facial nerve is done, it is usually done in the **labyrinthine part of the facial nerve** as ***the labyrinthine part of the facial nerve is the shortest and narrowest part of the facial nerve.***

NERVE STIMULATION TESTS OF FACIAL NERVE

There are 4–6 types of tests that can be carried out but the **best electrophysiological test is *electroneuronography also called evoked electromyography.*** This is the most valuable prognostic indicator in Bell's palsy.

However, this test has few drawbacks:

1. It is mainly useful in Bell's palsy and is NOT very useful in facial palsy due to other causes.
2. It is useful only if done between 3rd day and 14th day of palsy. It is not useful if done within 3 days and after 14 days of palsy.

TOPODIAGNOSTIC TESTS

Important topodiagnostic tests for facial are:

- Schirmer's test for greater superficial petrosal nerve
- Stapedial reflex for nerve to stapedius
- Electrogustometry for chorda tympani
- Salivary flow test for chorda tympani

RAMSAY HUNT SYNDROME

Ramsay Hunt syndrome is caused by reactivation of varicella zoster virus (VZV) in the geniculate ganglion of the facial nerve.

The classical presentation is erythematous vesicular rash on the ear with lower motor neuron palsy.

Important Differences between Bell's Palsy and Ramsay Hunt Syndrome

Bell's palsy	Ramsay Hunt syndrome
Is idiopathic/ no known cause	Caused by varicella zoster virus
Not painful	Excruciating pain may be present
Facial palsy with any rash	Facial palsy with erythematous vesicular rash
Electroneuronography helpful	Electroneuronography not helpful
Good to excellent prognosis	Prognosis is not as good
Main drug is prednisone	Acyclovir and prednisone
Surgical decompression may be required	Not required

TRAUMATIC FACIAL PALSY

The trauma could be

1. Accidental or
2. Iatrogenic/surgical

1. Accidental trauma causing fracture of the temporal bone can cause facial palsy.

   The fracture of the temporal bone could be

   - Longitudinal fracture: A more common type of fracture but chances of facial palsy is less common
   - Transverse fracture: A less common type of fracture compared to longitudinal fracture but it is a **more common cause of fracture causing facial palsy.**

2. Iatrogenic/surgical trauma: The most common surgery causing facial nerve palsy is **middle ear or mastoid surgery**. Second most common cause is **parotid surgery**.

   In order to avoid facial nerve damage during middle ear or mastoid surgeries, the facial nerve landmarks may be used.

Landmarks of facial nerve during ear surgery are
1. Cog/jog
2. Processes cochleariformis.

(Contd...)

PART 1: EAR

(Contd...)

3. Oral window
4. Bulge of lateral semicircular canal
5. Short process of incus
6. Digastric ridge
7. *Pyramidal eminence*

Management of facial palsy is same irrespective of the type of trauma. The treatment depends on the latent period between trauma and palsy.

1. When there is a gap of few hours to day between trauma and the onset of palsy- **Steroids are given. It is mainly conservative treatment.**
2. When the palsy is immediately after trauma- **Immediate surgical correction of the cause is done with repair of the facial nerve (if needed).**

Some important points related to facial palsy

- Most common tumor of the facial nerve is schwannoma
- Merkelson-Rosenthal syndrome includes:
  - Facial palsy
  - Lip/facial edema and swelling
  - Fissured tongue
- Ischaemia is most common in the labyrinthine part of facial nerve
- In supranuclear/upper motor neuron palsy
  - Ipsilateral side is normal and
  - Contralateral side has palsy with forehead spared
- In infranuclear/lower motor nuclear palsy
  - Ipsilateral side has complete palsy
  - Contralateral side is completely normal

Two interesting conditions related to nerve passing through temporal bones	
Crocodile tears also called Bogorad's syndrome	Usually follows Bell's Palsy or facial nerve trauma There is synkinesis between the parasympathetic fibres of submandibular/sublingual glands and fibres of lacrimal glands in the facial nerve. Tears flow down when patient begins to eat This is a typical case of synkinesis
Frey's syndrome or gustatory sweating	Usually happens after parotidectomy Auriculotemporal nerve is damaged during this case Parasympathetic fibres of inferior salivary nucleus travelling in glossopharyngeal nerve (IX nerve) and then in auriculotemporal are damaged These fibres cross connect with fibres supplying the sweat glands of cheek. As a result of this, Patient begins to sweat from the cheek while taking meals

IMPORTANT POINTS ABOUT INTRACRANIAL COMPLICATIONS OF CSOM

Pathogens from the middle ear reach intracranially through one of the following routes:

- Retrograde thrombophlebitis
- Direct spread by bony erosion
- Preformed pathway
  - ***Natural pathways***
  - ***Created by diseases, surgeries and trauma***

The common pathogens causing meningitis due to CSOM are:

Streptococcus pneumonia- most common

S. hemolyticus

Staphylococcus
Proteus
E. coli etc.
NOTE: Incident of *H. influenzae has reduced due to immunization.*
Lateral sinus thrombophlebitis/Sigmoid sinus thrombophlebitis:
Picket fence fever is the most typical presentation of lateral sinus thrombophlebitis.

Some of the Important Signs are:

- *Tobey Ayer sign or Queckenstedt sign*
- *Crowe beck sign*
- *Griesinger's sign*
- *Delta sign*

Investigation of Choice is Contrast Enhanced CT Scan

Treatment

- *Canal wall up MRM with drainage of abscess* in case lateral sinus thrombophlebitis is caused by ASOM
- *Canal wall down MRM with abscess drainage* in case lateral sinus thrombophlebitis is caused by CSOM.

Last minute revision

- *Most common intracranial complication of CSOM is meningitis*
- *Blue TM is seen in glue ear*
- *Mastoiditis may have reservoir sign and ironed out mastoid*
- *Bezold's abscess is the abscess in sternocleidomastoid muscle. This may cause torticollis*
- *Gradenigo's syndrome has*
  1. *Discharge*
  2. *Diplopia*
  3. *Deep seated pain/retrorbital pain*
- *Fistula sign may be positive in*
  1. *Labyrinthine fistula*
  2. *Tympanoplasty type V*
  3. *Stapedectomy*
- *Bell's palsy is the most common cause of facial palsy*
- *Steroids are the drug of choice in Bell's palsy*
- *Frey's syndrome is seen after parotidectomy when the auriculotemporal nerve gets damaged*
- *Second line of management for Bell's palsy is surgical decompression of facial nerve*

QUESTIONS

1. **Mastoid tip involved in:**
   a. Bezold abscess
   b. Luc's abscess
   c. Citelli's abscess
   d. Parapharyngeal abscess
2. **Infection of middle ear (otitis media) could lead to following complications, *except:***
   a. Loss of taste from anterior tongue
   b. Loss of salivation
   c. Complete facial paralysis
   d. Loss of lacrimation in the right eye
3. **A positive fistula test during Siegalisation indicates:**
   a. Ossicular discontinuity
   b. Para-labyrinthitis due to erosion of lateral semi-circular canal
   c. CSF leak through the ear
   d. Fixation of stapes bone
4. **Hyperacusis in Bell's palsy is due to the paralysis of the following muscle:**
   a. Tensor tympani b. Levator veli palatini
   c. Tensor veli palatini d. Stapedius
5. **Which part of the facial nerve is commonly exposed through natural dehiscence in the fallopian canal?**
   a. Horizontal part
   b. Upper half of the vertical part
   c. Lower half of the vertical part
   d. Labyrinthine part
6. **During otological examination all of the following will have positive fistula test, *except:***
   a. Dead ear
   b. Labyrinthine fistula
   c. Hypermobile stapes footplate
   d. Following fenestration surgery
7. **Which of the following statements best represents Bell's paralysis?**
   a. Hemiparesis and contralateral facial nerve paralysis
   b. Combined paralysis of the facial, trigeminal, and abducens nerves
   c. Idiopathic ipsilateral paralysis of the facial nerve
   d. Facial nerve paralysis with a dry eye
8. **All are true for Gradenigo's syndrome *except*:**
   a. It is associated with conductive hearing loss
   b. It is caused by an abscess in the petrous apex
   c. It leads to involvement of the Cranial nerves V and VI
   d. It is characterized by retro-orbital pain
9. **Features of Gradenigo's syndrome are all, except:**
   a. Otorrhea with deafness
   b. Trigeminal neuralgia
   c. Facial nerve palsy
   d. Retrobulbar pain
10. **A patient presents with facial nerve palsy following head trauma with fracture of the mastoid: Best intervention here is:**
    a. Immediate decompression
    b. Wait and watch
    c. Facial sling d. Steroids
11. **A case of Bell's palsy on steroids shows no improvement after 2 weeks; the next step in management should be:**
    a. Vasodilators and ACTH
    b. Physiotherapy and electrical stimulation
    c. Increase steroid dosage
    d. Electrophysiological nerve testing
12. **Which of the following is true regarding facial nerve palsy associated with temporal bone fractures:**
    a. Common with longitudinal fractures
    b. Common with transverse fracture
    c. Always associated with CSF otorrhea
    d. Facial nerve injury is always complete
13 **Recurrent facial palsy is a feature of:**
    a. Melkersson's syndrome
    b. Bell's palsy
    c. Diabetes d. All of the above
14. **Intratemporal lesion of chorda tympani nerve results in:**
    a. Loss of taste sensation from anterior 2/3rd of tongue
    b. Loss of secretomotor fibres to the submandibular salivary gland
    c. Loss of secretomotor fibres to the parotid gland
    d. Loss of taste sensations from posterior 1/3rd of tongue
15. **Patient presents with diplopia, fever and ear discharge. The most probable diagnosis is:**
    a. CSOM b. Meningitis
    c. Lateral sinus thrombophlebitis
    d. Petrositis
16. **All are true regarding 'Ramsay Hunt' syndrome is *except*:**
    a. Caused by virus
    b. Surgical removal gives excellent prognosis
    c. May involve 8th nerve
    d. Involve 7th nerve
17. **Which test can detect facial nerve palsy occurring due to lesion at the outlet of stylomastoid foramen?**
    a. Deviation of angle of mouth towards opposite side
    b. Loss of taste sensation anterior 2/3 of tongue
    c. Loss of sensation over right cheek
    d. Deviation of tongue towards opposite
18. **Facial nerve palsy at sternomastoid canal can cause:**
    a. Loss of corneal reflex at side of lesion
    b. Loss of taste sensation anterior 2/3 of ipsilateral tongue
    c. Loss of lacrimation at side of lesion
    d. Hyperacusis

19. A patient has hyperacusis, loss of lacrimation and loss of taste in the anterior 2/3 of tongue. Injury to the facial nerve is at what level?
   a. Horizontal part
   b. Vertical part proximal to nerve to stapedius
   c. Vertical part distil to nerve to stapedius
   d. Proximal to geniculate ganglion

20. Aetiology of facial nerve paralysis include all of the following *except*:
   a. Mumps
   b. Bell's palsy
   c. Acoustic neuroma
   d. MRM

21. Which fracture of the petrous bone will cause facial palsy more commonly?
   a. Longitudinal fracture b. Transverse fracture
   c. Mastoid d. Cribriform plate

22. The most common cause of CSF otorrhea:
   a. Rupture of tympanic membrane
   b. Fracture of petrous bone
   c. Fracture of mastoid air cells
   d. Fracture of parietal bone

23. Crocodile tear is due to:
   a. Cross innervations of facial nerve fibres
   b. Cross innervations of trigeminal fibres
   c. Improper regeneration of trigeminal nerve
   d. Cross innervations of auriculotemporal nerve

ANSWERS AND EXPLANATIONS

1. **a. Bezold abscess**

   In cases of mastoiditis, sometimes, the infections may spread through the the bone either
   1. By causing osteitis and osteomyelitis, or
   2. Through emissary veins

   And cause abscess around the mastoid and ear.
   Out of many such abscesses, two spread through mastoid process.
   1. The citelli's abscess spreads through digastric notch on the medial table of the mastoid process, and passes into the sheath of posterior belly of digastric muscle presenting as swelling in the submandibular area.
   2. The Bezold's abscess spreads through the mastoid tip and lateral table of mastoid process and spreads into the sternocleidomastoid muscle and may present as a swelling below the mastoid tip sometimes causing torticollis.

2. **d. Loss of lacrimation in the right eye**

   Lacrimation of the eye is controlled by the first branch of facial nerve namely greater superficial petrosal nerve. This nerve arises from the geniculate ganglion of facial nerve.
   Geniculate ganglion is present in the labyrinthine part of facial nerve which is proximal to the middle ear.

Route of Parasympathetic of Lacrimal Gland

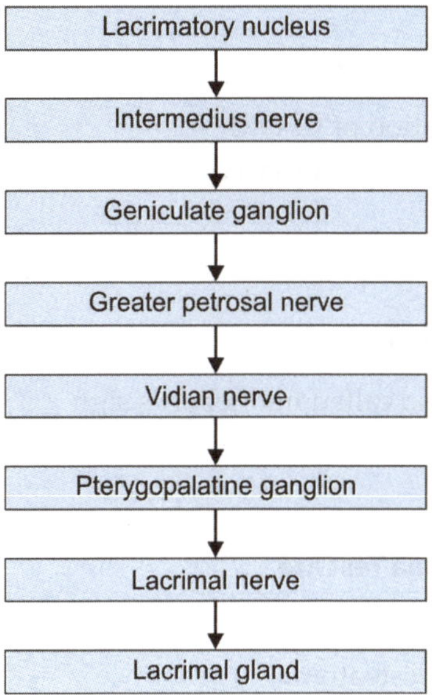

In the middle ear diseases like otitis media, the labyrinthine part is not involved and hence greater superior petrosal nerve will be spared and so patient will not have 'loss of lacrimation'.
Loss of taste of anterior 2/3 tongue and salivation by submandibular and sublingual glands are controlled by chorda tympani nerve which arises in the middle ear. Hence, the diseases of middle ear may damage the nerve.

Notice the Greater Superficial Nerve Arising before the Facial Nerve Enters the Middle Ear

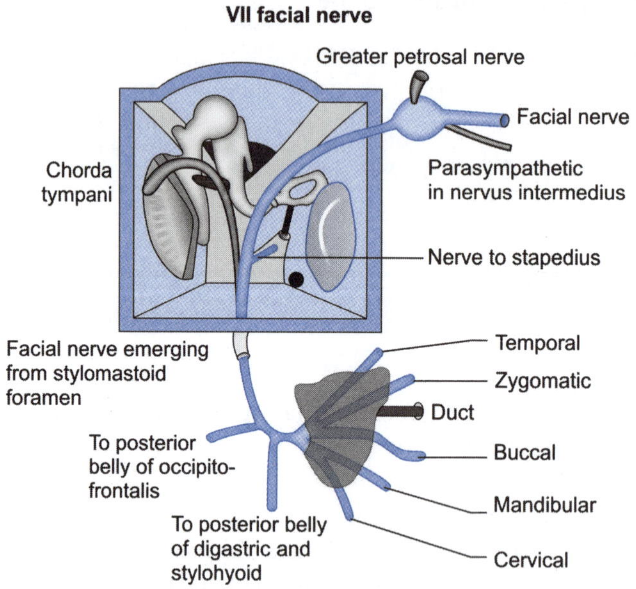

3. **b. Para-labyrinthitis due to erosion of lateral semi-circular canal**
Para-labyrinthitis due to erosion of lateral semi-circular canal is also called labyrinthine fistula.

Important causes of true positive fistula test are	Important causes of false positive fistula test are	Important causes of false negative fistula test are
1. Labyrinthine fistula, a complication of CSOM	1. Meniere's disease where it is also called Hennebert's sign	1. Dead labyrinth
2. Fenestration surgery or type V tympanoplasty	2. Congenital syphilis	2. Fistula which is blocked by cholesteatoma
3. Poststapedectomy	3. Hypermobile footplate	

Important Cause of True Positive Fistula Test are

- Labyrinthine fistula, a complication of CSOM
- Fenestration surgery or type V tympanoplasty
- Poststapedectomy
- Perilymph fistula

Important Causes of False Positive Fistula Test are

- Meniere's disease where it is also called hennebert's sign
- Congenital syphilis
- Hypermobile footplate

Important Causes of False Negative Fistula Test are

- Dead labyrinth
- Fistula which is blocked by cholesteatoma

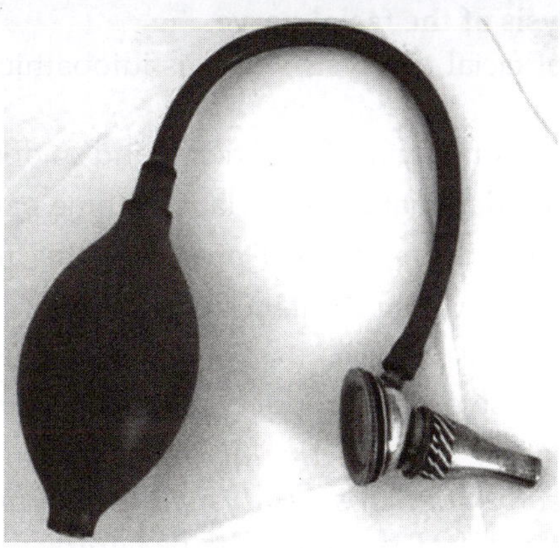

Siegel's speculum

4. **d. Stapedius**
   Of the four muscles mentioned, stapedius is the only one supplied a branch from facial nerve.
   The function of stapedius muscle is to dampen sound when they are very loud.
   Hence in patient of Bell's palsy, this muscle will be affected and will lead to hyperacussis.

5. **a. Horizontal part**
   The horizontal part is most commonly dehiscent.
   The temporal parts of facial nerve are:
   - Metal part
   - Labyrinthine part
   - Horizontal or tympanic part and
   - Vertical or mastoid part.
   - In the middle ear, the horizontal or tympanic part commonly has a natural dehiscent. As a result of this, facial nerve in this part may be exposed.
   - This part of the fallopian canal lies just over the oval window. Therefore, when it is dehiscent, the facial nerve may hang down and cover the oval window.
   - This anomaly is called ***overhanging facial nerve.***
   - This knowledge is important during middle ear surgeries or else facial nerve may be damaged during ear surgery. The commonest site of facial nerve trauma during middle ear surgery is the vertial part and not the horizontal part, despite the fact that horizontal part is the commonly exposed part.

6. **a. Dead ear**
   Fistula test is a type of ***vestibular function test.***
   In a fistula test, the patient begins to have nystagmus and vertigo on siegelisation of ear canal.
   The test is not positive in dead ear as the dead ear will not respond to any kind of stimulus.

Fistula Signs and Its Causes

Fistula sign	Causes of this sign
Fistula sign or true positive fistula sign	• Labyrinthine fistula • Perilymph fistula • Tympanoplasty type V • After stapedectomy/stapedotomy
False positive fistula sign or Hennebert's sign	• Meniere's disease • Congenital syphilis
	• Hypermobile footplate • Superior canal dehiscent syndrome
False negative fistula sign	• Dead labyrinth • Fistula blocked by cholesteatoma • Test not done properly

7. **c. Idiopathic ipsilateral paralysis of the facial nerve**
Bell's palsy is a specific type of facial paralysis which is idiopathic in nature *i.e.* where the cause of palsy is not known.
- Bell's palsy is idiopathic palsy of only the facial nerve and so does not have hemiparesis.
- In Bell's paralysis the site of inflammation is the labyrinthine part of the facial nerve.
Trigeminal nerve and abducens nerve are NOT present in this area and are very far away.
V^{th} nerve and VIth nerve are involved in ***Gradenigo's syndrome and NOT in Bell's paralysis.***
- Because of paralysis of the facial muscles, the eyelids are unable to close and so may lead to exposure keratitis. This may cause excessive tears production and NOT dryness of the eye.
- ***We know that the secretomotor fibres of the lacrimation for lacrimal glands travel through the facial nerve. If these fibres get involved in Bell's paralysis, then lacrimation may be affected and cause dryness of the eye. Therefore, dryness is NOT the rule of Bell's paralysis but may happen rarely.***

8. **a. It is associated with conductive hearing loss.**
Gradenigo's syndrome is a complication of CSOM where the disease spreads to the petrous apex. This may lead to forming of an abscess and involvement the V and VI cranial nerves.
Gradenigo's syndrome may be caused by the following conditions:
- Complication of CSOM, when the infection spreads to apex of petrous bone
- Abscess of the petrous bone
- Congenital cholesteatoma in the petrous bone.

Gradenigo's syndrome has three features. These features are:
1. ***Ear discharge***
2. ***Retro-orbital pain or deep pain***
3. ***Diplopia***

As we can see, ***hearing loss is NOT the part of this syndrome.***

Gradenigo's syndrome and hearing loss

It is interesting to note that Gradenigo's syndrome is caused because of middle ear diseases and therefore hearing loss is bound to be present in all cases of this syndrome.
But this conductive hearing loss (CHL) is NOT a part of the syndrome.

9. **c. Facial nerve palsy**
Gradenigo's syndrome is a complication of CSOM when the disease spreads to the petrous apex.
Petrous apex has two cranial nerves close to it. These nerves are:
1. Trigeminal and
2. Abducens
Facial nerve is not present near the petrous apex and so is NOT involved in this syndrome.
As a result of these nerves involvement, the following may be seen:
- Patient has trigeminal neuralgia where the pain is retro-orbital.
- Otorrhea is due to CSOM.
- The third feature of this syndrome is diplopia on lateral guaze, due to abducens palsy causing lateral rectus palsy.

Thus the three D's of Gradenigo's syndrome are:
1. ***Discharge***
2. ***Diplopia***
3. ***Deep pain (retro-oribtal pain).***

10. **a. Immediate decompression**
Mastoid fracture leading to facial nerve palsy is probably due to the fractured bone impinging on the facial nerve thus compressing it.
Hence, immediate surgery should be done to decompress the nerve to prevent degeneration of the nerve.
Treatment for traumatic facial nerve palsy depends on the latent period between the trauma and onset of palsy.

Treatment Policy for Traumatic Facial Nerve Palsy

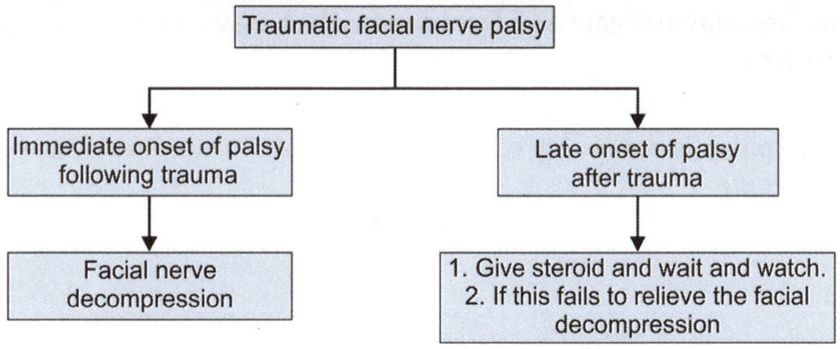

11. **d. Electrophysiological nerve testing**

In case of Bell's palsy the main drug is steroid.

If the patient does not respond to steroid for 2-3 weeks than surgical decompression may be required.

This is done only if the degeneration of the nerve has started.

Electrophysiological nerve test like electroneuronography is the best investigation to find out whether degeneration has started or not. Hence, this investigation is usually done before undertaking surgery.

Therefore if a patient of Bell's palsy does not respond to steroid, the next best management would be facial nerve decompression.

If this is NOT in the choice then the second acceptable answer is electrophysiological nerve test or electroneuronography.

Treatment Protocol for Bell's Palsy

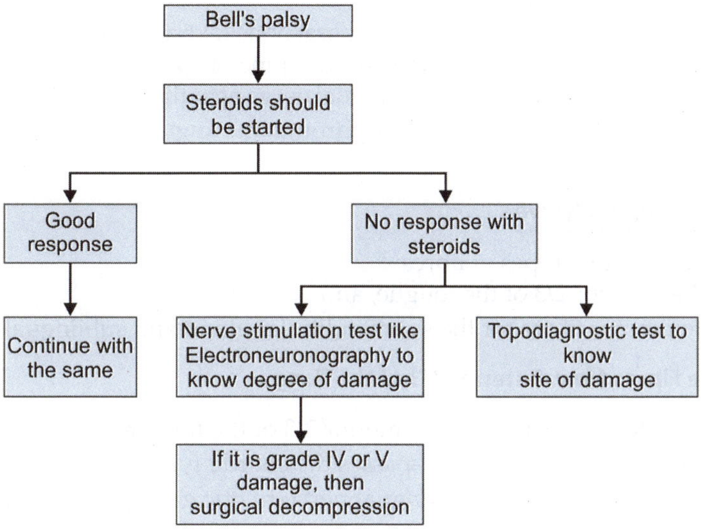

12. **b. Common with Transverse Fracture**

Temporal bone fractures are of three types:

1. Longitudinal fracture
2. Transverse fracture
3. Oblique fractures (not common)

Common fractures are:

Longitudinal fractures	Transverse fracture
• More common fracture	• Less common
• Middle ear has trauma	• Inner ear has trauma
• Hearing loss is conductive in nature	• Hearing loss is sensorineural in nature
• Findings in middle ear like hemotympanum common	• CSF otorrhea may be present
• Facial nerve palsy is less common	• Facial nerve palsy is more common

Temporal longitudinal fractures as well as transverse fracture may cause facial nerve palsy. But palsies are more common with transverse fracture of temporal bone as compare to longitudinal fracture.

Temporal bone fractures may not cause CSF rhinorrhea but may cause CSF otorrhea, and the palsy is usually partial and not complete.

13. **d. All of the above**

Recurrent facial nerve palsy is not a very common condition. It can, however, be seen in few conditions like:

- ***Melkersson's syndrome***
- ***Bell's palsy***
- ***Diabetes***
- ***Sarcoidosis,*** etc

Bilateral facial may also be seen in few conditions:

- ***Infective nerve diseases like leprosy, Guillain barre syndrome, etc***
- ***Few types of leukemias***
- ***Other conditions like sarcoidosis (this also causes recurrent facial nerve palsy), bulbar palsy, etc.***

14. **b. Loss of secretomotor fibres to the submandibular salivary gland**

Pathway of Chorda Tympani Nerve

- Chorda tympani is fourth branch of facial nerve. It arises in the temporal bone just after it comes out of the stylomastoid foramen.
- Chorda tympani then enters the middle ear through ***posterior canaliculi.*** Here it runs between the first two ossicles and travels anteriorly along the annulus of tympanic membrane.
- From the anterior part of the middle ear chorda tympani comes out through a canal in the ***petrotympanic fissure.*** This canal is called ***Huguier canal.***
- Now the chorda tympani nerve is outside the temporal bone (extra temporal part) and is in the infratemporal fossa. In the infratemporal fossa the nerve crosses the spine of sphenoid. It then runs between the mandible and the medial pterygoid muscle and joins the lingual nerve near the lower border of lateral pterygoid muscle.
- From here on the fibres of chorda tympani travel through the lingual nerve which, is a branch of mandibular division of trigeminal nerve.

Important Fibres in Chorda Tympani Nerve

Chorda tympani mainly has two types of fibres:

1. Taste fibres from the anterior 2/3 of the tongue, and
2. Preganglionic secretomotor fibres for the submandibular gland and sublingual gland.

Alternate Pathway for Taste Fibres from Anterior 2/3 of the Tongue

- There is however an alternate pathway for anterior 2/3 of the tongue.
- These alternate pathways of taste fibres by-passes the chorda tympbni nerve.
- The most important pathway is through lingual nerve to otic ganglion and thence to geniculate ganglion of the facial nerve.

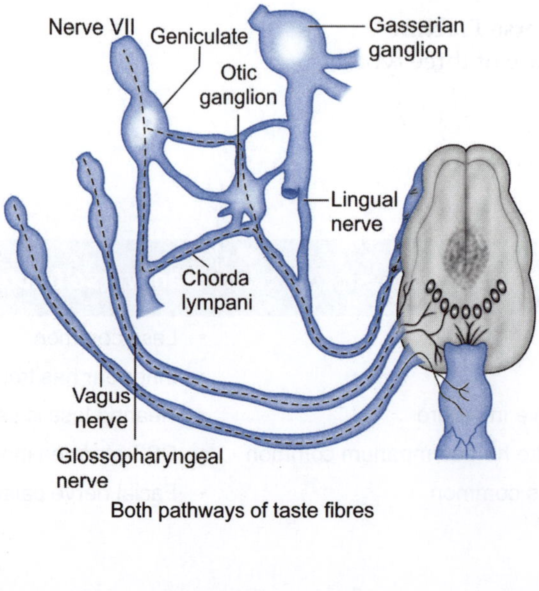

Both pathways of taste fibres

- Therefore trauma of chorda tympani nerve may spare these taste fibres from anterior 2/3 of the tongue but preganglionic secretomotor fibres will be damaged.
- Taste from posterior 1/3 of the tongue and circumvallate papillae are carried by glossopharyngeal (IXth) nerve.
- Secretomotor for parotid gland is from glossopharyngeal nerve.

In the same question, if the choices given are different, as shown below:

- Loss of taste sensation from anterior 2/3rd of tongue
- Loss of taste sensation from circumvallate papillae
- Loss of secretomotor fibres to the parotid gland
- Loss of taste sensations from posterior 1/3rd of tongue

In this, the answer is a. (loss of taste sensation from anterior 2/3rd of tongue)

15. **d. Petrositis**
    - Ear discharge with fever is a clear case of otitis media. A patient of otitis media having diplopia suggests that it has complicated to involving extra-auricular muscles.
    - This most commonly happens in petrositis that may lead to ***gradenigo's syndrome.***
16. **b. Surgical removal gives excellent prognosis**
    Ramsay Hunt syndrome is viral (Herpes zoster) infection of the geniculate ganglion of facial nerve.
    The most common presentations are:
    - Vesicles in the external ear
    - Facial palsy
    - Pain in the ear
    - In severe cases, VIIIth nerve may be involved.

Treatment

- Anti viral drugs like acyclovir and steroids are used
- Surgical excision is NOT an option.

17. **a. Deviation of angle of month towards opposite side**
18. **a. Loss of corneal reflex at side of lesion**

Brief Anatomy of Facial Nerve

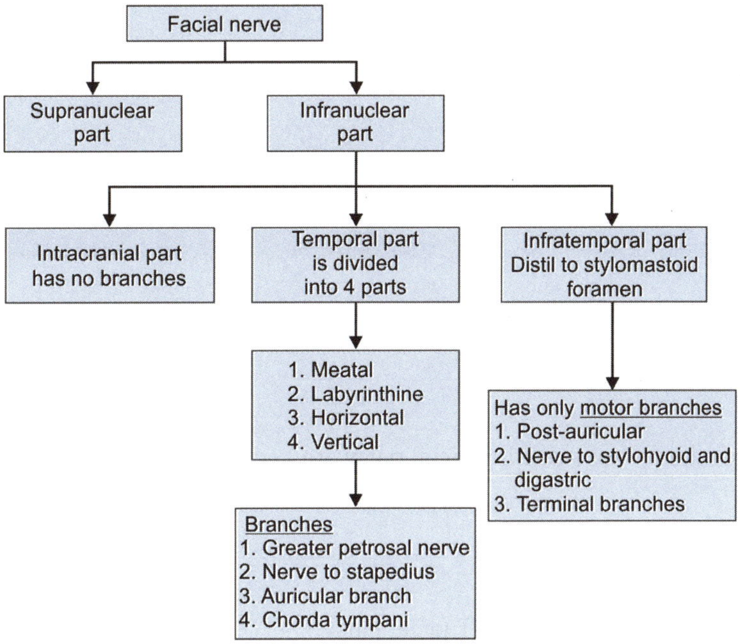

- Greater petrosal nerve arises in the temporal nerve and supplies lacrimal gland.
- Second branch is nerve to stapedius which supplies the stapedius muscle.
- Damage to this nerve may cause ***hyperacusis.***
- Auricular branch supplies canal skin
- Chorda tympani arises proximal to stylomastoid foramen and supplies taste in the anterior 2/3 tongue and secretomotor to submandibular and sublingual glands.
- Rest of the branches, arise after stylomastoid foramen and mainly supply facial muscles.
- Therefore, trauma at stylomastoid foramen will spare the branches in the temporal bones and affect only the motor of the face.

This may lead to:

- Loss of corneal reflex
- Deviation of angle of mouth to opposite side.
- Lacrimation will NOT be affected.
- Taste will NOT be affected
- Sensation on the cheek is supplied by trigeminal nerve and NOT facial nerve
- Muscle of the tongue is supplied by hypoglossal nerve and NOT facial nerve.

19. **d. Proximal to geniculate ganglion**

We know that the first branch of facial nerve is ***greater petrosal nerve*** and it arises from geniculate ganglion. This branch is responsible for lacrimation.

If the patient has loss of lacrimation then the lesion has to be proximal to the geniculate ganglion.

20. **a. Mumps**

Common Causes of Facial Palsy are:

Facial nerve palsy causes
1. Idiopathic/Bell's palsy- The most common cause of facial palsy
2. Infections-Most commonly CSOM/Cholesteatoma, herpes zoster, HIV, GB synd, EBV.
3. Tumours- Most commonly acoustic neuroma/parotid gland tumours
4. Trauma either accidental or iatrogenic
5. Systemic diseases like diabetes, sarcoidosis, etc.
6. Syndromes like Moebius syndrome, Melkersson-Rosenthal syndrome etc.
Causes of bilateral facial palsy (usually systemic diseases)
Guillain-Barre syndrome- most common causes
• Diabetes
• Sarcoidosis
• Leukaemias
• Lyme disease
• Infectious mononucleosis
• Moebius syndrome
Causes of recurrent facial nerve palsy
Bell's palsy
Diabetes
Melkersson-Rosenthal syndrome
Sarcoidosis

The four important viral infections causing facial palsy are:

1. Herpes zoster
2. HIV
3. GB syndrome
4. EBV

NOTE: Mumps may cause parotitis but NOT facial palsy.

21. **b. Transverse fracture**
Transverse fracture of the temporal bone can cause facial palsy more commonly as compared longitudinal fracture and fractures of mastoid and cribriform plate.
Cribriform plate fracture is the most common cause of CSF rhinorrhea.

22. **b. Fracture of petrous bone**
Petrous part of the temporal bone fracture is the most common cause of CSF otorrhea.

23. **a. Cross innervations of facial nerve fibres**
Crocodile tear is due to cross innervations of secretomotor fibres of lacrimal gland and secretomotor fibres of submandibular/sublingual gland. Both these are supplied by facial nerve.
In this the injury has to be ***proximal to the geniculate ganglion*** of the facial nerve.
One of the treatment options is injection of ***botilinium toxoid into the lacrimal gland.***

CHAPTER

6 Surgeries of the Middle Ear

In most of the infective diseases of the ear, medicinal treatment suffices. In unresponsive cases, surgeries may be needed. In few diseases like **active squamous COM (Unsafe CSOM or cholesteatoma); surgery is the first line of treatment.** Some non-infective diseases may also require surgical management, i.e **otosclerosis.**

All the ear surgeries are microscopic. The **focal length of the microscope during ear surgeries is 200–250 mm.**

Some of the important surgeries done in the middle ear are:
1. Myringotomy ± grommet insertion
2. Myringoplasty
3. Ossiculoplasty
4. Tympanoplasty
5. Mastoidectomy, and
6. Stapedectomy

1. **Myringotomy with/without grommet insertion**

   Myringotomy is like I and D of tympanic membrane in which a hole is made in the tympanic membrane.

   It is usually indicated in ASOM.

   The preferred quadrant of tympanic membrane for myringotomy is the ***posteroinferior quadrant. Anteroinferior quadrant is the second preferred site.***

   Grommet insertion is usually done in cases of:

   - *Glue ear and*
   - *Eustachian tube malfunction.*

   The quadrant for grommet are:

   - Anteroinferior quadrant in case of glue ear and
   - Anterosuperior quadrant in case of malfunctioning eustachian tube.

   NOTE: Never do myringotomy/grommet insertion in the posterosuperior quadrant. It is contraindicated in this quadrant.

   Complications of myringotomy are:

   - Permanent perforation
   - Trauma to middle ear structure
   - Spontaneous extrusion of grommet
   - Foreign body of middle ear (grommet falls inside the middle ear)
   - Cholesteatoma formation.

Important types of grommets are:

- Reuter Robbins
- Shepard
- Shea
- Paperella

Important differences between myringotomy and myringotomy+grommet insertion

Myringotomy	Myringotomy+grommet insertion
Common indication is bulging tympanic membrane with pain in ASOM	SOM/Glue ear is common indication
Preferred quadrant is posteroinferior	Preferred quadrant is anteroinferior
Preferred incision is circumferential	Preferred incision is radial
Usually adenoidectomy is not done along with it	Adenoidectomy is usually done with it
Complications are less common	More common complications seen.

2. **Myringoplasty**

It is repair of tympanic membrane done in case of tympanic membrane perforation.

Myringoplasty is done only for:

- ***Central perforation.***

It is contraindicated in:

- Marginal perforation and
- Attic perforation

Since central perforation is present in ***inactive mucosal COM;*** it can be inferred that:

- Myringoplasty is indicated in:
  1. **Inactive mucosal COM.**
  2. **Sometimes in Inactive squamous COM after excision of the retraction pocket**
- It is contraindicated in:
  1. **Active mucosal COM**
  2. **Active squamous COM (cholesteatoma)—absolute contraindication.**

In pinhole size permanent (very small) perforation; cauterization is done.
Trichloroacetic acid is used for cauterization of tympanic membrane.
NOTE: For cauterization of nasal septum done for Epistaxis; silver nitrate ($AgNO_3$) is used.
For small perforation (bigger than pin hole), FAT may be used as a graft material.
Traumatic perforation of tympanic membrane requires conservative management/ wait and watch.
Myringoplasty is very similar to Type I Tympanoplasty and therefore these two names mean the same.
Patch Test- A cigarette paper is used to cover the perforation. It is usually done before the Myringoplasty. It gives an idea of the hearing gain one will have after the surgery.

Temporalis fascia graft is most commonly used graft in myringoplasty. Other less commonly used grafts are:

- ***Temporalis fascia***
- *Vein graft*
- *Conchal cartilage*
- *Fat tissue/adipose tissue*
- *Perichondrium of tragus*
- *Dura.*

What are the advantages of temporalis fascia over other grafts?
1. It has a low basal metabolic rate (low BMR)
2. Easy to harvest during surgery
3. No separate incision needed. Can be harvested through the same incision as required for the main surgery
4. Very similar in thickness to a normal tympanic membrane
5. Behaves similar to the tympanic membrane.

The most common route employed during myringoplasty and other ear surgeries is the **post aural route and the incision given is *Wilde's incision.***

3. **Ossiculoplasty**

   Ossiculoplasty implies repair of ossicular chain usually done in case of traumatic disruption of ossicular chain. Sometimes the ossicles are damaged by the disease and all ossicles are not present. In such situations, prosthesis/ artificial ossicles may be required.

   Depending on the types of ossicular defects; the following classification is used:

	Austine and Kartush classification	
Group O	All ossicles intact	M+I+S+
Group A	Malleus and stapes present	M+ S+
Group B	Malleus present; stapes absent	M+ S-
Group C	Malleus absent; stapes present	M- S+
Group D	Malleus absent; stapes absent	M- S-
Group E	Intact chain but malleus head fixed	
Group F	Intact chain but stapes fixed	

Depending on the ossicles present, common prosthesis used are:

When incus and malleus are absent (Group A)	PORP (partial ossicular replacement prosthesis) is used
When all ossicles are absent (Group D)	TORP (Total ossicular replacement prosthesis) is used

The most common material used for these prosthesis is Hydroxyapatite.

NOTE: Prosthesis used during stapedectomy/stapedotomy is called piston. The most common material in this is Teflon.

The glue used for fixing PORP and TORP is the "fibrin glue".

4. **Tympanoplasty**

   Tympanoplasty has various definitions:

   - Repair of middle ear
   - Repair of the hearing mechanism
   - It is repair of tympanic membrane and ossicular chain at the same time.

Types of Tympanoplasty

There are five important types of tympanoplasties. A sixth type is also included in some books.

Tympanoplasty types	What is done in this
Type I	Also called *myringoplasty.* In this, the graft is placed over handle of malleus.
Type II	When we place graft over incus
Type III (columella)	Graft is placed over head of stapes. • This is also called *columella.* • *The third name is stapedomyringopexy/myringostapedopexy*
Type IV	Graft over round window and eustachian tube and oval window is left exposed • Creating a cavum minor and • Baffle effect
Type V	A fistula is created on **lateral semicircular canal.** This is also called *fenestration surgery.* *After this surgery; fistula test/sign may be positive.*
Type VI (Sino inversion, NOT accepted in most books)	It is reverse of type IV that's why it is called Sino inversion. Graft is placed over the round window NOT the oval window.

5. **Mastoidectomy**

Mastoidectomies are of three types. These are:

- Cortical mastoidectomy/Schwartz surgery/ Simple mastoidectomy
  - Complete mastoidectomy is a similar surgery
- Radical mastoidectomy
- Modified radical mastoidectomy (MRM)
  - Canal wall up mastoidectomy/intact wall surgery
  - Canal wall down mastoidectomy

- Cortical mastoidectomy/Schwartz surgery/ Simple mastoidectomy

  Simple mastoidectomy is like incision and drainage of mastoid antrum. In this, fluid/pus collection of the mastoid antrum is drained.

  When all the accessible air cell and antrum are exenterated, the surgery is called **complete mastoidectomy.**

  Common indications are:
  - Coalescent/Acute mastoiditis
  - Unresolving SOM/Glue ear
  - As an initial step for other surgeries.

The following serve as landmark for mastoid antrum:

a. ***McEwan's triangle or Suprameatal triangle***
b. ***Spine of Henle***
c. ***Cymba concha***

The surgeon should be aware of **Korner's septum**.

Korner's septum is ***persisting petrosquamous suture.***

All these surgeries are done under microscopic vision. The focal length of operating microscope during ear surgeries is **200–250 mm.**

- Radical mastoidectomy

  This is an extensive surgery of ear where *exteriorization* of middle ear cleft is done and everything, ***except footplate of stapes*** *is* removed.

  Indications of radical mastoidectomy:
  - Severe unsafe CSOM or Cholesteatoma
  - Tumors of ear
  - Cholesteatoma with *sensorineural hearing loss*.

Three essential steps of radical mastoidectomy:

- Exteriorization of mastoid, attic, mesotympanum, hypotympanum and protympanum
- Removal of everything EXCEPT foot plate of stapes, and
- Blockade/closure of eustachian tube.

- MRM (Modified radical mastoidectomy)

  MRM is exteriorization of mastoid antrum and attic.

  There are two main types of MRM:
  - Canal wall up MRM/ Intact wall mastoidectomy
  - Canal wall down MRM.

Differences between canal wall up and canal wall down mastoidectomies.

Canal wall up mastoidectomy	Canal wall down mastoidectomy
Posterior meatal wall is not broken. It is left intact Large meatoplasty is required	The posterior meatal wall is removed Meatoplasty not required
Done for less extensive disease	Done for more extensive disease

(Contd...)

(Contd...)

Large cavity is created giving rise to cavity problems	The cavity is relatively small. No cavity problem
Disease clearance is compromised.	Better disease removal is achieved
Hearing is better	Hearing is compromised/reduced
Recurrence and residual cholesteatoma is common	Recurrence and residual cholesteatoma is LESS common

In all the above mentioned mastoid surgeries the bone has to be cut. This can be achieved by one of the three instruments:

- **Mallet and gouge / hammer and gouge**
- **Motorized hand held drill, and**
- **Piezoelectric hand drill.**

Mallet and gouge is an old method where mastoid is cut like a chisel and hammer. It is not very precise and hence has a lot of complications.

Motorized hand held micro drill is the **most commonly** used method where a cutting drill is used to cut the bone. In this, two types of **burrs** are commonly used:

- **Cutting burr**—This is used to cut the bone rapidly and
- **Diamond burr**—In this diamond dust is attached to the drill. It is used for:
  1. *Fine cutting* and
  2. *To control bleeding during the surgery.*

During drilling, normal saline is sprayed/syringed at the drill site so as to keep the temperature down.

Piezoelectric drill is a very recent advancement in ENT surgery. In this drill, *ultrasonic vibrations* are used to cause *microfractures on the cortical bone.*

The main advantage of this is that ***the soft tissue is not damaged and only the mineralized bone is cut therefore complications are less common.***

To reduce the damage of facial nerve during mastoidectomy; the following precautions should be taken:

- Identify the various facial nerve landmarks (already mentioned above)
- Syringing with water should be done during drilling. This prevents thermal damage
- Use diamond drill when working near facial nerve
- Granulations from facial nerve should not be removed.

Few uncommon types of mastoidectomies:	
Atticotomy/Bondy's surgery	When disease confined to the attic/epitympanum
Racial recess approach/Posterior tympanotomy	• For removal of disease from middle ear • During cochlear implant

Last minute revision

- *Myringotomy is preferred in the posteroinferior quadrant of TM*
- *Myringotomy + grommet insertion is preferred in anteroinferior quadrant*
- *Most common graft for myringoplasty is temporalis fascia*
- *Temporalis fascia has a low BMR*
- *Ear prosthesis are made of hydroxyapatite*
- *Columella is type III tympanoplasty*
- *Fenestration surgery is type V tympanoplasty*
- *Macewen's triangle is the landmark for mastoid antrum*
- *The other name of Macewen's triangle is suprameatal triangle*
- *In Radical mastoidectomy, three steps done are:*
  - *Exteriorization*
  - *Removal of everything except footplate of stapes*
  - *Closure of eustachian tube*
- *Focal length of microscope used for ear surgery is 200-250 mm*
- *Diamond burr can be used for stopping bleeding during mastoidectomy.*

QUESTIONS

1. In central safe perforation the treatment of choice is:
a. Clearance and antibiotics
b. Myringoplasty
c. Radial mastoiditis
d. Modified mastoidectomy

2. Cortical mastoidectomy is indicated in:
a. CSOM with brain abscess
b. Coalescent mastoiditis
c. Perforation in pars flaccida
d. Cholesteatoma

3. Deafness associated with atticoantral perforation is treated with:
a. Instillation of drops
b. Modified radical mastoidectomy
c. Wait and watch
d. Simple mastoidectomy

4. In CSOM with cholesteatoma with vertigo, treatment of choice is:
a. Antibiotics and labyrinthine sedative
b. Myringoplasty
c. Immediate mastoid exploration
d. Labyrinthectomy

5. A 30-year-old male is having attic cholesteatoma of left ear with lateral sinus thrombophlebitis. Which of the following will be the operation of choice?
a. Intact canal wall mastoidectomy
b. Simple mastoidectomy with tympanoplasty
c. Canal wall down mastoidectomy
d. Mastoidectomy with cavity obliteration

6. In CSOM with attic cholesteatoma, treatment of choice is:
a. Modified radical mastoidectomy
b. Myringoplasty
c. Simple mastoidectomy
d. Antibiotics

7. Radical mastoidectomy is indicated in:
a. ASOM
b. CSOM
c. Acute mastoiditis
d. Masked mastoiditis

8. An incision lateral side of the temporal bone to reach the antrum through:
a. Trautman's triangle
b. Temporal line
c. Suprameatal line of Macewen's
d. Notch of Rivinus

9. Myringotomy is done in:
a. CSOM
b. Middle ear effusion
c. Otosclerosis
d. Barotraumas

10. Medical treatment is NOT effective in which type of suppurative otitis media?
a. Tuberculous OM
b. Secretory OM
c. Acute suppurative OM
d. Chronic suppurative OM

11. A patient of CSOM has cholesteatoma and presents with vertigo. Treatment of choice would be:
a. Antibiotics and labyrinthine sedative
b. Myringoplasty
c. Immediate mastoid exploration
d. Labyrinthectomy

12. Primary treatment of middle ear cholesteatoma is:
a. Surgical treatment
b. Medical and Surgery
c. Radiotherapy
d. Chemotherapy

13. A 5-year-old boy been diagnosed to have posterior superior retraction pocket cholesteatoma. All would constitute part of the management, *except:*
a. Audiometry
b. Mastoid exploration
c. Tympanoplasty
d. Myringoplasty

14. All of the following techniques are used to control bleeding from bone during mastoid surgery *except*:
a. Cutting drill over the bleeding area
b. Diamond drill over the bleeding area
c. Bipolar cautery over the bleeding area
d. Bone wax

15. Which focal length in the objective piece of microscope is commonly used for ear surgery?
a. 100 mm
b. 250 mm
c. 450 mm
d. 950 mm

16. For acute coalescent mastoiditis, treatment of choice is:
a. Simple mastoidectomy
b. Radical mastoidectomy
c. Extended mastoidectomy
d. Antibiotics and steroids

17. Fistula test will be positive in:
a. Cochlear otosclerosis
b. Cholesteatoma
c. Secretory otitis media
d. Early malignant otitis externa

18. To do myringotomy in ASOM, incision is given in posteroinferior region. This is the preferred region for all of the following reasons *except:*
   a. It is easily accessible
   b. Damage to ossicular chain does not occur
   c. Damage to cauda tympani is avoided
   d. It is very vascular region

19. Most difficult site of removal of cholesteatoma in the sinus tympani is related to:
   a. Anterior facial ridge
   b. Post facial ridge
   c. Epitympanum
   d. Hypotympanum

20. In radical mastoidectomy all the following are done *except:*
   a. Lowering of facial ridge
   b. Mucosa and middle ear muscles removed
   c. All ossicles removed except stapes footplate
   d. Maintains patency of eustachian tube

IMAGE BASED QUESTION

21. Which of the following is true of the picture given:

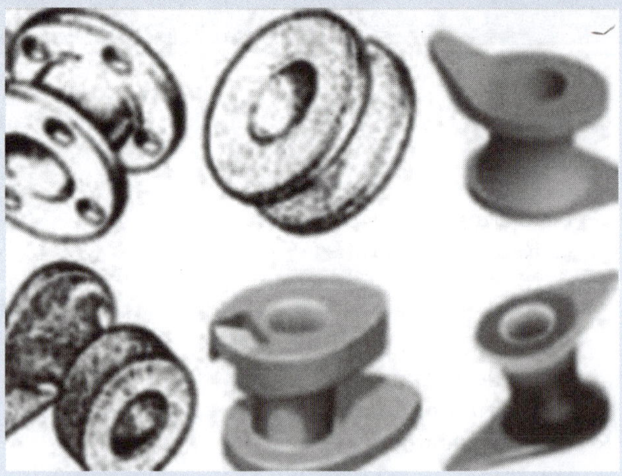

   a. These are different types of tracheostomy tubes
   b. These are types of buttons used por perichondritis
   c. These are septal buttons used for septal perforation
   d. These are grommets used for glue ear

ANSWERS AND EXPLANATIONS

1. **b. Myringoplasty**
2. **b. Coalescent mastoiditis**
3. **b. Modified radical mastoidectomy**
4. **c. Immediate mastoid exploration**

   Chronic suppurative otitis media (CSOM) can be divided into four types. If untreated they may lead to a number of complications like coalescent mastoiditis.

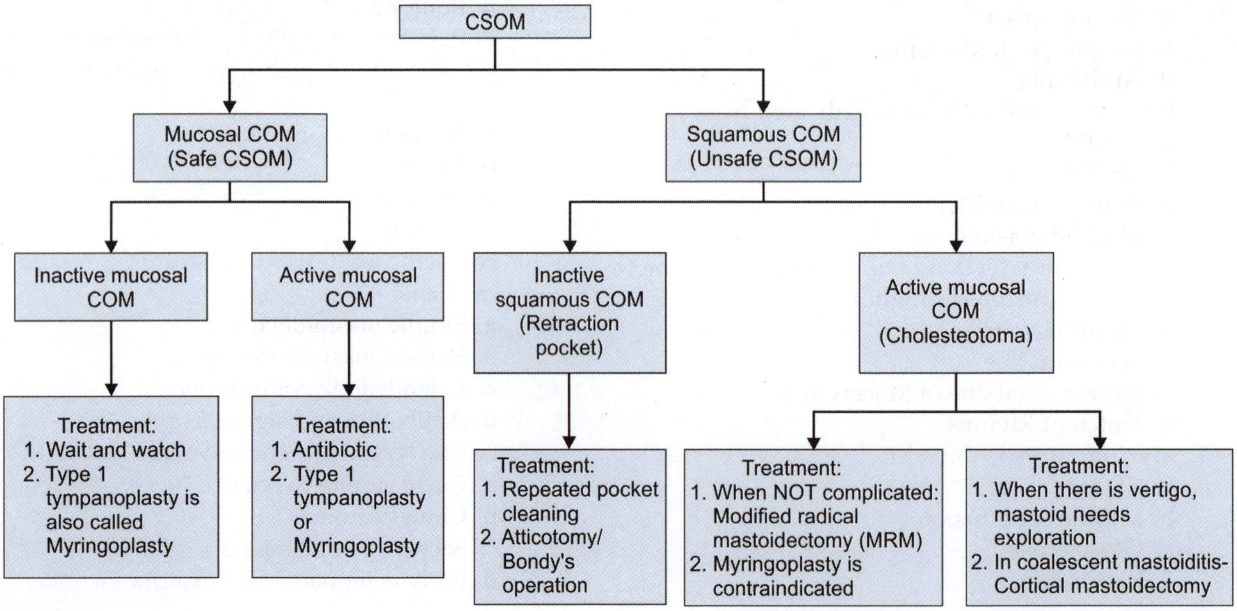

Highlights

- ***Tympanoplasty is done for Safe CSOM. Type 1 tympanoplasty is also called Myringoplasty.***
- ***Wait and watch is an alternate option when NOT active but not preferred.***
- ***In unsafe CSOM, surgery is a must.***
- ***MRM is the surgery of choice in Unsafe CSOM.***
- ***Myringoplasty is contraindicated in Unsafe CSOM.***
- ***Antibiotics can be given to all patients of CSOM, especially when the disease is active.***
- ***Cortical mastoidectomy is done for mastoiditis.***
- ***In vertigo with cholesteatoma, the site of fistula has to be explored and close/blocked.***

5. **c. Canal wall down mastoidectomy**

6. **a. Modified radical mastoidectomy**

The presence of cholesteatoma suggests that the disease is of the unsafe type.
The treatment of cholesteatoma anywhere in the middle ear is MRM.
In severe cases of cholesteaotoma, radical mastoidectomy may be done.
Modified radical mastoidectomy (MRM) are of various types, like:

- Canal wall up or intact wall
- Canal wall down
- Bondy's mastoidectomy or atticotomy
- Posterior tympanotomy or facial recess approach
- Combined approach surgery.

In the case of CSOM with attic cholesteatoma, disease has to be removed from the attic/epitympanum.
This type of mastoidectomy is called **Atticotomy (a type of MRM).**

Types of Mastoidectomies:

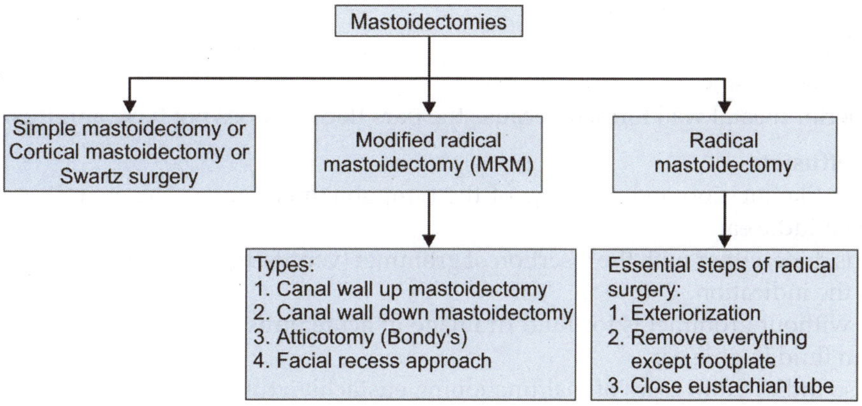

7. **b. CSOM**

Radical mastoidectomy is the ear surgery where the middle ear cleft is:

- Exteriorized
- Removal of almost everything from the ear **(except the stapes footplate)**
- Closure the eustachian tube opening.

The main aim of this surgery is to eradicate the disease from the ear.
The main disadvantage is that hearing is poor.
Such a radical surgery cannot be done for acute diseases like ASOM and mastoiditis.
Therefore, the main indication of radical mastoidectomy is extensive cholesteatoma or unsafe CSOM.
Some of the important indications of radical mastoidectomy are:

- Severe/extensive cholesteatoma or unsafe CSOM
- Failed initial surgery/Revision mastoid surgery
- CSOM with high SNHL
- Ear tuberculosis not responding to medication
- Ear tumors
- Approach to petrous apex etc.

Treatment for CSOM

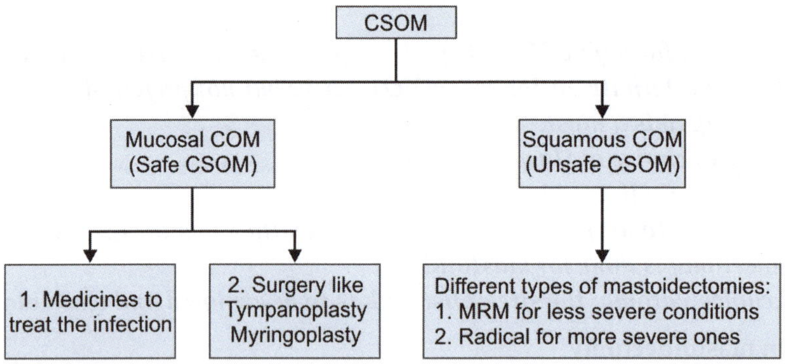

8. **c. Suprameatal line of Macewen's**

The landmark of mastoid antrum is Macewen's triangle which is also called suprameatal triangle.

In case these two are not given in the choices, then '***Spine of Henle***' is the accepted answer.

The Macewen's triangle has three boundaries. These are:

1. ***Posterosuperior meatal wall also called the Spine of Henle.***
2. ***Temporal line also called suprameatal line, and***
3. ***Tangent drawn*** between the above two.

During the mastoid surgery, incision is given here and the mastoid is opened by drilling on the Macewen's triangle.

The mastoid antrum is approximately 12–15 mm deep from this point.

- **Trautman's triangle** is a triangle which is seen after opening the mastoid. This is bounded by:
  - Anteriorly by the bony labyrinth
  - Posteriorly by the sigmoid sinus, and
  - Superiorly by the dural plate.
- **Notch of Rivinus** is a gap between:
  - The pars flaccida and
  - The superior meatal wall formed because the pars flaccida does not have annulus.

9. **b. Middle ear effusion**

Myringotomy is like incision and drainage of the tympanic membrane. This is indicated to drain the fluid collected in the middle ear.

Myringotomy is done, either with the insertion of grommet (ventilating tube) or without insertion of grommet, depending on the indication.

Myringotomy without grommet is for fluid drainage in acute otitis media and myringotomy with grommet is done to drain fluid in glue ear.

Grommet is also indicated in cases of malfunctioning eustachian tube.

Myringotomy is usually done in the posteroinferior quadrant of tympanic membrane and grommet is inserted in the anteroinferior quadrant.

Myringotomy	Myringotomy with grommet insertion
• Is indicated in ASOM	• Is indicated in Glue ear/SOM
• Incision is preferred in the posteroinferior quadrant of tympanic membrane	• Is preferred in anteroinferior quadrant
• Adenoidectomy is not done along with it	• Adenoidectomy is usually done along with it

10. **d. Chronic suppurative OM**

Chronic suppurative OM can be either of:

- Tubotympanic (safe type) or
- Atticoantral (unsafe) type.

In both types of CSOM, tympanic membrane perforation is seen. Hence, surgical repair of tympanic membrane will be required. In unsafe CSOM, mastoidectomy may be required. Hence, the main treatment in case of CSOM is surgical.

Treatment for CSOM

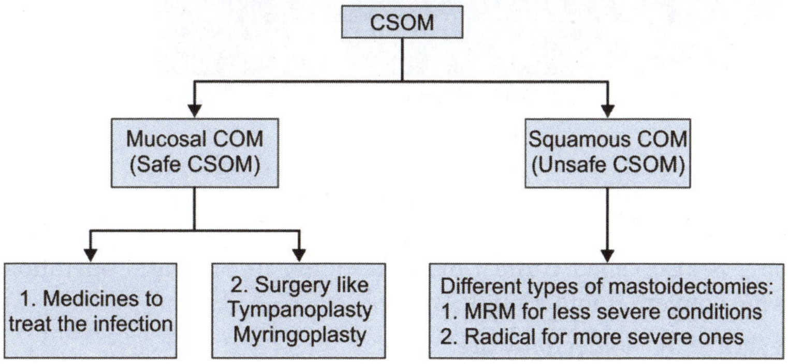

11. **c. Immediate mastoid exploration**

This is a case of complicated cholesteatoma with labyrinthine fistula. Complications happen in unsafe CSOM.

The treatment of choice for labyrinthine fistula is immediate exploration of mastoid and closure of fistula.

- Antibiotics and sedatives will not work in a patient of cholesteatoma with complications.
- Myringoplasty is done in safe CSOM. It is ***contraindicated in cholesteatoma (Unsafe CSOM).***
- Labyrinthectomy is the end stage surgery when the hearing is also completely gone.

12. **a. Surgical treatment**

Cholesteatoma is not a malignant and hence RT or chemotherapy is not used. Although it is not a malignant disease it is an aggressive disease and so needs removal.

Surgery is the primary treatment but medicines may be added.

We have already discussed this before.

13. **d. Myringoplasty**

The above mentioned patient with posterosuperior retraction pocket cholesteatoma has unsafe CSOM (***Inactive squamous COM***).

- Myringoplasty is indicated only for permanent central perforation (safe CSOM/mucosal COM).
- The above given case is a patient with unsafe CSOM where either mastoidectomy or tympanoplasty is done. Sometimes both the procedures may be combined depending on the requirement.
- Audiometry is done to assess hearing of the patient.

14. **a. Cutting drill over the bleeding area**

Mastoid surgery is done by cutting the mastoid bone with a cutting drill. If cutting drill were to control bleeding then it would not cause bleeding in the first place.

Cutting drill is not used to control bleeding, rest of the mentioned choices are all used to control bleeding during mastoid surgery.

- Bipolar cautery and bone wax are very commonly used to stop bleeding during surgeries.
- Special note should be made about the diamond drill which is used to cut as well as control the bledding.

Mastoidectomy drill has three types of burr that is used for cutting:

- Cutting burr: This cuts the bone very fast but can cause bleeding.
- Policing burr: This cut slowly and is used for smoothening the mastoid cavity
- Diamond burr: This cuts very slowly and precisely.

15. **b. 250 mm**

Microscopes are integral part of ENT surgeries. They are used for the surgeries of ear, nose as well as throat. However, microscopic nasal surgeries are not done anymore.

During the surgeries of different area; the lens with different focal lengths are used.

The various focal lengths are:

Surgeries	Focal lengths
Ear surgeries	200–250 mm
Nasal surgeries	300 mm
Throat surgeries	400 mm

16. **a. Simple mastoidectomy**

Simple mastoidectomy is also called cortical mastoidectomy or Schwartz operation, in which the mastoid antrum and air cells are converted into a single cavity.

Other indications of simple mastoidectomy are:
- Acute otitis media not responding to medication
- As an approach to other surgeries etc.

Macewen's triangle is the land mark for mastoid antrum during mastoidectomy.

17. **b. Cholesteatoma**

Important causes of ***true positive fistula test*** are:
- ***Labyrinthine fistula, a complication of CSOM***
- ***Fenestration surgery or Type V tympanoplasty***
- ***Post stapedectomy***
- ***Perilymph fistula***

Important causes of **false positive fistula** test are:
- ***Meniere's disease where it is also called hennebert's sign***
- ***Congenital syphilis***

Important causes of **false negative fistula** test are:
- ***Dead labyrinth***
- ***Fistula which is blocked by cholesteatoma***

Labyrinthine fistula is a complication of cholesteatoma and so fistula sign may be positive in ***cholesteatoma that complicates***.
- Cochlear otosclerosis is otosclerosis of inner ear and fistula sign is NOT present.
- Secretory otitis media is a safe type of middle ear infection. No fistula sign in this.
- Malignant otitis externa is an external ear disease. No fistula sign in this.

18. **d. It is very vascular region**
- The angulation of the tympanic membrane and the shape of external auditory meatus is such that the posteroinferior quadrant is the most accessible area of the tympanic membrane during myringoplasty.
- The ossicular chain and chorda tympani are predominantly in the posterosuperior quadrant of the middle ear and tympanic membrane and therefore they do not get damaged during myringoplasty.
- The most vascular part of the tympanic membrane is the ***posterosuperior quadrant and NOT postero-inferior quadrant.***
- ***Because the posteroinferior quadrant in NOT very vascular, bleeding is not a problem during myringoplasty in this quadrant.***

19. **a. Anterior facial ridge**

Posterior wall of the middle ear has two important recesses. These are:
- Facial recess
- Sinus tympani

They are on either side of facial ridge and facial nerve (facial nerve runs inside the facial ridge).
Facial ridge (with facial nerve) is lateral to sinus tympani and is medial to facial recess.

Sinus Tympani

The two important boundaries of sinus tympani are:
1. Ponticulus is superior
2. Subiculum is inferior

This is the most difficult area of the middle for removal of cholesteatoma.
This is made difficult by the anterior part of the facial ridge.

- Epitympanum is also called attic. This is the most common site of cholesteatoma. However, cholesteatoma removal from this area is easy. The surgery needed for this area is ***atticotomy (Bondy's mastoidectomy).***
- Hypotympanum is usually disease free area.

20. **d. Maintains patency of eustachian tube**

Radical mastoidectomy is a type of mastoidite surgery it also controls mastoid bleeding . This surgery is done in cases of unsafe CSOM (active squamous COM or cholesteatoma).
The three essential steps of radical mastoidectomy are:

1. ***Exteriorization of the ear.*** This is achieved by:
   a. Breaking the bridge and
   a. Lowering the facial ridge
2. ***Removal of every thing from the cavity (mucosa, muscles, ossicles etc) EXCEPT foot plate of stapes***
3. ***Closure of the eustachian tube.*** Patency of the eustachian tube is NOT maintained.

IMAGE BASED ANSWER

21. **d. These are grommets used for glue ear**

These are pictures of grommets which are inserted into the tympanic membrane in patients suffering from glue ear.

CHAPTER 7

Tests and Investigations for Ear Diseases

The two primary functions of ear are:

1. Hearing, and
2. Balancing.

We all know that the entire ear or hearing pathway is used for hearing.

For balancing, external ear and middle ear are NOT used, and rest of the pathway is used.

Therefore in ear diseases, we must investigate different parts of ear and different types of investigations for both, hearing as well as balancing.

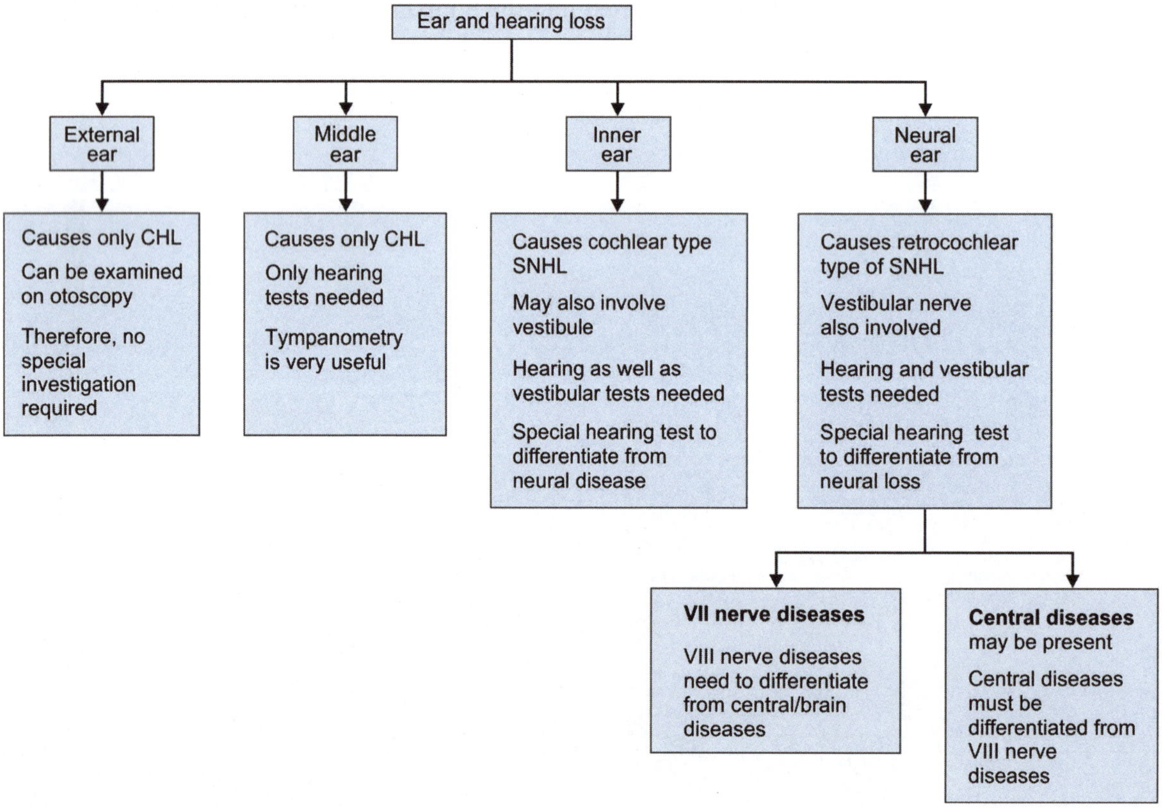

Working Classification of Hearing Loss

0–25 db	Normal hearing
26–40 dB	Mild hearing loss
41–55 dB	Moderate hearing loss
56–70 dB	Moderately severe hearing loss
71–90 dB	Severe hearing loss
>91 dB	Profound hearing loss

Some important tests in case of EAR DISEASES

Tests	Types
Tuning fork tests	Rinne's test Weber's test Schwabach's test/ABC test Bing test Gelle's test, etc.
Audiometry and Special audiometry tests	Pure tone audiometry (PTA) Recruitment test (ALBL) Short increment sensitivity index (SISI) Tone decay test Rollover curve Speech discrimination score (SDS), etc.
Tympanometry and Stapedial reflex	Tympanometry and Acoustic reflex/stapedial reflex
Evoked physiological tests	Electrocochleography/Cochlear microphonics (CM) Otoacoustic emission (OAE) Brainstem-evoked response audiometry (BERA) Central evoked response audiometry (CERA)
Vestibular function tests	Caloric test Electronystagmography (ENG)/video ENG Optokinetic test Galvanic test Posturography Fistula test Vestibular evoked myogenic potential (VEMP) Dix-Hallpike manoeuvre, etc.

Main Differences between CHL and SNHL Findings

Tests	Conductive hearing loss	Sensorineural hearing loss
Rinne's test	BC > AC	AC > BC
Weber's test	Lateralizes to same side	Lateralizes to opposite side
Absolute bone conduction (ABC)	Same as examiner	Reduced than examiner
Schwabach's test	Increases	Decreases
Gelle's test	Negative test	Positive test
Bing test	No change in loudness	Loudness increases
Audiometry (PTA)	A-B gap is more than 10 dB (some accept 15 dB)	A-B gap less than 10-15 dB

Differences between Cochlear Diseases and Retrocochlear Diseases

Tests	Cochlear diseases	Retrocochlear diseases
Stapedial/acoustic reflex	Present	Absent
Recruitment	Present	Absent
Short increment sensitivity index (SISI)	Present	Absent
Bekesy audiometry	Type II graph	Type III or Type IV graph
Tone decay phenomena of one minute	Seen at < 25 dB above threshold	At > 25 dB above threshold
Rollover curve	Not seen	Seen

(Contd...)

(Contd...)

Tests	Cochlear diseases	Retrocochlear diseases
Speech discrimination score (SDS)	Slightly reduced	Severely reduced
Cochlear microphonics (CM)	Absent	Present
Otoacoustic emission (OAE)	Affected	Not affected
BERA	Latency is normal between wave I and wave V	Increased latency between wave I and wave V

TUNING FORK TEST

The most commonly used frequency during tuning fork test is **512 Hz.**

Although the common tuning fork tests and their interpretations are already discussed, few more points about the two most important tuning fork tests are as follows:

Rinne's Test

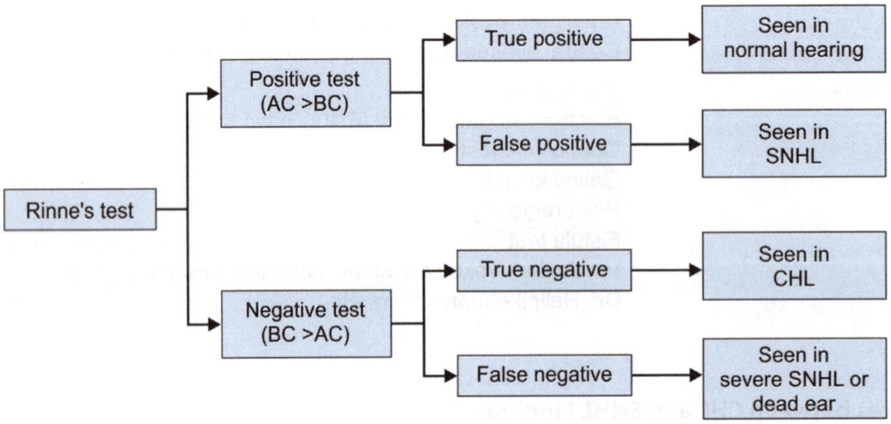

Weber's Test

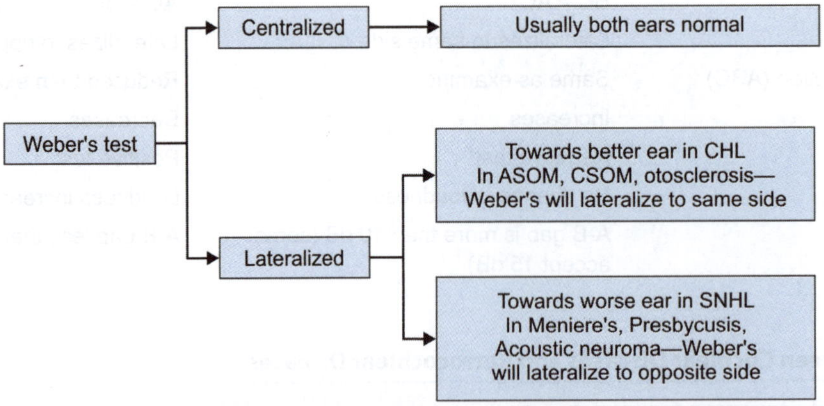

- *What is false negative Rinne's*
- *When Rinne's is negative (BC >AC) and Weber's is lateralized to the opposite side*

While checking air conduction (AC) in one side; it may be heard/lateralized to the other ear when the threshold of sound is >40 dB

While checking bone conduction (BC) in one ear, it will lateralize to other ear when the threshold is 5 dB

Therefore, bone conduction is very sensitive

This makes Weber's test the most sensitive tuning fork test

Some points to remember about tuning fork

The most commonly used frequency during tuning fork test is 512 Hz.

For Gelle's test, Siegel's speculum is required
Gelle's test used is considered as a diagnostic tuning fork test for:
- Otosclerosis and
- Ossicular chain disruption

False negative Rinne's test is seen in Dead ear/Severe sensorineural hearing loss
There are few more types of outdated types of tuning fork tests. Do NOT waste time on them.

AUDIOMETRY/PURE TONE AUDIOMETRY (PTA)

Audiometry is done using single frequency at a time and is, therefore, called pure tone audiometry.
It is a **subjective type of investigation, unlike tympanometry, which is an objective type.**

Aim of audiometry is to know the following:

1. Whether or not hearing loss is present
   - When threshold is above 25 dB, it suggests hearing loss and
   - When threshold is below 25 dB, it suggests normal hearing
2. Degree of hearing loss
3. Type of hearing loss. Whether
   - Conductive (CHL), or
   - Sensorineural (SNHL)
4. Side of hearing loss
5. Sometimes, it may also be used to know the cause of hearing loss. This can be known depending on the shape of the audiogram.

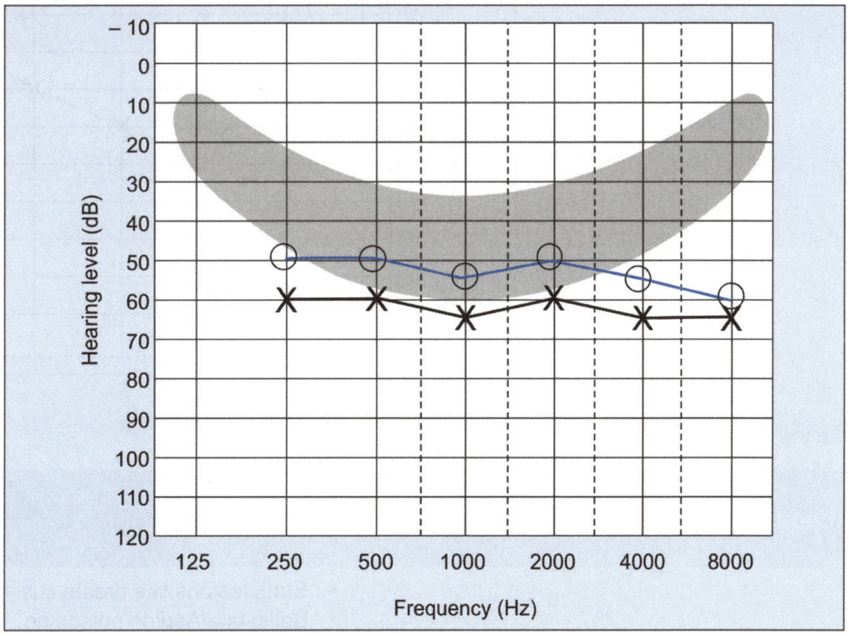

A typical audiogram may look like the above diagram

Kindly note that the audiogram is a **graph between frequency and hearing level.**

1. When we increase the loudness of sound to check hearing level, the loudness is increased in the multiples of 5 dB.
2. **The frequencies that are usually checked are 125 Hz, 250 Hz, 500 Hz, 1000 Hz, 2000 Hz, 4000 Hz and 8000 Hz.**

3. **When we check frequencies > 8000 Hz, it is called "high-frequency audiometry".**
4. **High frequency audiometry is indicated in suspected case of *Ototoxicity*.**
5. **In case, some thresholds are less than 25 dB and some are more than 25 dB, the average of *250 Hz, 500 Hz, 1000 Hz and 2000 Hz* is usually calculated.**
6. **When this value is ≥ 25 dB, it suggests normal hearing**
7. **When this value is > 25 dB, it suggests hearing loss**

IMPORTANT TYPES OR SHAPES OF AUDIOGRAMS AND THEIR DIAGNOSIS

For conductive hearing loss

Types/shapes of graph	Diagnosis
1. Upward sloping/left sloping (more loss at lower frequency)	• Otosclerosis
2. Downward sloping/right sloping (loss at higher frequency)	Conditions with increased mass in middle ear • Serous otitis media (SOM) • Ossicular chain damage
3. Dip at 2000 Hz/Carhart's notch	• Otosclerosis

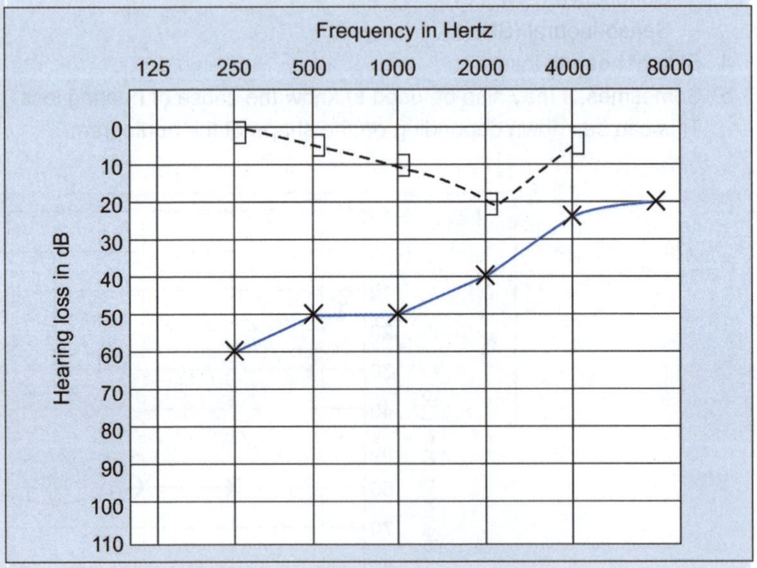

For sensorineural hearing loss

Types/shapes of graph	Diagnosis
1. Flat graph	• Strial lesions like presbycusis • Salicylate/Aspirin poisoning
2. Downwards sloping/right sloping More loss at higher frequencies	Problems of organ of Corti, e.g. • Ototoxicity • Noise-induced hearing loss (NIHL)
3. Upwards sloping/left sloping More loss at lower frequency	When membranes stiffens, e.g • Early stage of Meniere's disease • Other causes of hydrops

Types/shapes of graph	Diagnosis
4. Trough-shaped or "U"-shaped	• Congenital hearing loss
5. Dip at 4000 Hz	• Acoustic neuroma • Sometimes NIHL

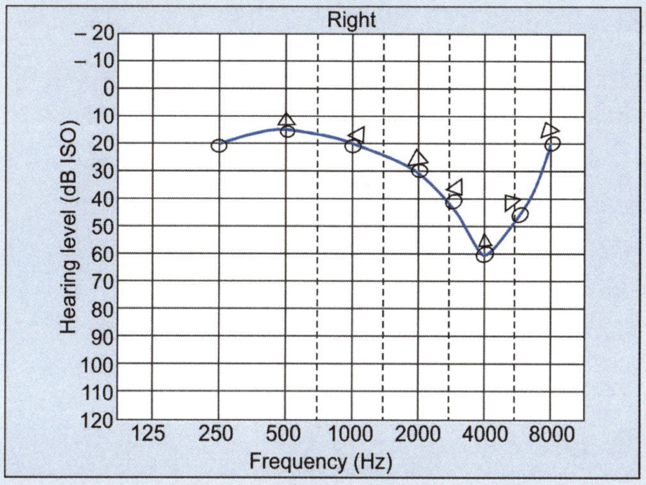

MASKING DURING AUDIOMETRY

As discussed under the topic of tuning fork:

1. AC lateralizes to other ear when the threshold is >40 dB, and
2. BC lateralizes to other ear when the threshold is 5 dB

This means that when one ear is checked with above-mentioned thresholds, the sound may be heard on the other ear also and give wrong result of audiometry.

In order to avoid this confusion, **masking of the other ear/nontesting ear** is advised.

Therefore:

1. During AC testing, masking is required when the threshold of sound is >40 dB, and
2. During BC testing, masking is required when the threshold is 5 dB or more. For practical reason, masking is always done during bone conduction (BC)

Tympanometry

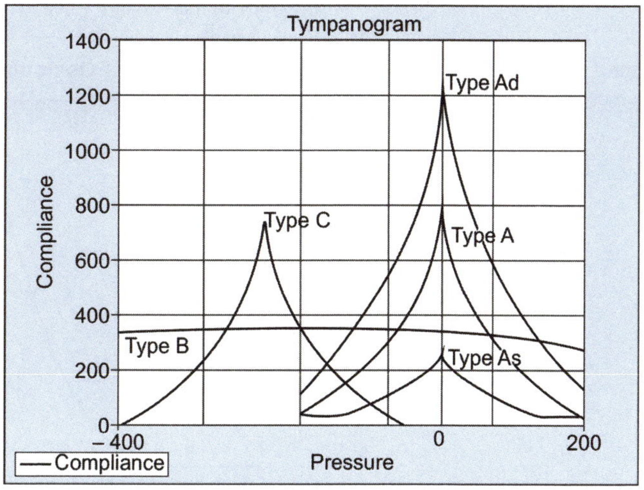

Tympanogram showing all types of graphs

TYMPANOMETRY IS ALSO CALLED IMPEDANCE AUDIOMETRY

In tympanometry, we look for the ***compliance** of middle ear.*

Tympanometry is done dusing the probe of the following frequencies:

- 220 Hz frequency probe.
- Some times 226 Hz probe is also used
- In infants < 4-6 months old, the probe of 1000 Hz is used

Tympanometry is an **objective type of investigation**

Based on compliance of middle ear, tympanograms are of five main types. They are given below.

Type A	Compliance is normal	**Normal middle ear** 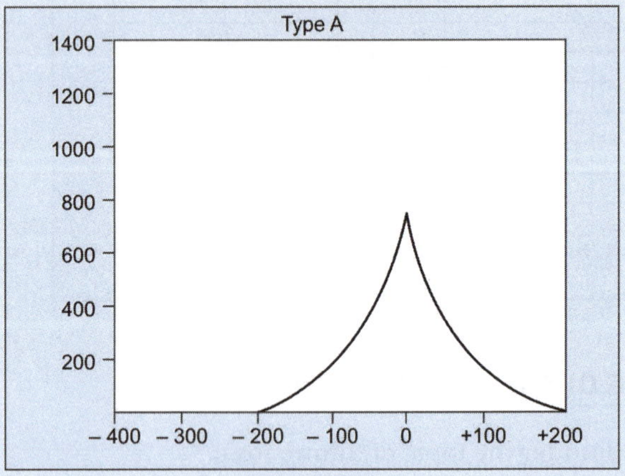
Type As	Compliance is reduced	Otosclerosis 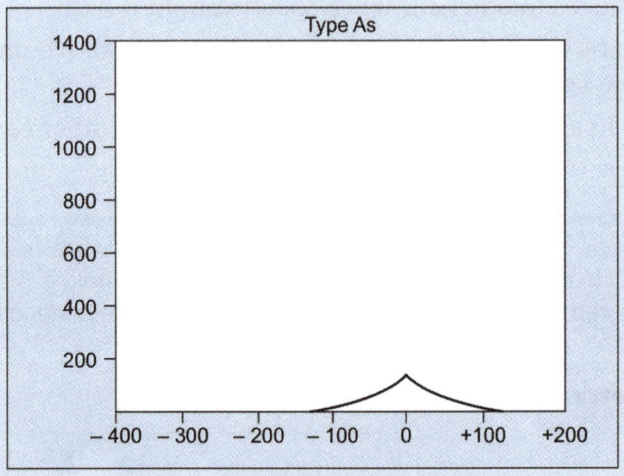
Type Ad	Compliance is increased	**Disruption of Ossicular Chain** 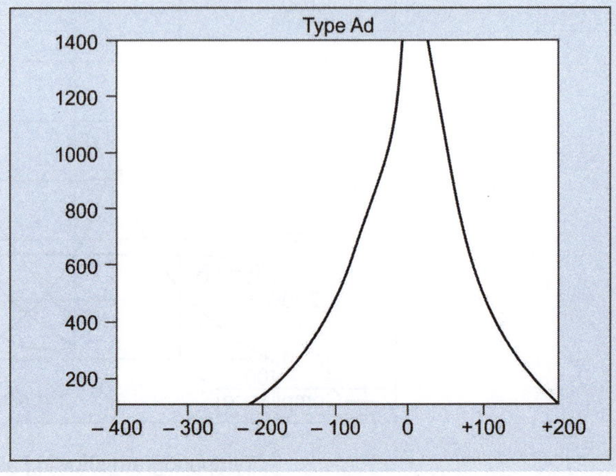

(Contd...)

(Contd...)

Type B	Also called flat tympanogram	**1. Low flat** in case of **fluid in ear like:** ASOM and Glue Ear 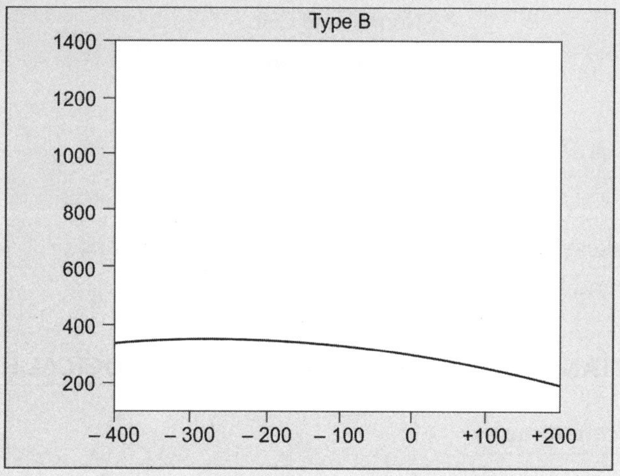
		2. High flat in case of perforation, like • CSOM
Type C	Also called negative tympanogram	**Glue Ear and ET dysfunction** 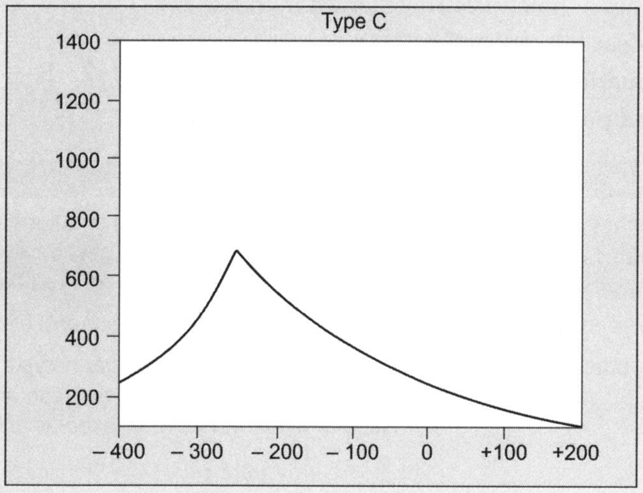

From the above given points, we can see that tympanogram is usually used for

- **Make diagnosis of *middle ear diseases***
- ***Check the stapedial reflex/acoustic reflex***
- ***Check the functioning of eustachian tube***

To check the function of the eustachian tube, these are the common tests:

1. Tympanometry/impedance reflux
2. Politzerization
3. Toynbee test

Among the above-mentioned tests, **tympanometry is the best.**

Comparison between Audiometry and Tympanometry

Audiometry	Tympanometry
Checks the threshold of hearing	Based on compliance or impedance of middle ear
Subjective investigation	Objective investigation
Used for disease in any part of the hearing path	Used only for middle ear disease
Mainly to know about hearing status of ear	Mainly to make diagnosis for middle ear disease

Bekesy Audiometry

Bekesy audiometry curves are of five types. They are as follows:

Type I	Normal and CHL
Type II	Cochlear disease
Type III	Retrocochlear disease
Type IV	Retrocochlear disease
Type V	Malinger

NOTE: Bekesy audiometry is an outdated investigation.
Do not spend too much time studying it

IMPORTANT POINTS ABOUT EVOKED PHYSIOLOGICAL HEARING TESTS

Electrocochleography

We already know that the function of cochlea is **transduction.**
Which means: The cochlea converts mechanical energy of sound into the electrical potential.
This electrical potential of the cochlea is graphed in this test
Three types of potentials are obtained in this:

1. **Cochlear microphonics (CM)**
2. **Summation potential (SP), and**
3. **Action potential (AP)**

Electrocochleography	
1. Cochlear microphonics	• This is AC potential (AC) of outer hair cell • Produced when hair cell gets depolarized during transduction • Therefore, it is absent in hair cell damage or cochlear diseases
2. Summation potential	• It is DC potential (direct current) of outer hair cell
3. Action potential	• This is potential of cochlear nerve Note: In Meniere's disease, the ratio of SP/AP increases Ratio SP/AP > 0.4–0.45 is taken as diagnostic of Meniere's

Otoacoustic Emission (OAE)

Otoacoustic emission is the potential produced due to mechanical lengthening (electromotility) of outer hair cells.
It can be of many types:

1. Spontaneous OAE
2. Evoked OAE
3. Distortion OAE

Like the cochlear microphonics, OAE is also affected in cochlear diseases

NOTE: Otoacoustic emission (OAE) is used:

- For screening of hearing loss in newborn and infants (first line investigation)
- For diagnosis of hearing loss due to cochlear pathology.

In every child who has to be admitted in NICU, OAE should be done.

Brainstem-Evoked Response Audiometry (BERA)

This is an objective type of investigation for hearing.
It is a complex graph produced as the electrical potential travels from cochlea into the eighth nerve.
BERA graph ideally has **seven waves/peaks.** Each peak is produced by different part of the hearing path.

Waves of BERA	Their causes
Wave I	• Distal part of VIII nerve This part of the nerve is in the internal acoustic meatus. This part of the nerve is myelinated The 1st BERA wave corresponds with cochlear microphonics Because both are produced by close by areas. Therefore, both will be affected by similar diseases
Wave II	• Proximal part of VIII nerve This part of the nerve is unmyelinated The nerve is about to enter the brainstem
Wave III	• Cochlear nucleus
Wave IV	• Superior olivary nucleus (SON) SON receives nerve from both the side of cochlea
Wave V	• Lateral lemniscus. Partly contributed by inferior colliculus This is most constant and most reliable wave of BERA, therefore This is the most important wave of BERA It may be delayed in acoustic neuroma
Waves VI and VII	• Inferior colliculus

The main advantages of BERA are:

1. It is objective test and can be used test or screen hearing in uncooperative patient.
2. ***This is second most common investigation to check hearing in infants and children.***
3. It is used to differentiate a cochlear disease from a retrocochlear disease.
4. It can tell site of disease in retrocochlear disease.

Note: The two good investigations for screening and diagnosis of hearing loss in infants/newborns are:

1. Best option is to carry out both the investigations, i.e OAE and BERA.
2. Otherwise, otoacoustic emission (OAE) is done first.
3. If required, we can follow up with BERA

Central-Evoked Response Audiometry (CERA)

This wave is obtained by evoking the central auditory pathway in the brain.
It can be used in cases of central cause of hearing defects.

IMPORTANT VESTIBULAR FUNCTION TEST

Caloric Test

Caloric test is one of the most commonly done test to check the vestibule.
Caloric test has many types and therefore has many names.
Some common examples are:

Names of caloric tests
• Bithermal caloric test • Fitzgerald-Hallpike test • Modified Kobrak test • Dundas grant test or cold air caloric test
NOTE: 1. *Dundas grant test or cold air caloric test is done in patients who have perforation of the tympanic membrane* 2. Tube is used for this. This tube is called dundas grant tube 3. ethyl chloride is used as coolant in this tube

In this test, water/saline of two different temperatures is used.

The temperature of saline used is:

- ***30° C and 44° C (normal body temperature, i.e. 37° ± 7°)***

During caloric test:

- ***The horizontal canal has to be aligned in vertical canal.***
- This can be achieved by changing position of patient. Patient can be placed in one of the two positions
  1. Supination with head raised by 30°.
  2. Sitting down with head bent backwards by 60°.

In caloric test, when the ear canal is syringed with either 30 degree or 44 degree water, the following happens:

- "Convection current/thermoconvection" is set up in the fluid of horizontal semicircular canal
- This will stimulate the cristae ampullaris of the horizontal semicircular canal
- This will start "nystagmus" along with vertigo/nausea
- Besides convection current, caloric test causes another effect resulting in nystagmus. This alternate physiology is:

Expansion of endolymph caused by heat
↓
Asymmetric stimulation of canal ring
↓
Volume displacement towards the cupula
↓
Causes nystagmus

- The duration of nystagmus can tell us the following two things:
  1. Canal Paresis and/or
  2. Direction Preponderance
- This can be used to diagnose the functional status of the vestibule
- *When syringing is done in both the ears at the together; endolymph movement in the two ears will take place in opposite direction and neutralize each other. Therefore nystagmus will NOT be induced.*

Syringing with *cold water or 30° causes nystagmus of the opposite side,* whereas *warm water or 44° syringing causes nystagmus of the same side.*

This can be remembered by a very commonly used mnemonic **"COWS".**

Eye movement vs nystagmus	
Hypoactive disease of vestibule *and* *cold water (30 degrees) syringing of canal*	*Causes eye movement on the same side, but* *Nystagmus of the opposite side*
Hyperactive/irritative disease of vestibule and *Syringing with warm water (44 degrees)*	*Causes eye movement of the opposite side, but* *Nystagmus of the same side* *Note: Since most diseases are hypoactive lesions; Nystagmus in most cases is on the opposite side* *Note: as discussed above, nystagmus is opposite to the eye movement caused by syringing*

Differences between peripheral and central nystagmus

Peripheral nystagmus	Central nystagmus
Peripheral diseases are diseases of vestibule	These are diseases of central pathway
Usually horizontal nystagmus	Usually vertical or rotatory nystagmus, i.e. • *Downbeating nystagmus is present in Arnold-Chiari disease*

(Contd...)

(Contd...)

Peripheral nystagmus	Central nystagmus
Has latency of few a seconds	No latency
Short lasting	Long lasting
Fatigable	Not fatigable
Direction dependent	Not dependent
Associated with nausea/vomiting	No nausea/vomiting

Important points about other vestibular function tests

- Stimulation of lateral canal causes horizontal nystagmus
- Stimulation of posterior canal causes upbeating nystagmus

- End organs of vestibule (macula and crista ampullaris) are stimulated in all types of vestibular function test EXCEPT the "Galvanic test", where the vestibular nerve is stimulate
- Therefore, galvanic test can be used to differentiate *end organ disease vs vestibular nerve disease.* This can be compared to BERA (for VII nerve disease) and OAE (for end organ or hair cell disease).
- VEMP is caused by *saccule and inferior vestibular nerves of ear*
- Therefore, the disease of any of these (saccule and inferior vestibular nerve) can diminish this potential.

REVIEW OF EAR DISEASES AND THEIR INVESTIGATIONS

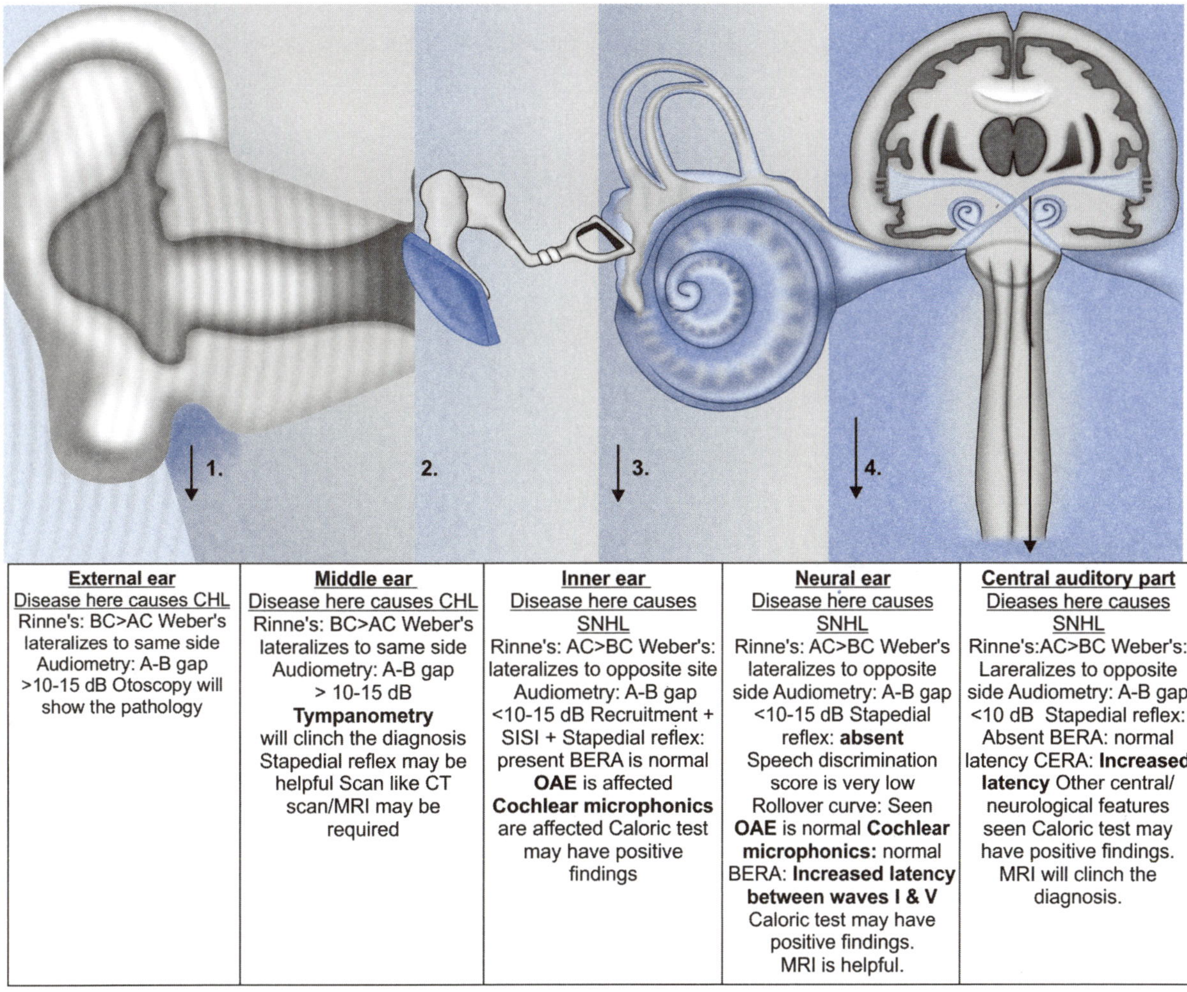

External ear	Middle ear	Inner ear	Neural ear	Central auditory part
Disease here causes CHL Rinne's: BC>AC Weber's lateralizes to same side Audiometry: A-B gap >10-15 dB Otoscopy will show the pathology	Disease here causes CHL Rinne's: BC>AC Weber's lateralizes to same side Audiometry: A-B gap > 10-15 dB **Tympanometry** will clinch the diagnosis Stapedial reflex may be helpful Scan like CT scan/MRI may be required	Disease here causes SNHL Rinne's: AC>BC Weber's: lateralizes to opposite site Audiometry: A-B gap <10-15 dB Recruitment + SISI + Stapedial reflex: present BERA is normal **OAE** is affected **Cochlear microphonics** are affected Caloric test may have positive findings	Disease here causes SNHL Rinne's: AC>BC Weber's lateralizes to opposite side Audiometry: A-B gap <10-15 dB Stapedial reflex: **absent** Speech discrimination score is very low Rollover curve: Seen **OAE** is normal **Cochlear microphonics:** normal BERA: **Increased latency between waves I & V** Caloric test may have positive findings. MRI is helpful.	Dieases here causes SNHL Rinne's:AC>BC Weber's: Lareralizes to opposite side Audiometry: A-B gap <10 dB Stapedial reflex: Absent BERA: normal latency CERA: **Increased latency** Other central/ neurological features seen Caloric test may have positive findings. MRI will clinch the diagnosis.

Last minute revision

- *In conductive hearing loss like CSOM, otosclerosis, Weber's will lateralize to the same side*
- *In sensorineural hearing loss like Meniere's, presbycusis, it will lateralize to opposite side*
- *Severe sensorineural hearing loss may give false negative Rinne's test*
- *Audiometry is a subjective type of investigation*
- *Meniere's disease has more loss at lower frequencies*
- *Otosclerosis shows Cahart's notch*
- *Noise-induced hearing loss has dipped at 4000 Hz*
- *High frequency is done in ototoxicity*
- *"As" tympanogram is seen in pregnant ladies with hearing loss due to otosclerosis*
- *Best test for screening of hearing in newborns is evoked OAE*
- *Second best test of screening is BERA*
- *The fifth peak of BERA is formed by lateral lemniscus*
- *Cold air caloric test is called dundas grant test*
- *Caloric test with cold water causes nystagmus to opposite side*
- *Caloric test with warm water causes nystagmus to the same side.*

QUESTIONS

1. **A positive fistula test during Siegalization indicates:**
   a. Ossicular discontinuity
   b. Para-labyrinthitis due to erosion of lateral semicircular canal
   c. CSF leak through the ear
   d. Fixation of stapes bone
2. **Use of siegel's speculum during examination of the ear provides all except:**
   a. Magnification.
   b. Assessment of movement of the tympanic membrane.
   c. Removal of foreign body from the ear.
   d. As applicator for the powdered antibiotic of ear.
3. **Otoacoustic emissions (OAE) are derived from which of the following:**
   a. Outer hair cells b. Basilar membrane
   c. Oral window d. Tympanic membrane
4. **In conductive deafness, Weber's test is lateralized to the**
   a. Deaf ear b. Normal ear
   c. Both ears d. None
5. **A child was treated for H. influenzae meningitis for 6 month. Most important investigation to be done before discharging the patient is:**
   a. MRI
   b. Brainstem evoked auditory response
   c. Growth screening test
   d. Psychotherapy
6. **In 'cold caloric stimulation test', the cold water induces movement of the eyeball in the following direction:**
   a. Towards the opposite side
   b. Towards the same side
   c. Upwards d. Downwards
7. **Carhart's notch is seen at dip at:**
   a. 0.5 Hz b. 1 Hz
   c. 1.5 Hz d. 2 Hz
8. **Weber test is best elected by:**
   a. Placing the tuning fork on the mastoid process and comparing the bone conduction of the patient with that of the examiner
   b. Placing the tuning fork on the vertex of the skull and determining the effect of gently occluding the auditory canal on the threshold of low frequencies.
   c. Placing the tuning fork on the mastoid process and comparing the bone conduction in the patient
   d. Placing the tuning fork on the forehead and asking him to report in which ear he hears it better.
9. **Impedance audiometry is for the pathology of the:**
   a. External ear b. Middle ear
   c. Mastoid cell extension
   d. Inner ear
10. **All are subjective test for hearing EXCEPT:**
    a. Tone Decay
    b. Impedance audiometry
    c. Speech audiometry
    d. Puretone audiometry
11. **Otoacoustic emission arises from:**
    a. Inner hair cells
    b. Outer hair cells
    c. Both inner and outer hair cells
    d. Organ of Corti
12. **Conductive deafness occurs in:**
    a. Travelling in aeroplane or ship
    b. Trauma to labyrinth
    c. Stapes abnormal at oval window
    d. High noise
13. **In Fitzgerald and Hallpike differential caloric test, cold-water irrigation at 30 degrees centigrade in the left ear in a normal person will include:**
    a. Nystagmus to the right side
    b. Nystagmus to the left side
    c. Direction changing nystagmus
    d. Positional nystagmus
14. **Which is the investigation of choice in assessing hearing loss in neonates:**
    a. Impedance audiometry
    b. Brainstem Evoked Response Audiometry (BERA)
    c. Free field audiometry
    d. Behavioral audiometry
15. **Hearing in infants can be tested by:**
    a. Schwabach's test
    b. Acoustic reflex impedance audiometry
    c. Threshold tone decay test
    d. Pure tone audiometry
16. **In right middle ear pathology Weber`s test will be:**
    a. Normal
    b. Centralized
    c. Lateralized to right side
    d. Lateralized to left side
17. **Investigation of choice for eustachian tube dysfunction:**
    1. Politzer 2. Vemp
    3. Tympanometry 4. Rhinomanometry
18. **According to the WHO definition of hearing loss, what is the value to classify as profound hearing loss?**
    a. 61-71 dB b. >81 dB
    c. >91 dB d. >101 dB
19. **A child was treated for H. influenzae meningitis for 6 months most important investigation to be done before discharging the patients:**
    a. MRI
    b. Brainstem evoked auditory response
    c. Growth screening test
    d. Psychotherapy

20. **Acoustic reflex decay test is positive in:**
    a. VIII rerve lesion
    b. Cerebellar lesion
    c. Midbrain lesion
    d. Auditory cortex lesion
21. **A patient presents to your clinic for evaluation of hearing defect. Rinne's test shows air conduction greater than bone conduction on both sides with Weber's test lateralized to right side. What is the next logical step:**
    a. This is normal test
    b. Schwabach's test
    c. Repeat Rinne's test on right side
    d. Wax removal
22. **Which is the recommended test for neonatal screening of hearing:**
    a. Automated auditory brainstem response
    b. Spontaneous OAE
    c. Evoked OAE
    d. Distorted OAE
23. **Gelle's test is done for:**
    a. Otosclerosis
    b. NHL
    c. Sensorineural hearing loss
    d. Retrocochlear disease
24. **Carhart's notch in audiometry is deepest at which of these frequencies:**
    a. 0.5 KHz
    b. 1 KHz
    c. 2 KHz
    d. 4 KHz
25. **What should be the loss of hearing at least for Weber's test to lateralize?**
    a. 5 dB
    b. 10 dB
    c. 15 dB
    d. 20 dB

IMAGE BASED QUESTIONS

26. **The graph below shows what type of hearing test?**

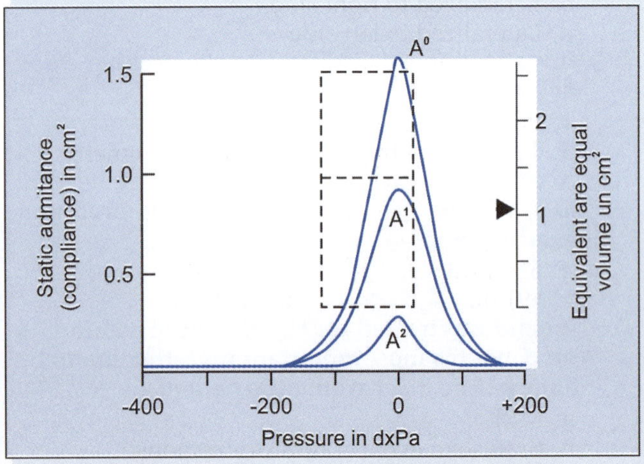

a. Audiogram
b. Tympanogram
c. BERA graph
d. Electrocochleography

27. **In this picture, which of the following tests is being done?**

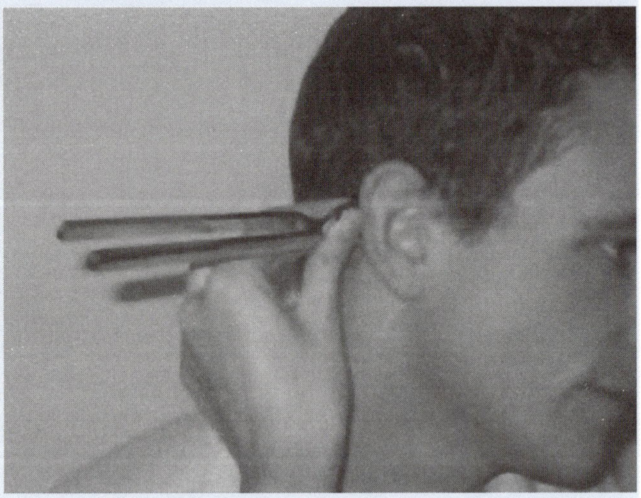

a. Fistula test
b. Brown's test
c. Air conduction with tuning fork
d. Bone conduction with tuning fork

28. **From the picture given above, which of these can be inferred:**
    a. If cold water is used, nystagmus will be on left side
    b. If cold water is used, nystagmus will be on right side
    c. It is used to remove foreign body from ear
    d. It is used to remove cholesteotoma from ear
28. **A 46-year-man complains of hearing loss. The audiogram is shown below. Which of the following is true in this case?**

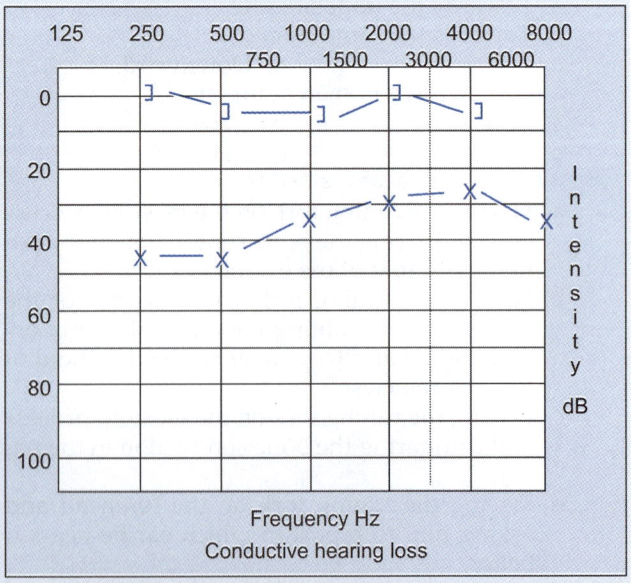

What does this show?
a. Left conductive loss
b. Left sensorineural loss
c. Right conductive loss
d. Right sensorineural loss

29. From the picture given below, which of these can be inferred?

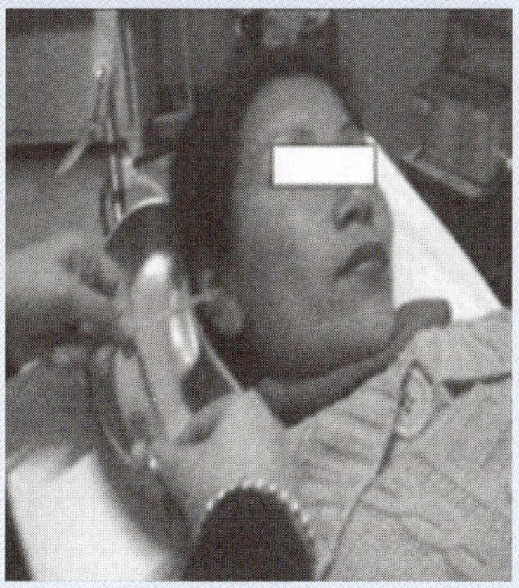

a. If cold water is used, nystagmus will be on left side
b. If cold water is used, nystagmus will be on right side
c. It is used to remove foreign body from ear
d. It is used to remove cholesteatoma from ear

30. Look at the picture and answer the following:

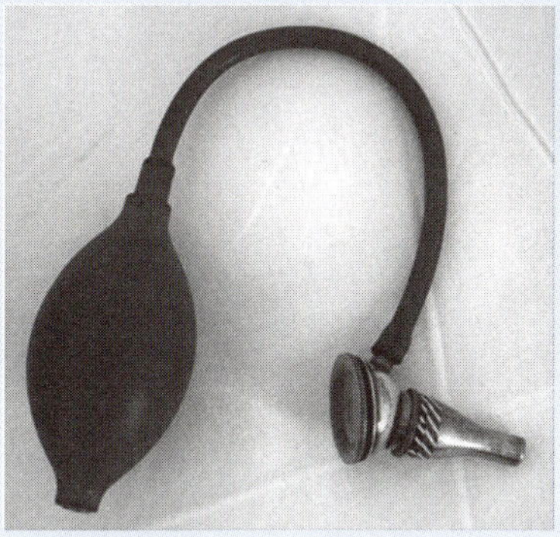

a. It is used for opening the eustachian tube
b. It is used to check the mobility of tympanic membrane
c. It can be used for removing foreign body from ear
d. It can be used to remove foreign body from nasal cavity

31. Which of the following is NOT true about this picture?

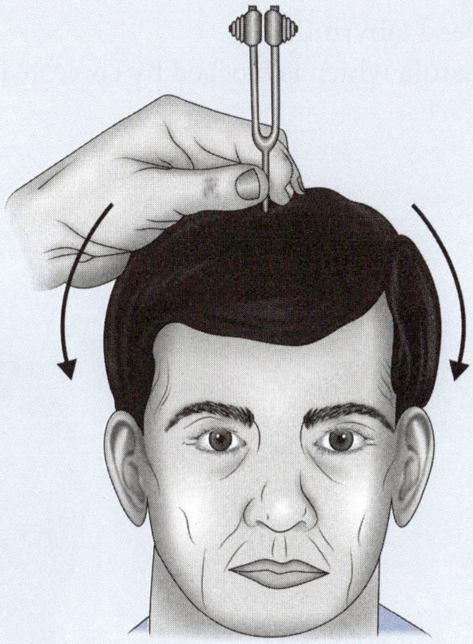

a. Rienne's test is being done
b. Weber's test is being done
c. In conductive hearing loss, it will lateralize to the diseased side
d. In sensorineural loss, it will lateralize to the better side

ANSWERS AND EXPLANATIONS

1. **b. Para-labyrinthitis due to erosion of lateral semicircular canal**
Para-labyrinthitis due to erosion of lateral semicircular canal is also called labyrinthine fistula.

Important causes of true positive fistula test are	Important causes of false positive fistula test are	Important causes of false negative fistula test are
1. Labyrinthine fistula, a complication of CSOM	1. Meniere's disease, where it is also called Hennebert's sign	1. Dead labyrinth
2. Fenestration surgery or type V tympanoplasty	2. Congenital syphilis	2. Fistula which is blocked by cholesteatoma
3. Post-stapedectomy	3. Hypermobile footplate	

IMPORTANT CAUSES OF TRUE POSITIVE FISTULA TEST ARE

1. Labyrinthine fistula, a complication of CSOM
2. Fenestration surgery or type V tympanoplasty

3. Post-stapedectomy
4. Perilymph fistula

IMPORTANT CAUSES OF FALSE POSITIVE FISTULA TEST ARE

1. Meniere's disease where it is also called Hennebert's sign
2. Congenital syphilis
3. Hypermobile footplate

IMPORTANT CAUSES OF FALSE NEGATIVE FISTULA TEST ARE

1. Dead labyrinth
2. Fistula which is blocked by cholesteatoma

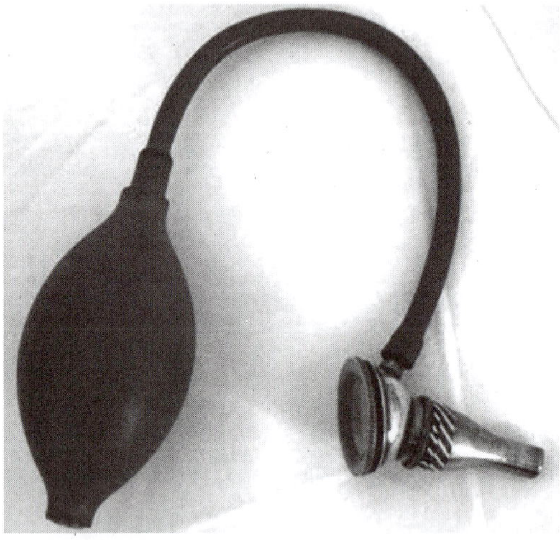

Siegel's speculum

2. **c. Removal of foreign body from the ear.**

Seigel's speculum is a very important instrument in the hand of an ENT surgeon. It is widely used for

1. Assessment of TM mobility
2. Application of powered medication in the canal
3. To elicit brown sign
4. To elicit fistula sign
5. For tuning fork test like Gelle`s test
6. It can be used for magnification, though otoscope is better, but foreign bodies cannot be removed.

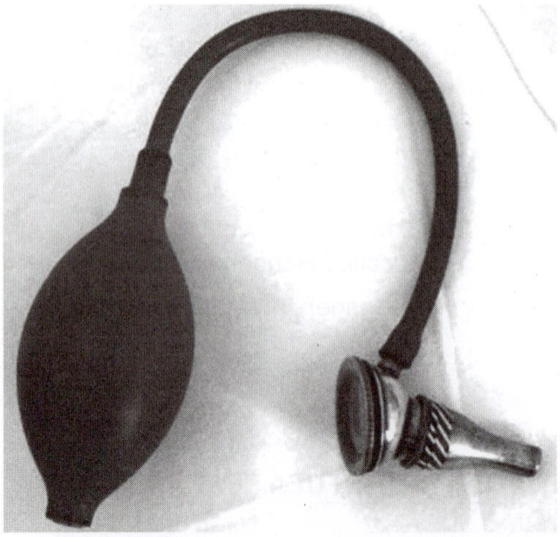

Siegel's speculum

3. **a. Outer hair cells**

Otoacoustic Emission (OAE) is low-intensity sound produced by movements of the outer hair cell of a normal cochlea and can be elicited by a very sensitive microphone placed in the external ear canal and then analyzed by a computer.

This emission is produced due to ***electromotility (contraction and relaxation) of hair cells.***

PHYSIOLOGY OF OAE PRODUCTION

Sound vibration enters the inner ear
↓
Vibration of basilar membrane
↓
Friction between the stereocilia of hair cell and tectorial membrane
↓
Opening of voltage-gated channels on the hair cell
↓
Influx of K^+ ions
↓
Depolarization
↓
Production of cochlear microphonics

These can either be of two types:

- Spontaneous or
- Induced/evoked.

After being produced from the outer hair cells in the cochlea, it travels in a reverse direction, i.e.

Outer hair cells
↓
Basilar membrane
↓
Perilymph
↓
Oral window
↓
Ear ossicles
↓
Tympanic membrane
↓
External ear

OAEs are used as an investigating tool for hearing loss due to cochlear disease.

It is a very important investigation to confirm hearing loss in newborns and infants.

Otoacoustic emission should be differentiated from ***cochlear microphonics.***
Cochlear microphonics are produced as a result of ***depolarization of the hair cell.***

PHYSIOLOGY OF COCHLEAR MICROPHONICS

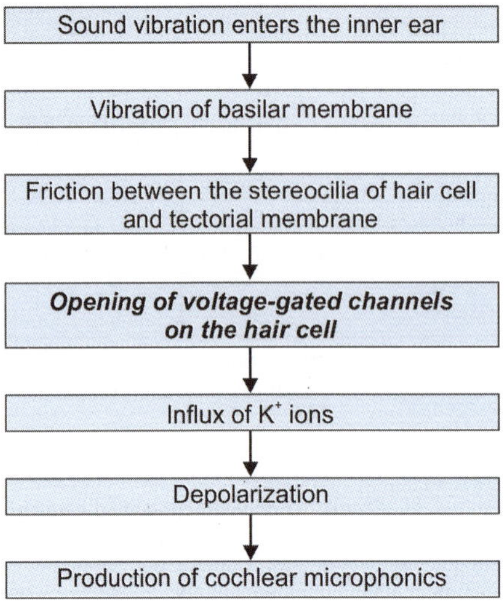

Otoacoustic emission (OAE) is the screening test for hearing of a new born child.
It should be done as a routine in every new born and infants who are admitted in the NICU.

4. **a. Deaf ear**
In conductive hearing loss the Rinne's test is negative.
Whereas, Weber's is lateralized to the diseased side.
In case of bilateral conductive hearing loss, it is lateralized to the worse side.

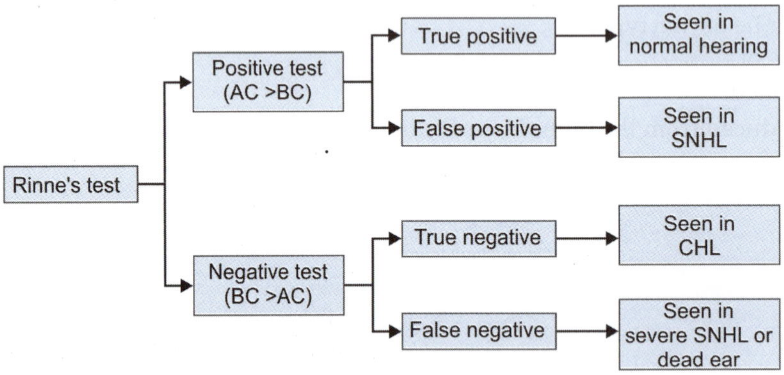

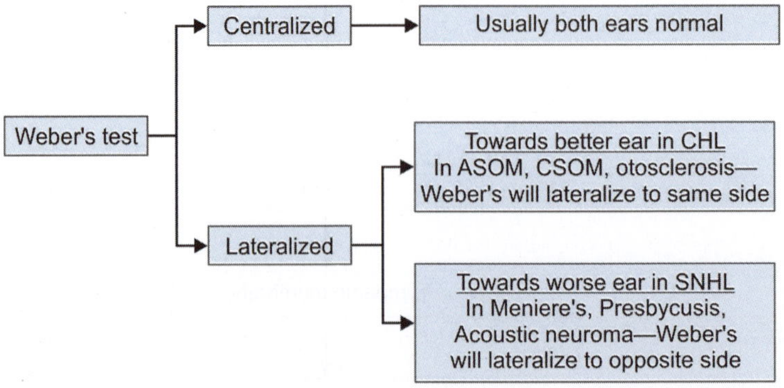

5. **b. Brainstem-evoked auditory response**
One of the advantages of Brainstem evoked auditory response (BERA) is that it is an objective type of test and so can be done in children.

A child on treatment for influenza for 6 months may have sensorineural hearing loss.

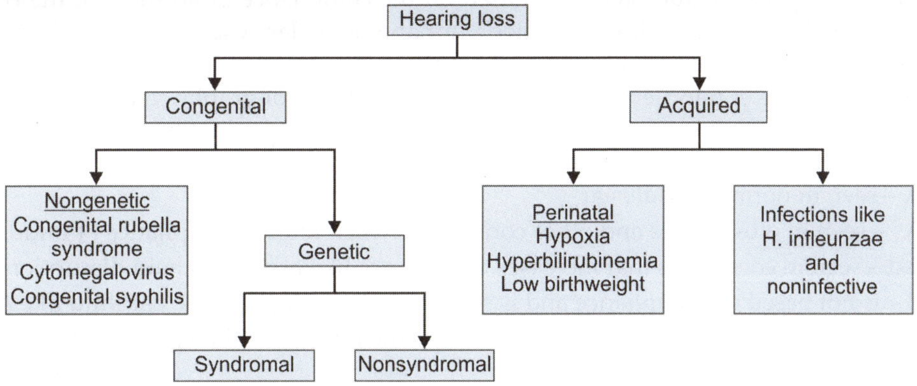

This is a very important cause of perinatal infection causing hearing loss.
In such a condition, one of the two may be done:

- Otoacoustic emission (OAE), or
- Brainstem-evoked response audiometry (BERA), or
- Both.

6. **b. Towards the same side**
This is a very tricky question.
There is a difference between eye movement and nystagmus.
During nystagmus, the eye moves in both the directions.

Slow component of nystagmus	This component is caused: • Disease of the ear or • Caloric test
Fast component	This is the correction or compensation done by the brain. Direction of nystagmus is defined by the direction of fast component.

From the above table we can see that caloric test causes slow component. This is always opposite the fast component. Fast component defines the direction of nystagmus.

Therefore, direction of eye movement is opposite to the direction of nystagmus.

Cold caloric stimulation test causes the nystagmus to the opposite side of caloric test. This can be easily remembered by the mnemonic COWS.

Therefore, in cold caloric stimulation test, the cold water induces eye ball movement to the same side and, hence, the nystagmus will be opposite of this.

If the question had asked the direction of nystagmus, then the answer would have been 'towards the opposite side'.

7. **d. 2 Hz**
Carhart's notch is an audiogram finding and is a very important feature in patients of otosclerosis.

In this,

- There is a sudden dip at 2000 Hz seen in the bone conduction curve.
- The total depth of the dip is approximately 15 dB.
- The Carhart's notch disappears after stapedectomy.

Other important findings in audiogram in otosclerosis are:

- Cookie bite curve
- Significant air-bone gap (A-B gap)

8. **d. Placing the tuning fork on the forehead and asking him to report in which ear he hears it better.**
Weber's test is a very useful tuning fork test, which is commonly done to assess hearing of the patient. In this test, the tuning fork is placed on the forehead of the patient and is asked to report in which ear he hears it better. In sensorineural hearing loss. Weber's is lateralized to the better ear and in conductive hearing loss, it is lateralized to the worse ear.

9. **b. Middle ear**

The principle of impedance audiometry is based on the compliance or stiffness of the tympanic membrane and the ossicular chain of the middle ear called tympano-ossicular system.

Hence, it is mainly used for diagnosis of middle ear diseases.

Depending on the type of middle ear pathology five main types of graphs called tympanograms can be seen in impedance audiometry.

They are as follows:

- Type A—seen in normal middle ear
- Type As—seen in otosclerosis and other conditions which reduce compliance of middle ear
- Type Ad—seen in conditions that increases compliance like ossicular chain disruption
- Type B—is not based on compliance and is seen in cases having middle ear fluid like AOM
- Type C—seen in cases having negative pressure in the middle ear like glue ear.

10. **b. Impedance audiometry**

Impedance audiometry, also called tympanometry, is an objective test for hearing.

The uses of impedance audiometry are:

- *Diagnosis of middle ear diseases causing conductive hearing loss*
- *Differentiating conductive hearing loss from sensorineural hearing loss*
- *Differentiating cochlear hearing loss from neural hearing loss*
- *Evaluating stapedial reflex*
- *Measurement of middle ear pressure*
- *Evaluating function of eustachian tube, etc.*

11. **b. Outer hair cells**

Otoacoustic emissions (OAE) are low-intensity sounds produced by the outer hair cells in a normal person. They are absent when outer hair cells are damaged. Therefore they are used to find out the function of cochlea.

12. **c. Stapes abnormal at oval window**

Conductive deafness may be caused in some patients travelling in aeroplane but never in ship.

Trauma to labyrinth and noise will cause sensorineural hearing loss.

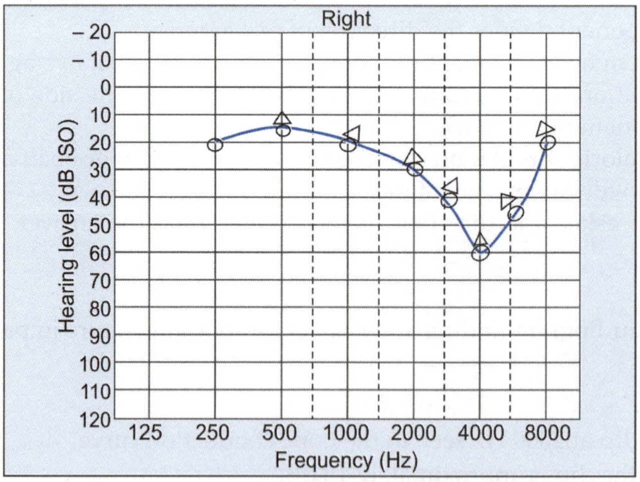

Audiogram of noise-induced hearing loss showing dip at 4000 Hz.

13. **a. Nystagmus to the right side**

Fitzgerald-Hallpike caloric test also called bithermal caloric test is done to find out the vestibular function. In this, ear is syringed with water of two different temperatures, i.e. 30 degrees and 44 degrees.

Irrigation with 30 degrees water produces nystagmus to the opposite side and irrigation with 44 degrees produces nystagmus to the same side. This can be remembered easily by remembering the mnemonic COWS, where

- 'C' stands for cold water,
- 'O' stands for opposite side,

- 'W' stands for warm water and
- 'S' stands for same side.

Hence, cold water irrigation will produce nystagmus to the opposite side.

In Fitzgerald-Hallpike test, the position of the patient is supination with head raised by 30 degrees and the procedure stimulates the lateral (horizontal) semicircular canal to produce nystagmus.

14. **b. Brainstem-Evoked Response Audiometry (BERA)**

BERA, free field audiometry and behavioral audiometry are all used to assess hearing of an infant.

BERA has the following advantages

- It is an objective test
- It provides an ear specific information
- It can differentiate cochlear disease from retrocochlear disease
- In case of retrocochlear disease, it can localize the site of problem.

15. **b. Acoustic reflex impedance audiometry**

Hearing in infants can be tested by a test which is objective in nature as a child cannot respond or cooperate during a subjective test.

Acoustic reflex impedance audiometry is the only objective test in the choices and rest of the mentioned tests are subjective type of investigations.

The other hearing test which can be done in children is otoacoustic emission (OAE) and BERA. These can be ***used for screening of neonate, specially OAE.***

16. **c. Lateralized to right side**

In case of conductive hearing loss; Weber's is lateralized to the diseased ear and in sensorineural hearing it is lateralized to the opposite ear.

Middle ear pathology will cause conductive type of hearing loss. Hence, in right middle ear pathology, Weber's will be lateralized to the right side.

17. **3. Tympanometry**

Politzer is an instrument which is used to open the eustachian tube when it is closed. It is mainly for treatment purpose. However, sometimes it can also be used to diagnose when the eustachian tube is functioning or not.

Rhinomanometry is used to measure the nasal airflow and its driving pressure. It measures the narrowest part of the nasal cavity.

Rhinostereometry is microscopic examination of the inferior turbinate. It is done to see the changes in the diameter/size of this turbinate.

VEMP stands for ***vestibular evoked myogenic potential.*** VEMP is used to diagnose problems of saccule and inferior vestibular nerve.

Tympanogram is usually used to:

- **Make diagnosis of *middle ear diseases.***
- ***Check the stapedial reflex/acoustic reflex***
- ***Check the functioning of eustachian tube***

The function of the eustachian tube can be checked by the following investigations:

1. ***Tympanometry/impedance reflex***
2. ***Politzerisation***
3. ***Toynbee test***

Among the above mentioned tests, **tympanometry is the best.**

18. **b. >81 dB**

There are many classifications for hearing impairment, of which the WHO classification is given below:

World Health Organization Grades of Hearing Impairment (WHO, 2008)			
Grade of impairment	**Corresponding audiometric ISO value**	**Performance**	**Recommendations**
0 - No impairment	25 dB or better (better ear)	No or very slight hearing problems. Able to hear whispers.	

(Contd...)

(Contd...)

1 - Slight impairment	26-40 dB (better ear)	Able to hear and repeat words spoken in normal voice at 1 meter.	Counselling. Hearing aids may be needed.
2 - Moderate impairment	41-60 dB (better ear)	Able to hear and repeat words spoken in raised voice at 1 meter.	Hearing aids usually recommended.
3 - Severe impairment	61-80 dB (better ear)	Able to hear some words when shouted into better ear.	Hearing aids needed. If no hearing aids available, lip-reading and signing should be taught.
4 - Profound impairment including deafness	81 dB or greater (better ear)	Unable to hear and understand even a shouted voice	Hearing aids may help in understanding words. Additional rehabilitation needed. Lip-reading and sometimes signing essential

However, the WHO classification is NOT used in practice. The more practical classification especially for interpretation of pure tone audiometry is given below:

0–25 db	Normal hearing
26–40 dB	Mild hearing loss
41–55 dB	Moderate hearing loss
56–70 dB	Moderately severe hearing loss
71–90 dB	Severe hearing loss
>91 dB	Profound hearing loss

19. B. Brainstem-evoked auditory response

Meningitis in a small child due to H. influenza may affect the VIII cranial nerve.
This has to be diagnosed before the child is discharged.
The best investigation for VIII nerve in infants is BERA (Brainstem evoked auditory response)
NOTE: The first screening test for hearing in infants is otoacoustic emission (OAE).
Every newborn who has to be admitted in NICU must undergo OAE and, if possible, BERA.

20. A. VIII nerve lesion

The auditory pathway is given below:

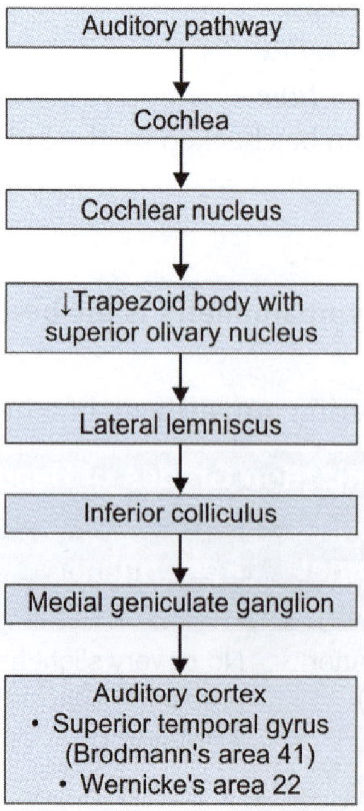

ACOUSTIC REFLEX ARCH IS GIVEN BELOW

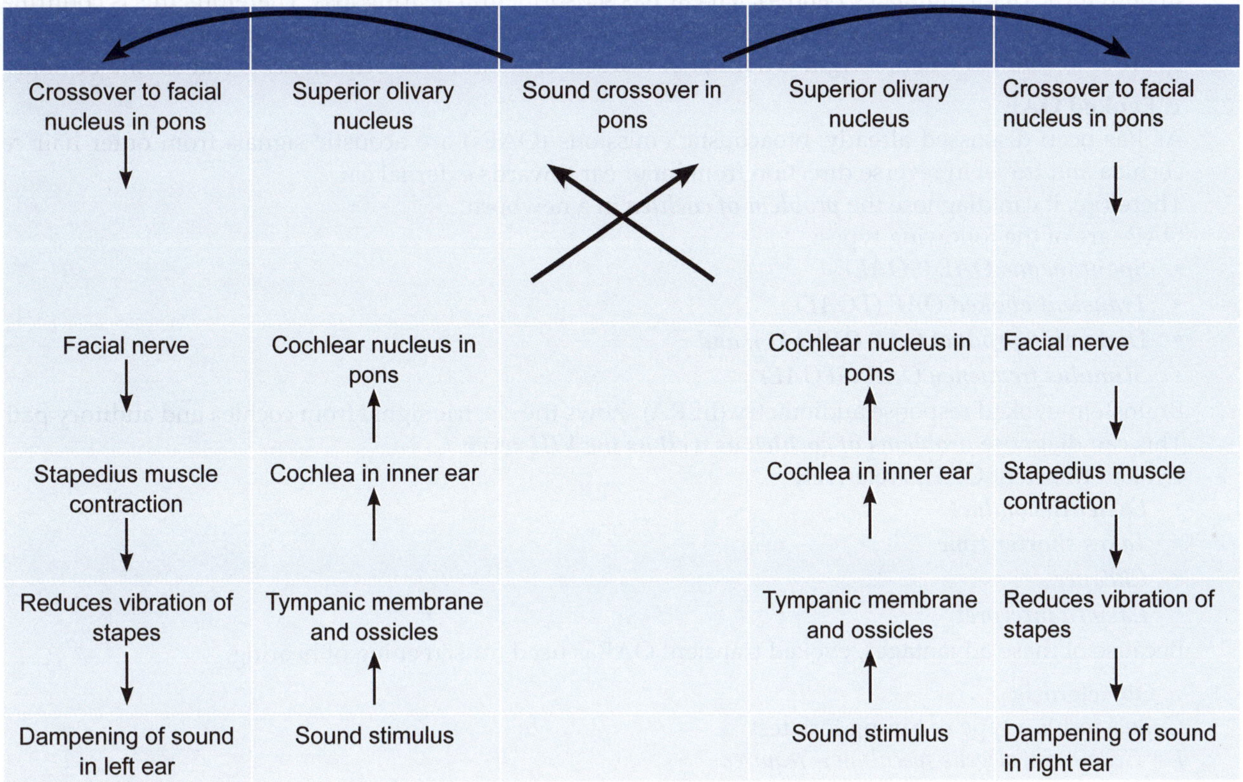

From the above information, we understand that the structures needed for normal acoustic are:

- Tympanic membrane
- Ossicles
- VIII nerve
- Cochear nucleus and pons
- VII nerve nucleus
- VII nerve
- Stapedius muscle

Higher centers of auditory pathway do not contribute to acoustic reflex.

Hence, damage/lesion of any of the above mentioned structures will decay the acoustic reflex. Lesion of higher centers does NOT decay the reflex.

From the choices given, VIII nerve is the correct answer.

21. **b. Schwabach's test**

If Weber's test is lateralized to right side, there are five possibilities:

Possibilities	Right side	Left side
1	• Normal side and	• Sensorineural hearing loss
2	• Conductive hearing loss and	• Normal side
3	• Conductive hearing loss and	• Sensorineural hearing loss
4	• Less sensorineural hearing loss and	• More sensorineural hearing loss
5	• More conductive hearing loss and	• Less conductive hearing loss

- Because both sides have air conduction greater than bone conduction, they either have:
  - Normal hearing or
  - Sensorineural hearing loss

Therefore, conductive hearing is NOT possible on any side (because AC > BC).

This means possibilities no. 2, 3, and 5 cannot be seen in this patient (because they have conductive hearing loss). So, either possibility on 1 or 4 is possible.
In both these cases (numbers 1 and 4), left ear has sensorineural hearing loss. Therefore, this is confirmed.
But right is either normal as shown in possibility no. 1 or sensorineural hearing loss as shown in no. 4.
In order to confirm whether right is normal or has sensorineural loss, ***Schwabach's test should be done.***

22. **c. Evoked OAE**
As has been discussed already, otoacoustic emissions (OAEs) are acoustic signals from outer hair cells of cochlea and travel in reverse direction from inner ear towards external ear.
Therefore, it can diagnose the ***problem of cochlea*** in a newborn.
OAEs are of the following types:
- ***Spontaneous OAE (SOAE)***
- ***Transient evoked OAE (TOAE)***
- ***Distortion product OAE (DPOAE), and***
- ***Stimulus frequency OAE (SFOAE)***

Brainstem-evoked response audiometry (BERA) shows the electric signal from cochlea and auditory pathway. This can diagnose ***problems of cochlea as well as the VIII nerve.***
Evoked transient OAE is relatively:
- ***Easier to conduct***
- ***Takes shorter time***
- ***Cheaper***
- ***Easy to interpret***

Because of these advantages, evoked transient OAE is used for screening of hearing.

23. **a. Otosclerosis**
Gelle's test is a type of tuning fork test
For Gelle's test, siegel's speculum is required
Gelle's test used is considered as a diagnostic tuning fork test for:
- Otosclerosis and
- Ossicular chain disruption

It is negative in a patient of otosclerosis.

24. **c. 2 KHz**
Carhart's notch is an audiogram finding as shown below:

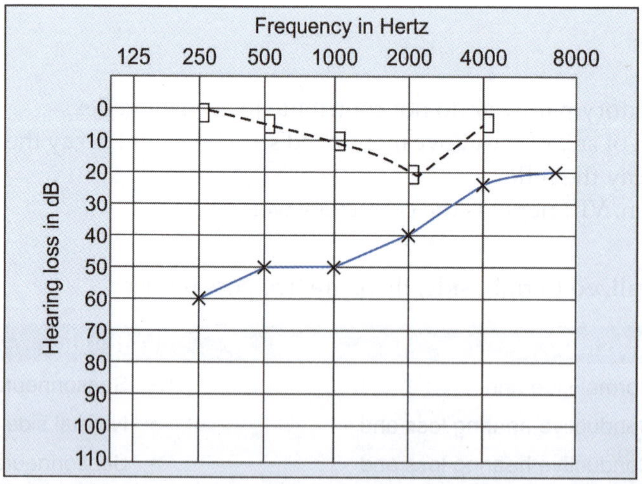

As you can see, the notch or dip starts at 500 Hz and is deepest at 2000 Hz (2 KHz). At 2 KHz , it deeps by 15 dB.

25. **a. 5 dB**
Rinne's test is negative in conductive hearing loss. The minimum hearing loss must be 15-20 dB for it to be negative.
Weber's lateralizes when in sensorineural hearing loss or conductive hearing loss is 15-25 dB. However, Weber's can lateralize with as little as **5 dB** difference between the two ears.

IMAGE BASED ANSWERS

26. **b. Tympanogram**
The above investigation is a tympanogram, which is showing:
A type tympanogram, A_s tympanogram and A_d type tympanogram.

27. **d. Bone conduction test with tuning fork**
As you can see, the base of the tuning fork is placed on the mastoid bone. This is done during bone conduction.

28. **a. Left conductive loss**
The symbols used during audiometry are:

Symbols	Right ear	Left ear
AC	O	X
BC	<	>

If we know these symbols, we can easily know that the upper graph (above 25 dB), is left ear bony conduction (BC) graph.
The lower graph depicts air conduction (AC) below 25 dB (threshold is more than 25 dB).
- If only AC audiogram shows threshold of more than 25 dB (i.e, below the 25 mark), then it suggests conductive hearing loss. This is shown in this graph.
- If both AC and BC graphs below the 25 mark but the gap between the two (A-B gap) is less than 15 dB, than it is sensorineural loss.
- If both AC and BC graphs below the 25 mark but the gap between the two (A-B gap) is more than 20 dB, than it is mixed loss.

29. **a. If cold water is used, nystagmus will be on left side**
In this picture, caloric test is being done on the right side.
If you remember the mnemonics COWS, right side syringing with cold water should give nystagmus to the left side.

30. **b. It is used to check the mobility of tympanic membrane**
This is a picture of siegle's speculum.
It can be used to check the mobility of tympanic membrane.
Other uses are:
- Carry out Gelle's tuning fork test
- Carry out Brown's test and Fistula test etc.
  - To open the eustachian tube, politzer is used

31. **a. Rienne's test is being done**
The picture shows Weber's test being done.
- The Weber's test will lateralize to the diseased side in conductive hearing loss.
- It will lateralize to the better side in sensorineural loss.

CHAPTER 8

Non-infective Diseases of the Middle Ear

GLOMUS TUMOR

Glomus Tumor is Most Common Tumor of Middle Ear

Glomus tumor is a type of paraganglioma. Paraganglioma is a type of neural crest tumour

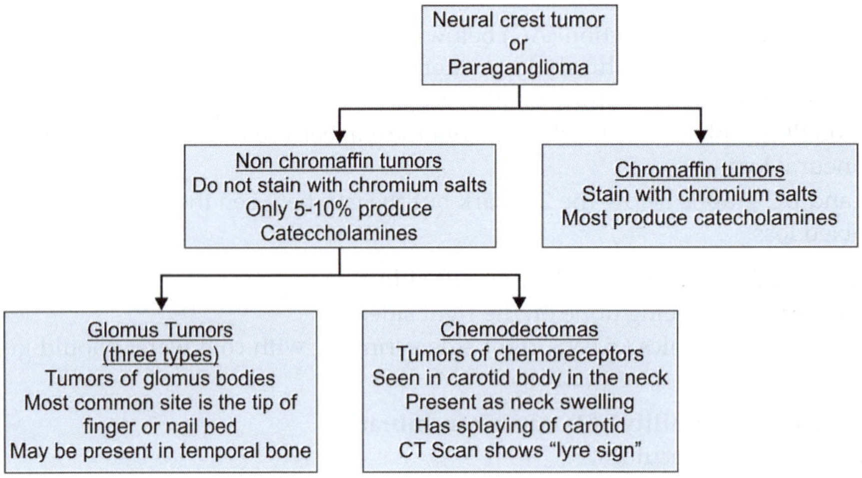

Glomus tumors could be of three main types:

	Three types of Glomus Tumors	
Glomus tympanicum (most common type)	Glomus jugulare	Glomus vagale (very rare and not discussed)
Arises from *Tympanic plexus*	Arises from *Jugular Vein*	Arises from *Vagus Nerve*
Present on • Promontory and • Hypotympanum	Present near the jugular fossa	

Glomus tumor is *non capsulated, very slow growing benign tumor* which is **vascular** in nature.

The blood supply is through **ascending pharyngeal artery.**

It is usually unilateral and is more common in female. (female : male, **5 : 1**)

The most important presentation is **"pulsatile tinnitus with conductive hearing loss"**.

Although "**feeling of mass in the ear" could be more common** feature of glomus tumor; the more diagnostic presentation is ***"pulsatile tinnitus"*.**

Pulsatile tinnitus may be present in few other conditions. They are:

- Glomus tumor
- A-V malformations
- High jugular bulb
- Aberrant internal carotid artery

CT scan can diagnose these conditions as shown in this flow chart:

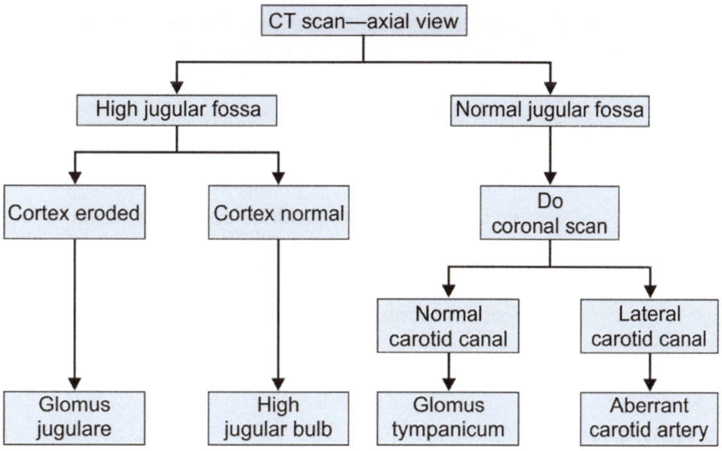

Less Common Presentation of Glomus Tumors are:

- Tympanic membrane appear blue in color due to glomus jugulare spread in the middle ear.

Causes of blue-colored tympanic membrane
• Glue ear/Serous otitis media
• Old hemotympanum also called • Cholesterol granuloma
• Glomus jugulare

- Four important features in glomus tumour are:
  1. Rising sun sign
  2. Brown sign
  3. Phelp sign
  4. Aquino sign
- Cranial nerves may be involved
  VII, IX, X, XI, XII, etc.

Signs in glomus tumor		Seen in which tumor
1. Rising sun sign	A red vascular tumour in the hypotympanum of middle ear gives a look of rising sun.	Glomus tympanicum
2. Brown sign	On Siegelization of the ear canal, the tumor pulsates and then blanches.	Glomus tympanicum
3. Phelp's sign	It is a radiological sign. In this, erosion of bony crest between carotid artery and jugular vein is seen on a scan.	Glomus jugulare
4. Aquino's sign	On compressing the jugular vein of the same side, the pulsatile tinnitus disappears.	Seen in both tumours but more prominent in Glomus tympanicum

Nerve involved	Name of syndrome	Which tumour
Facial nerve (VII)	Most common nerve involved	Glomus tympanicum
IX, X, XI	Vernet syndrome	Glomus jugulare
IX, X, XI, and XII	Collet-Sicard syndrome	Glomus jugulare

INVESTIGATION OF CHOICE IS CONTRAST-ENHANCED CT SCAN

Combination of HRCT and Gd MRI	Investigation of choice
Four-vessel angiography	• Carotid and circle of Willis angiography • Jugular venography • Vertebral angiography
Histopathology	Zellballen cells/chief cells may be seen.
24 hours urinary VMA	• 5-10% tumours produce catecholamines • If present, can raise blood pressure • Sudden and extreme rise of BP may be encountered during surgery.
18F DOPA PET and 18FDG glucose PET	Recent mode of investigation, especially to detect multiple site tumours.

CLASSIFICATION OF GLOMUS TUMOR

Many types of classification are available for glomus tumour.
The most acceptable is the **Fisch classification.**

NOTE: Fisch classification is used for
- Glomus tumour and
- Juvenile Angiofibroma of the nasopharynx

Treatment

Treatment of choice is ***surgery***.
However, *Radiotherapy* or embolization may also be done in this patient.

OTOSCLEROSIS AND PAGET'S DISEASE OF TEMPORAL BONE

Otosclerosis is a disease of **endochondral layer of the otic capsule/ bony labyrinth**.
Otic capsule is different from rest of bone in two aspects:
1. It has almost NO remodeling, i.e. absence of osteoclastic and osteoblastic activities
2. Endochondral layer has immature cartilaginous areas called ***"globuli interossei"***

In case of otosclerosis
1. **There is resorption of endochondral bone with enlargement of perivascular spaces and vascular proliferation which is followed by deposition of immature or *woven bone—this stage is called Otospongiosis or Active stage.***
2. **Later on, active resorption and remodelling continue in this area, leading to production of mature or *lamellar bone—this stage is called Otosclerosis or Passive stage.***

Otosclerosis is Therefore Divided into Two Steps

1. ***Otospongiotic stage* or active stage**, and
2. ***Otosclerotic stage* or passive stage**

The most common site of otosclerosis is **fistula ante fenestram,** which is present on the medial wall of middle ear just anterior to the oval window.

Patient Profile in Otosclerosis
• usually starts in young age (22-40 yrs) • seen in females • usually bilateral but starts in one ear • flares up during pregnancy • autosomal dominant • is hereditary

	Aetiology
• Genetics	Defect in expression of COL1A1 may be the cause
• Virus	Measles may be the cause
• Unknown causes	

	Types of otosclerosis
Clinical otosclerosis	Presents with gradually progressive, conductive hearing loss in a young lady with positive family history and normal membrane
Cochlear otosclerosis	Presents with purely sensorineural hearing loss
Histological otosclerosis	No clinical presentation (most common type)

Differences between clinical otosclerosis and cochlear otosclerosis:

Clinical otosclerosis	Cochlear otosclerosis
Has conductive hearing loss	Has sensorineural hearing loss
Happens when otosclerotic focus involves footplate of stapes	Happens when focus reaches endosteum of cochlea
Is due to fibrous fixation of footplate	Is due to hyalinization of the spiral ligament, leading to imbalance of metabolites and ions
Typical features of otosclerosis are seen	Not seen
Relatively easy to improve hearing with surgical treatment	Difficult to improve hearing/Treat the disease

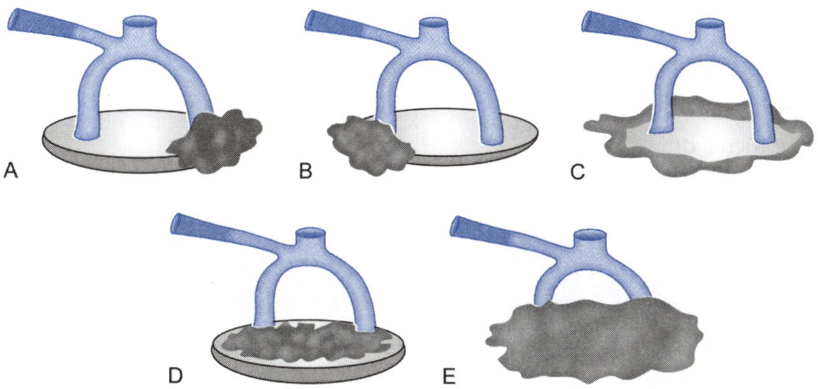

Different types of clinical otosclerosis

Three important features of otosclerosis are:

	Important features
1. Schwartz sign	*Tympanic membrane has* ***flamingo pink*** *coloration.* It is seen only in the *active stage* and is not seen in the passive stage. Most patients present in the passive stage of disease, Schwartz sign is usually **not** seen.
2. Paracusis Willisii	Patient of otosclerosis hears better in noisy environment
3. Carhart's notch	This is *audiological finding*. This notch has the following: 1. There is dip at *2000 Hz*. 2. It is seen in *(BC) bone conduction curve*. 3. It shows false or apparent SNHL. 4. After stapedectomy, the Carhart's notch disappears. Note: Carhart's notch may be seen in most conditions having conductive hearing loss.

Investigations

Tests	Findings
Tuning fork finding	*Rinne's shows BC > AC* *Weber's is lateralized to the same side* *Gelle's test is negative/there is no change. This used to be diagnostic for otosclerosis*
Audiometry	Shows 1. An upward sloping curve 2. A-B gap >15 dB 3. Carhart's notch at 2000Hz
Tympanometry	**"As" type of tympanogram** – this could be diagnostic of otosclerosis
Acoustic reflex	**Absence of acoustic reflex or biphasic on-off pattern. This could be:** **1. The earliest sign of otosclerosis** **2. Pathognomonic of otosclerosis**
HRCT	**It may be useful in differentiation active and passive phases of otosclerosis**

TREATMENT OF OTOSCLEROSIS

1. Medicinal

The only useful drug is ***Sodium fluoride****.*

Indications of Sodium fluoride in otosclerosis are:

1. Active stage of otosclerosis which is shown by either **positive Schwartz sign or HRCT.**
2. Cochlear otosclerosis with **SNHL.**

The most important contraindication of sodium fluoride is:

- Passive stage of otosclerosis

Hence **Sodium fluoride** is given if at least one of the three is present.

- Positive Schwartz sign
- HRCT showing active focus, or
- Audiometry shows SNHL

In otosclerosis, sodium fluoride may act in one of the following ways
• It reduces the osteoclastic activities
• It increases the osteoblastic activities
• It inhibits cytotoxic enzymes in the cochlea

2. Hearing Aid

Hearing aid is an instrument whose main function is amplification of sound.

3. Stapedectomy or Stapedotomy

These are the important surgeries done in cases of otosclerosis.

Indication of stapedectomy and stapedotomy
• Passive stage of otosclerosis

Selection criteria for these surgeries
• Hearing threshold of >30 dB • A-B gap of 10-20 dB • Young age

Contraindications of stapedectomy and stapedotomy
1. Active otosclerosis
2. Cochlear otosclerosis
3. Extreme age of patient
4. Medical disease
5. Middle ear infection
6. Only hearing ear
7. Second ear surgery
8. Having Meniere's disease

About prosthesis

- Most common material used is "Teflon". If you may recall, hydroxylapatite is used in TORP and PORP
- The length of this piston is 4.5-4.75 mm
- About 0.25 mm of this crosses the undersurface of footplate/0.25 mm should be inside the inner ear
- In stapedotomy, hole on the footplate is either 0.4 mm or 0.6 mm
- This perforation can be created with:
  1. Laser
  2. Micro drill
  3. Perforator

Complications of Stapedectomy/Stapedotomy
1. Failed surgery where surgery shows no significant hearing improvement or conductive hearing loss. This is due to displacement of prosthesis from hole of the footplate
2. Sensorineural hearing loss (SNHL). This can be either: – Immediate onset SNHL, or – Late onset SNHL.
3. Perilymph or CSF gusher
4. Persisting vertigo
5. Positive fistula sign
6. Foreign body of inner ear also called "floating foot plate"
7. Facial nerve palsy when there is "overhanging" facial nerve
8. Excessive bleeding due to persisting stapedial artery.

Paget's Disease of the Temporal Bone

Paget's disease is very uncommon in the temporal.
When present; the aetiology and pathology are quite similar to Otosclerosis.

Comparison between otosclerosis and Paget's disease

Otosclerosis	Paget's disease of temporal bone
Seen in endochondral layer of otic capsule	Mainly pelvis. It is uncommon in ear
Pathophysiology already discussed	There is increase in osteoclastic activities causing reabsorption followed by architecturally unsound bone deposition
May be caused by measles	May be caused measles or paramyxovirus
Mainly conductive hearing loss	Mainly sensorineural hearing loss
Hearing loss is due to stapes footplate fixation	Hearing loss is mainly due to "narrowing of internal acoustic meatus"
Tinnitus and vertigo very uncommon	Tinnitus and vertigo may rarely be present
Sodium fluoride is the main drug	Bisphosphonates are the main drug

Van der Hoeve Syndrome

This important syndrome may be associated with *otosclerosis*. In this syndrome, patient may have the following:

1. *Osteogenesis imperfecta*
2. *Blue sclera, and*
3. *Otosclerosis*

Last minute revision

- The most common site of glomus tumour is nailbed/fingertip
- The most common tumour of middle ear is glomus tumour
- Pulsatile tinnitus is a very important presentation of glomus tumour
- Three special features of glomus tumour are:
  1. Rising sun sign
  2. Brown's sign
  3. Phelp's sign
- Most common site of otosclerosis is fissula ante fenestram
- It causes hearing loss in pregnant females
- Special features are:
  1. Schwartz sign
  2. Paracusis Willisii
- Tympanogram shows "As" type
- Audiometry shows Carhart's notch
- Sodium fluoride is given in active stage
- Stapedectomy is done in passive stage
- Complications of stapedectomy are sensorineural hearing loss, perilymph fistula, facial palsy, etc.
- Van der Hoeve syndrome has:
  1. Osteogenesis imperfecta
  2. Blue sclera
  3. Otosclerosis

QUESTIONS

1. **A 25-year-old woman was suffering from bilateral hearing loss for 6 years, which became profound with pregnancy. On tympanogram, which of the following curves is obtained:**
   a. Ad
   b. As
   c. B
   d. A
2. **Schwartz sign is seen in:**
   a. Otosclerosis
   b. Glomus jugulare
   c. Meniere's disease
   d. Acoustic neuroma
3. **Brown sign is seen in:**
   a. Glomus tumor
   b. Meniere's disease
   c. Acoustic neuroma
   d. Otosclerosis
4. **A 30-year-old woman with family history of hearing loss from her mother's side developed hearing problem during pregnancy. Hearing loss is bilateral, slowly progressive, with bilateral tinnitus that bothers her at night. Pure tone audiometry shows conductive hearing loss with an apparent bone conduction hearing loss at 2000 Hz. What is the most likely diagnosis?**
   a. Otosclerosis
   b. Acoustic neuroma
   c. Otitis media with effusion
   d. Sigmoid sinus thrombosis
5. **True statement about glomus jugulare tumor is:**
   a. Malignant neoplasm
   b. Benign non-encapsulated vascular tumor
   c. May involve V to VII cranial nerve
   d. Arises from the promontory of middle ear
6. **A 31-year-old female patient complains of bilateral impairment of hearing for the past 5 years. On examination, tympanic membrane is normal and audiogram shows a bilateral conductive deafness. Impedance audiometry shows As type of curve and acoustic reflexes are absent. All constitute part of treatment, except:**
   a. Hearing aid
   b. Stapedectomy
   c. Sodium fluoride
   d. Gentamicin
7. **Most common site for the initiation of otosclerosis is:**
   a. Foot plate of stapes
   b. Margins of stapes
   c. Fissula ante fenestram
   d. Fossula post fenestram
8. **Most common tumour of middle ear is:**
   a. Adenocarcinoma
   b. Squamous cell carcinoma
   c. Glomus tumour
   d. Acoustic neuroma
9. **Common age for otosclerosis is:**
   a. 5-10 years
   b. 10-20 years
   c. 20-30 years
   d. 30-45 years
10. **Earliest symptom of glomus tumour is:**
    a. Pulsatile tinnitus
    b. Deafness
    c. Headache
    d. Vertigo
11. **In otosclerosis during stapes surgery prosthesis is used:**
    a. Teflon piston
    b. Grommet
    c. Total ossicular replacement
    d. All of the above
12. **Soldier's helmet with deafness is seen in:**
    a. Paget's disease
    b. Osteosclerosis
    c. Osteogenesis imperfecta
    d. Otospongiosis
13. **In otosclerosis, the most common structure of the inner ear that is involved in:**
    a. Saccule
    b. Spiral ganglion
    c. Stria vascularis
    d. Spiral ligament
14. **Which of the following is not resected in stapedotomy:**
    a. Anterior crus of stapes
    b. Posterior crus of stapes
    c. Stapedial ligament
    d. Lenticular process of incus
15. **Otospongiosis is inherited as:**
    a. Autosomal dominant
    b. Autosomal recessive
    c. X-linked dominant
    d. X-linked recessive
16. **All the following statements about sodium fluoride in otosclerosis are true except:**
    a. It acts by inhibiting proteolytic enzymes
    b. It acts by inhibiting osteoblastic activities
    c. It is contraindicated in chronic nephritis
    d. It is indicated in patients with a positive Schwartz sign.
17. **Following operations are done in otosclerosis:**
    a. Stapedectomy
    b. Stapedotomy
    c. Fenestration surgery
    d. Sacculotomy
18. **Fisch classification is used for:**
    a. Juvenile angiofibroma
    b. Nasopharyngeal carcinoma
    c. Vestibular schwannoma
    d. Glomus tumour

19. Glomus tumour invading the vertical part of carotid canal is which type according to Fisch classification?
a. Type A
b. Type B
c. Type C1
d. Type C2

20. A patient presents with bleeding from ear, pain, tinnitus and progressive deafness. On examination, there is red swelling behind the intact tympanic membrane, which blanches on pressure with pneumatic speculum. Management includes all *except:*
a. Radiotherapy
b. Surgery
c. Interferons
d. Preoperative embolization

IMAGE BASED QUESTION

21. A 38 years lady has hearing loss and feeling of mass in the ear. On examination a red mass was present in the middle ear. The mass was surgically excised and the histopathological slide of the mass is shown. Which is true?

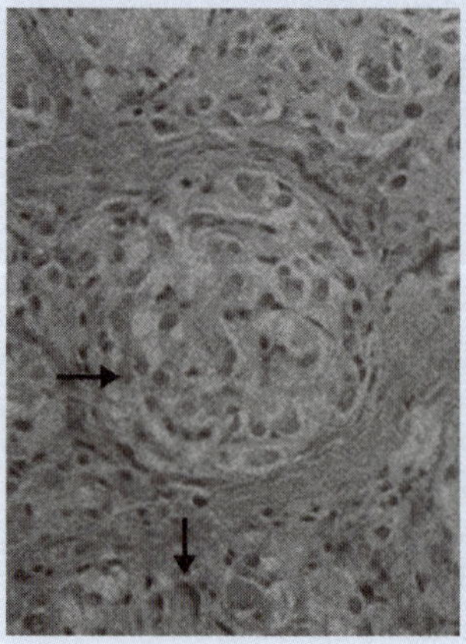

a. This is zellballen cell of glomus tumour
b. This histopathological finding is diagnostic of paragangliomas
c. Pulsatile tinnitus may be seen in these patients
d. All are true

ANSWERS AND EXPLANATIONS

1. **b. As**
The above given case is a typical patient of otosclerosis and in otosclerosis, impedance audiometry will show **"As" curve**.
• Ad curve is seen in ossicular disruption
• B curve is seen in case of middle ear fluid
• A curve is seen in normal person

2. **a. Otosclerosis**
Schwartz sign is a very important sign in a patient of otosclerosis. In this, the tympanic membrane has a ***flamingo pink blush on the tympanic membrane***.
A very important point about this sign is that it is seen only in the active stage (also called otospongiotic stage) of the disease and is not seen in the passive stage of the disease. Most patients of otosclerosis who report to the clinician are in the passive stage; hence this sign is not seen in most patients of otosclerosis.
The other important features of otosclerosis are:
• Paracusis willisii and
• Carhart's notch
NOTE- Whenever a question describes a patient as ***"a young female patient with bilateral hearing loss which is conductive in nature, the question is referring to a patient of otosclerosis".***

3. **a. Glomus tumor**
When siegelization of ear canal with glomus tumour is done, the glomus tumour pulsates vigorously and then blanches. This is called Brown sign. Some of the important signs of glomus tumour are:
• ***Brown's sign***
• ***Rising sun sign***
• ***Phelp's sign***
• ***Aquino sign***

4. **a. Otosclerosis**
Otosclerosis is a disease of middle ear which is more common in middle-aged females with positive family history and the disease flares during pregnancy. The patient usually presents with gradually progressive B/L conductive hearing loss. Pure tone audiometry which shows apparent bone conduction hearing loss is called Carhart's notch.

5. **b. Benign non-encapsulated vascular tumor**
Glomus jugular is a type of paraganglioma which arise from glomus bodies of jugular vein.
It is a very slow growing, capsulated benign tumour which is more common in females.
Since it arises in the jugular fossa, the last four cranial nerves, i.e. IX-XII nerves are involved.
The other glomus body tumour called glomus tympanicum which arises from tympanic plexus, arises from the promontory and not glomus jugular.
Glomus tympanicum presents as pulsatile tinnitus and hearing loss.
Between 1-5% of these tumours secrete catecholamines.

6. **d. Gentamicin**
The above mentioned patient has otosclerosis. This is confirmed by "As" curve in impedance audiometry.
Treatments of otosclerosis are the following:
   1. Medicinal—The drug given is ***sodium fluoride***.
      This is useful only in the active stage.
   2. Surgical treatment—***Stapedectomy*** is the surgery of choice
   3. Hearing aid—This is an option when the first two cannot be used.

   Gentamicin is an ototoxic drug and hence will not be given.

7. **c. Fissula ante fenestram**
Otosclerosis most commonly starts at the fissula ante fenestram. This site is very close to (just anterior to) the footplate of stapes and hence the disease spreads to this area causing hearing loss.
Hence the anterior part of footplate is the commonly involved part of footplate.
The three important sites of otosclerosis are:
   1. ***Fissula ante fenestram***
   2. ***Fossula post fenestram***
   3. ***Oval window***

8. **c. Glomus tumour**
It is a very slow-growing, noncapsulated benign vascular tumour which is more common in females.
The glomus body tumour of middle ear is called glomus tympanicum and it arises from tympanic plexus, on promontory.
It presents as pulsatile tinnitus and hearing loss.

9. **c. 20-30 years**
Otosclerosis is a disease of young females which presents as gradually progressive conductive hearing loss in both the ears with positive family history. It usually presents between the ages of 20 and 30 years.

10. **a. Pulsatile tinnitus**
Glomus tumour is glomus body tumour often seen on the promontory in the middle. The other common site is the jugular fossa in the skull base.
When the tumour is present in the middle ear, it causes hearing loss and pulsatile tinnitus.
Since patient usually complains of pulsatile tinnitus, this becomes the earliest symptom, although almost all these patients also has conductive hearing loss.
However, some books will consider hearing loss as the first symptom.

11. **a. Teflon piston**
Stapedectomy is a surgery of stapes done in patients of otosclerosis. In this, the stapes suprastructure is removed along with a part of stapes footplate.
This is replaced by a Teflon piston, which takes over the function of the stapes.

PROSTHESIS MATERIAL DURING STAPEDECTOMY AND TYMPANOPLASTY

Stapedectomy prosthesis	Tympanoplasty prosthesis
• Piston	• Total ossicular replacement prosthesis (TORP) • Partial ossicular replacement prosthesis (PORP)
Prosthesis materials • Teflon. Most common material • Platinum • Steel • Alloys, etc.	Prosthesis materials • Hydroxyapatite. This is most common material

- Grommet is a ventilating tube used in myringotomy which is done for glue ear.
- Total ossicular replacement prosthesis (TORP) is used for reconstruction of ossicular chain usually during tympanoplasty.

12. **a. Paget's disease**

Paget's disease is also called "osteitis deformans".

In this disease, there is remodelling and deposition of the bone leading to enlargement of the bone. If it happen in the skull bone, the skull gets enlarged and hence the name ***soldier's helmet.***

If the problem spreads to the labyrinthine bone, hearing may be affected.

COMPARISON BETWEEN OTOSCLEROSIS AND PAGET'S DISEASE

Otosclerosis	Paget's disease of temporal bone
Seen in endochondral layer of otic capsule	Mainly pelvis. It is uncommon in ear
There is resorption of endochondral bone with enlargement of perivascular spaces and vascular proliferation which is followed by deposition of immature or *woven bone–this stage is called Otospongiosis or Active stage* Later on, active resorption and remodelling continues in this area leading to production of mature or *lamellar bone—this stage is called Otosclerosis or Passive stage.*	There is increase in osteoclastic activities causing reabsorption followed by architecturally unsound bone deposition. This leads to fragile and enlarged bone
May be caused by measles	May be caused measles or paramyxovirus
Mainly conductive hearing loss	Mainly sensorineural hearing loss
Hearing loss is due to stapes footplate fixation	Hearing loss is mainly due to **"narrowing of internal acoustic meatus"**
Tinnitus and vertigo very uncommon	Tinnitus and vertigo may rarely be present
Sodium fluoride is the main drug	Bisphosphonates are the main drug

13. **d. Spiral ligament**

The most commonly involved structure of inner ear in otosclerosis is the spiral ligament.

This happens when the otosclerotic focus reaches the endosteum of cochlea. This leads to ***atrophy and hyalinization of spiral ligament***.

The hair cells, spiral ganglion and stria vascularis are normal.

14. **d. Lenticular process of incus**

The name of the surgery is ***"stapedotomy"***

Why would a part of incus (lenticular process), be removed in the surgery of stapes (stapedotomy).

During stapedotomy every part of stapes are removed except footplate. A fistula or hole is drilled on the footplate through which the prosthesis will pass into the inner ear.

15. **a. Autosomal dominant**

Otospongiosis is the active stage of otosclerosis. We know that otosclerosis (otospongiosis) transmits as autosomal dominant disease. It is therefore seen in families.

16. **b. It acts by inhibiting osteoblastic activities.**

*The most useful drug is **Sodium fluoride**.*

Indications of Sodium fluoride in otosclerosis are:

1. Active stage of otosclerosis which is shown by either **positives Schwartz sign or HRCT.**
2. Cochlear otosclerosis with **SNHL**.

Hence **Sodium fluoride** is given if at least one of the three is present.

- Positive Schwartz sign
- HRCT showing active focus, or
- Audiometry shows SNHL

In otoclerosis, sodium fluoride may act in one of the following ways

- It reduces the osteoclastic activities
- It increases the osteoblastic activities
- It inhibits cytotoxic enzymes in the cochlea

17. **d. Sacculotomy**
In otosclerosis when surgery is indicated, the following surgeries can be done:
    - Stapedectomy
    - Stapedotomy
    - Fenestration surgery (this surgery is NOT done anymore).

    Sacculotomy introduced by Cody and Fick is done for Meniere's disease.

18. **d. Glomus tumour**
Fisch classification is used for glomus tumour.
However, there is also a Fisch classification for juvenile angiofibroma, but is NOT used in practice.

19. **d. Type C2**
Fisch classification of glomus tumour:

1. Type A tumor	Tumor limited to middle ear (carries the best prognosis)
2. Type B tumour	Tumor limited to the tympanomastoid area with no infralabyrinthine compartment involvement
3. Type C tumor This is divided into three types:	Tumor involving the infralabyrinthine compartment of temporal bone with extension to petrous apex
Type C1	Tumor with limited involvement of the vertical portion of the carotid canal
Type C2	Tumor invading the vertical portion of the carotid canal
Type C3	Tumor invasion of the horizontal portion of the carotid canal
4. Type D tumor has 2 types (D1)	Tumor with an intracranial extension less than 2 cm in diameter
Type D2	Tumor with an intracranial extension greater than 2 cm in diameter

20. **c. Interferons**
This is clearly a case of glomus tumour.
Treatment of glomus tumour is:
Preoperative embolization followed by surgical excision.
Radiotherapy is indicated where surgery is not indication.
Note: Interferons have NO role in glomus tumour.

IMAGE BASED ANSWER

21. **d. All are true**
Zellballen cell are large loose clusters of cells enveloped by thin vascular channels. The thin vascular channels separate the clusters of cells giving a well defined nest like appearance (as shown in the picture). This histopathologic findings is diagnostic of paragangliomas.
    - Glomus tumor is a type of paraganglioma.
    - The other important type of paraganglioma is *chemodectoma*.

CHAPTER

9 Diseases of the Inner Ear/ Labyrinthine Diseases

Inner ear diseases are diseases affecting the labyrinth.

Therefore they will have the "**cochlear features**" in contrast to "**retrocochlear features**" which seen in diseases of the eight cranial nerve.

Let us recall the important cochlear features seen in cochlear diseases:

Cochlear features/features seen in disease of labyrinth
• Recruitment phenomena may be present
• Short increment sensitivity index (SISI) is better
• BERA has normal latency between wave I and wave V • Stapedial reflex/acoustic reflex may be present

Important inner diseases discussed are:

Inner ear diseases
Meniere's disease
Benign paroxysmal positioning vertigo (BPPV)/Cupulolithiasis/canalolithiasis
Superior semicircular canal dehiscent syndrome/ Minor's syndrome
Vestibular neuronitis

MENIERE'S DISEASE

Meniere's disease is a disease of membranous labyrinth or membranous sac wherein there is ***increase in the quantity of endolymph in the membranous labyrinth.***

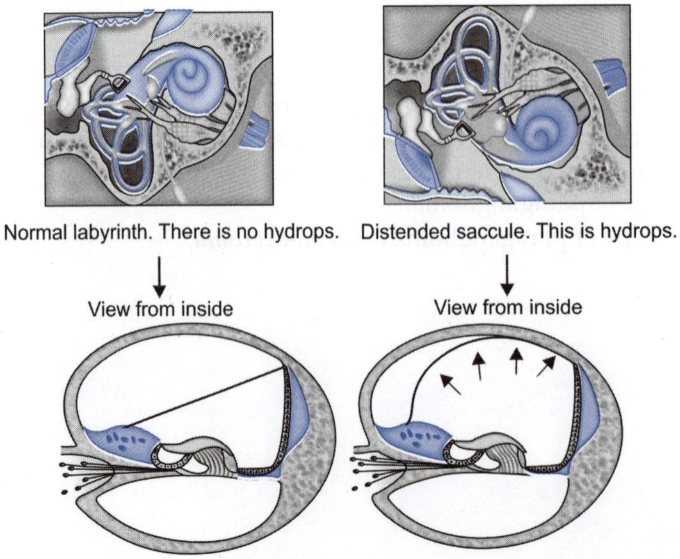

This is either due to:
- Increase production of endolymph or
- Reduced drainage of endolymph or
- Both.

The result of this increase in endolymph leads in the distension of endolymphatic sac/development of hydrops. This is called **endolymphatic hydrops.**

Endolymphatic hydrops is the most important feature of Meniere's disease.

One of the probable cause of this condition is mutation of gene in short arm of chromosome 6.

Depending on the cause of Meniere's disease, it can be divided into two types:

Primary Meniere's disease	Meniere's syndrome/ secondary Meniere's disease
Is idiopathic in nature May be caused by mutation of gene in short arm of chromosome 6	• Caused by other conditions like 1. Syphilis 2. Mumps 3. Cogan's syndrome 4. Hypothyroidism, etc

This condition is usually seen in *middle aged male and is usually unilateral.* It is autosomal dominant disease and is hereditary.

Presenting Features

The cardinal triad of Meniere's disease are
1. Episodic vertigo. – Vertigo is associated with nausea/vomiting and nystagmus – Duration of vertigo may last from *24 minutes to 24 hrs.*
2. Fluctuating hearing loss – It is sensorineural hearing loss – Initially it affects lower frequencies (*this gives UPWARD SLOPING audiogram)* – Later it may involve lower as well as higher frequencies *(gives FLAT audiogram)*
3. Fluctuating tinnitus
• Less important symptoms are:
– Ear fullness
– Monural diplacusis – Sweating, diarrhoea, bradycardia, etc • When there are tinnitus, hearing loss and vertigo are present together; it is called *meniere's triad.*

Variants of Meniere's disease	
Cochlear hydrops	*Has mainly cochlear symptoms*
Vestibular hydrops	*Mainly has vestibular symptoms*
Lermoyez disease or Reverse Meniere's or Inverse Meniere's	*Symptoms appear in reverse order.* *Hearing loss and tinnitus start and is progressive, followed by an attack of vertigo.* *After vertigo, all the symptoms subside.*
Tumarkin otolithic drop attacks	*In this the patient falls down as if he/she has been PUSHED*

Some Special Features Seen in Meniere's Disease

1. **Recruitment**
   Recruitment is a feature of cochlear disease and therefore may be present in other cochlear diseases as well
2. **Short increment sensitivity index (SISI).**
   SISI is also a feature of cochlear diseases

3. **Hennebert's sign**

   This is also called **false positive fistula sign.**

   This sign may be seen in few other diseases also.

Fistula sign	Causes of this sign
Fistula sign or True positive fistula sign	• Labyrinthine fistula • Perilymph fistula • Tympanoplasty type V • After stapedectomy/stapedotomy
False positive fistula sign or Hennebert's sign	• Meniere's disease • Congenital syphilis • Hypermobile footplate • Superior canal dehiscent syndrome
False negative fistula sign	• Dead labyrinth • Fistula blocked by cholesteatoma • Test not done properly

4. **Tullio's *phenomena***

   When there is a loud noise of low frequency it produces nystagmus and vertigo.

Tullio's phenomena is seen in many conditions like
1. Meniere's disease 2. Labyrinthine fistula 3. Tympanoplasty type V/Fenestration surgery 4. Stapedectomy/stapedotomy 5. Hypermobile footplate 6. Superior semicircular canal dehiscent syndrome/ Minor's syndrome, etc
NOTE: In all these conditions fistula test/sign may also be present

Investigations

1. **Audiometry**

   – Audiometry in the initial stage will show higher loss at lower frequencies **(upwards sloping graph)** and later on loss at all frequencies **(flat graph).**

   – It may also show special features like recruitment, SISI, etc which have been discussed already.

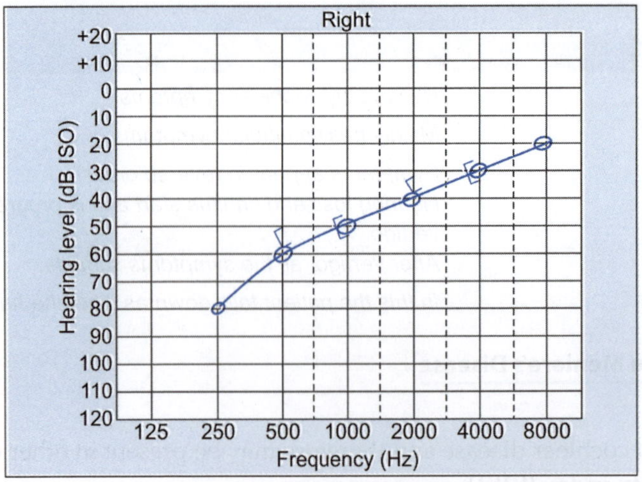

Audiogram showing upward slope

2. **Caloric Test**

   Most commonly shows ***canal paresis.*** Some times may show ***direction preponderance to the opposite side.***

3. **Glycerol Test**
   - Glycerol is given orally.
   - Glycerol is an osmotic diuretic agent and therefore causes dieresis.
   - This leads to loss of body fluid along with endolymph.
   - Loss of endolymph causes in the improvement of symptoms in the patient.
   - Improvement is also seen in the various investigation results.

4. **Reverse Glycerol Test**

   Acetazolamide is given to the patient and the symptoms worsen.

5. **Electrocochleography**

   This is the ***most sensitive and most specific investigation for Meniere's disease.***

   Therefore, it is also the ***most diagnostic test*** for Meniere's disease.

   Electrocochleography can pick up three things
   1. **Cochlear microphonics (CM):** This is electrical potential of the outer hair cell.
   2. **Summation potential (SP):** This is electrical potential of the outer hair cell.
   3. **Action potential (AP):** This is action potential of the VIIIth nerve in the cochlea.

   The most important thing is the ratio between summation potential (SP)and action potential (AP).

   The normal ratio of SP:AP is **0.3 or 30%.**

   In Menieres disease this ratio is **0.40-0.45 or 40%-45%.**

6. **Vestibular Evoked Myogenic Potential (VEMP)**
   - VEMP is the potential that can be recorded in the sternocleidomastoid muscle when the vestibule (Saccule) is stimulated with the sound energy.
   - This potential is dependant on saccule and inferior vestibular nerve.
   - In Meniere's disease, since the saccule is distended, this potential is not normal.

TREATMENT OF MENIERE'S DISEASE

1. **Restrict fluid, salt,** tea, coffee, tobacco, etc. Patient should be careful during driving and swimming, traveling.
2. **Medicines**
   - *In acute stage* of the disease, we use

     Vestibular sedatives and other drugs like dimenhydrinate, antiemetics and sedatives like diazepam are used.

     Vasodilators like inhalation of carbogen and parenteral histamine are also useful
   - *In chronic phase other* drugs may be added. Important among these drugs are

     Steroids-Steroids may also be given through ***intratympanic instillation.*** This avoids the systemic complication of steroids.

     Betahistine *may also be used.*

Betahistine in Meniere's disease

- It is a histamine analogue
- It is H1 and H2 agonist
- It acts as a central vasodilator and improves microcirculation of stria vascularis in the cochlea. This will treat/prevent atrophy
- Controls the asymmetry of the vestibules in Meniere's disease, thereby controlling vertigo
- It inhibits the activity in the vestibular nucleus and therefore has vestibular sedative type action

   Diuretic can be used

3. **Surgeries**
   - Endolymphatic sac decompression
   - This was one of the first surgery done for Meniere's disease and was done by P**ortmann.**

- Therefore this surgery is also called ***Portmann surgery.***
- During this surgery, a very important landmark for endolymphatic sac is used. This landmark of endolymphatic sac is called **"Donaldson's line"**
- Cody's tack and Fick's operation.
- It is also called **Sacculotomy.** A hole is created in the saccule so that extra endolymph drains out.
- Shunt surgery
- A shunt is created in the labyrinth to drain out the fluid
- **Vestibular nerve resection**
- **Ultrasound destruction of vestibule**
- **Vestibulectomy**

This can be either chemical vestibulectomy or surgical vestibulectomy.

Chemical vestibulectomy/Intratympanic gentamicin/ITG

- This is done by using ototoxic drugs like *gentamycin.*
- The procedure is called chemical vestibulectomy or *Intratympanic gentamicin or ITG.*
- During this surgery *microwicks/microcannulas/microtubules* for controlled and sustained release of gentamicin.
- The microwicks are placed near the ROUND WINDOW.
- The gentamycin enters the inner ear through the secondary tympanic membrane of the round window by the process of endocytosis.
- Gentamicin being an ototoxic drug will damage the vestibule. This gentamicin will NOT damage the cochlea.
- When gentamicin is given parenterally (intravenous); it may damage the cochlea along with the vestibule.
- NOTE: As mentioned above, steroid can also be instillated through the same method. This avoids the systemic complications of steroid.

4. ***Cooksey-Cawthorne exercises***

   Also called **vestibular exercise.**

   It helps in better and faster compensation usually done along with surgeries of the vestibule.
5. ***Meniett's device***

   This is a special device used for Meniere's disease.

   In this, ***intermittent low pressure pulse therapy*** used.
6. ***Alternobaric oxygen with continuous variations in pressure*** is also an option.
7. ***Gene therapy.*** In this therapy, segment of nucleic acid is transferred into the cell.

BENIGN PAROXYSMAL POSITIONAL VERTIGO (BPPV)

It is also called cupulolithiasis and canalolithiasis

In BPPV, patient has sudden and momentary attacks of vertigo and nausea precipitated by sudden change of head position.

The duration of vertigo and nausea is **momentary or for few seconds (10-20 sec.) only.**

This is important because on the basis of this, the cause of vertigo can be identified.

NOTE: In case of Meniere's disease, the duration of vertigo is between 24 minutes to 24 hours.

Diseases causing vertigo	Duration of vertigo
• Phobic postural vertigo's	< 5 seconds
• BPPV	10-20 seconds
• TIA and Migraine	Less than 20 minutes
• Meniere's disease	20 min – 24 hours
• Perilymph fistula	20 min – 24 hours
• Vestibular neuronitis	> 24 hours (one day)
• CNS diseases.	> 24 hours (one day)

This happens due to ***otoliths/otoconia which dislodges from macula and gets deposited in posterior semicircular canal.***

Therefore, the nystagmus is vertical torsional.

The cause of this could be varied:

- Following trauma.
- Drug induced.

An important test done in this patient is **Dix Hallpike test.**

For treatment of BPPV an important manoeuvre is done called ***Epley's manoeuvre.***

Some less common manoeuvres that can be used in BPPV are:

- Brandt-Daroff maneouvre
- Semont manoeuvre

Since, the duration of vertigo is very short, *antivertigo drugs* do not have much important in this disease.

The other mode of treatment is **Singular Neurectomy.**

In this surgery, the singular nerve is resected.

NOTE: Singular nerve is a branch of inferior vestibular nerve and it supplies posterior semicircular canal.

Inner ear nerve resection	Indications
Vestibular neurectomy	Meniere's disease
Singular neurectomy	Benign paroxysmal positional vertigo

SUPERIOR SEMICIRCULAR CANAL DEHISCENT SYNDROME

This condition is sometimes referred to as "**Minor's Syndrome".**

As the name suggests, bony part of the superior semicircular canal is dehiscent.

It is usually congenital condition and is often bilateral.

Presentation

- Dizziness/imbalance
- **Hennebert's sign may be present**
- **Tullio's phenomena may be present**
- **Autophony.**

  In autophony, patients his/her own body sounds clearly. This sound usually transmits through bony conduction.

Few conditions that give rise to " autophony" are:
Patulous eustachian tube Superior semicircular canal dehiscent syndrome

- Hearing loss.

Hearing loss in case of superior semicircular canal, may show a condition called **"third window effect"**

Third window effect

Third window effect is a condition in which the patient has conductive hearing loss, although the pathology is present in the labyrinth/inner ear.

Such an effect occurs because the dehiscent part of the superior semicircular canal acts as the third window, an additional window to

1. Oval window and
2. Round window.

This situation may be present in few other conditions like

- Dilated endolymphatic duct
- Fistulas of cochlea

Management

- CT Scan will diagnose this condition.
- **VEMP** may be elicited in this condition
- **No treatment** required in most cases
- In severe cases**, surgical repair** may be needed.

Last minute revision

- *Meniere's disease is called endolymphatic hydrops*
- *It is caused by genetic defect on mutation on long arm of chromosome 14*
- *Lermoyez disease is reverse Meniere's disease*
- *Tumarkin's causes drop attacks*
- *Features of meniere's disease are*
  1. *Recruitment*
  2. *Tulio's phenomena*
  3. *Diplacusis*
  4. *Hennebert's sign, etc*
- *Electrocochleography is the gold standard investigation*
- *Hennebert's sign is false positive fistula sign*
- *It is seen in*
  1. *Meniere's*
  2. *Congenital syphilis*
  3. *Hypermobile footplate*
- *Ratio of summation potential and action potential is more than 40%*
- *Drugs are main treatment option. Drugs like betahistine which is a central vasodilator*
- *Intratympanic gentamicin is a treatment option*
- *In this microwicks/microtubules are used, which ar placed near round window*
- *BPPV is a problem of posterior semicircular canal*
- *In this vertigo is for 10-20 seconds*
- *Dix-hallpike maneuver can be used for diagnosis*
- *Epley's maneuver can be used for treatment of BPPV*
- *Superior canal dehiscent syndrome can cause third window effect*
- *Superior canal dehiscent syndrome can present similar to meniere's disease*

QUESTIONS

1. **Recruitment test is positive in:**
   a. Otosclerosis
   b. Meniere's disease
   c. Chronic mastoiditis
   d. Otitis externa
2. **Meniere's disease is characterized by:**
   a. Conductive hearing loss and tinnitus
   b. Vertigo, ear discharge, tinnitus and headache
   c. Vertigo, tinnitus, hearing loss and headache
   d. Vertigo, tinnitus and hearing loss
3. **Meniere's disease is characterized by all *except:***
   a. Vertigo
   b. Sensorineural hearing loss
   c. Tinnitus
   d. Ear discharge
4. **Which of the following is not a typical feature of Meniere's disease?**
   a. Sensorineural deafness
   b. Pulsatile tinnitus
   c. Vertigo
   d. Fluctuating deafness
5. **Differential diagnosis of Meniere's disease are all *except*:**
   a. Acoustic neuroma
   b. CNS disease
   c. Labyrinthitis
   d. Suppurative otitis media
6. **In classical Meniere's disease which one of the following is true?:**
   a. Carhart's notch is characteristic feature in pure tone audiogram
   b. Schwartz's sign is seen on tympanic membrane
   c. Low frequency sensorineural deafness is often seen in audiogram
   d. Decompression of fallopian canal is treatment of choice
7. **Chromosome responsible for hereditary Ménière's disease is:**
   a. 6 b. 9
   c. 11 d. 14
8. **Initial mechanism of action of intratympanic gentamicin microwick catheter inserted into inner ear in treatment of Menier's disease:**
   a. Damage outer hair cell
   b. Binds to hair cell Na^+-K^+ ATPase channel
   c. Acts on melanoreceptors of outer hair cell
   d. Bind to Mg^{2+} channel
9. **Vasodilatation of internal ear for Meniere's disease is:**
   a. Nicotinic acid b. Histamine
   c. Serotonin d. Both a and b
10. **Which of the following is true of Meniere's disease:**
    a. Surgery is the mainstay of treatment
    b. Electrocochleography is the gold standard investigation for diagnosis
    c. Semont's maneuver is used for treatment
    d. In initial stage, inverted "V" shaped audiogram is seen
11. **Third window effect:**
    a. Perforated tympanum
    b. Dehiscent superior semicircular canal
    c. Round window d. Oval window
12. **Endolymphatic decompression is done in:**
    a. Tinnitus b. Acoustic neuroma
    c. Meniere's disease d. Perilymph fistula
13. **What is the treatment for BPPV ?**
    a. Vestibular exercise
    b. Intralabyrinthine streptomycin
    c. Antihistamines
    d. Canalith repositioning procedure

IMAGE BASED QUESTION

14. **The following audiogram is most likely seen in which of these diseases:**

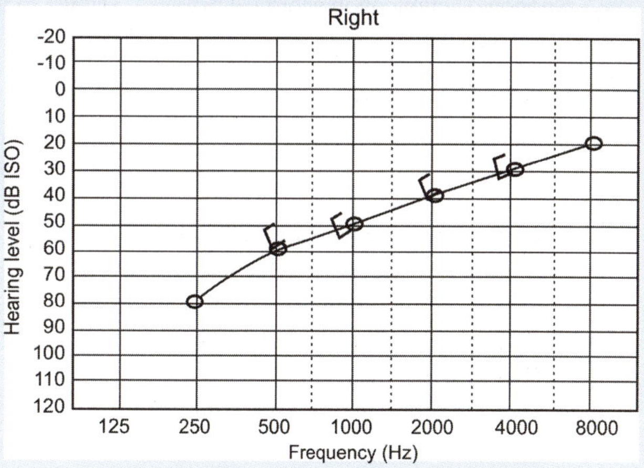

    a. Meniere's disease b. Ototoxicity
    c. Noise induced hearing loss
    d. Acoustic neuroma

ANSWERS AND EXPLANATIONS

1. **b. Meniere's disease**

Recruitment test is positive in cochlear disease and is used to differentiate cochlear from retrocochlear disease. Alternate binaural loudness balance (ABLB) is used to check the presence of recruitment.

In this the threshold of hearing increases due to SN loss but once he/she starts hearing, the loudness of hearing increased abnormally as the intensity is increased. Which means that once the patient begins to hear the sound, if the intensity of the sound is kept increasing; the subjective sensation of hearing increases more than the increase in the intensity of sound.

Other hearing tests that can differentiate cochlear hearing loss from retro-cochlear loss are:
- Short increment sensitivity index (SISI)
- Threshold tone decay test
- Speech discrimination score with roll over test
- Bekesy audiometry
- BERA, etc.

DIFFERENCES BETWEEN COCHLEAR DISEASES AND RETROCOCHLEAR DISEASES

Tests	Cochlear diseases	Retrocochlear diseases
Stapedial/acoustic reflex	Present	Absent
Recruitment	Present	Absent
Short increment sensitivity index (SISI)	Present	Absent
Bekesy audiometry	Type II graph	Type III or Type IV graph
Tone decay phenomena of one minute	Seen at < 25 dB above threshold	At > 25 dB above threshold
Roll over curve	Not seen	Seen
Speech discrimination score (SDS)	Slightly reduced	Severely reduced
Cochlear microphonics (CM)	Absent	Present
Otoacoustic emission (OAE)	Affected	Not affected
BERA	Latency is normal between wave I and wave V	Increased latency between wave I and wave V

2. **d. Vertigo, tinnitus and hearing loss**

Meniere's disease is the disease of labyrinth and so will cause sensorineural hearing and will not have ear discharge. These patients will have tinnitus, vertigo and hearing loss.

The typical triad of meniere's disease are:
1. *Fluctuating tinnitus*
2. *Fluctuating hearing loss, and*
3. *Episodic vertigo*

The fourth important feature is ear fullness.

3. **d. Ear discharge**

Meniere's disease is the disease of inner ear and hence will have symptoms of inner ear. Ear discharge is a feature of middle ear disease.

4. **b. Pulsatile tinnitus**

Pulsatile tinnitus is a feature of glomus tumor whereas fluctuating tinnitus is a feature of meniere's disease.

5. **d. Suppurative otitis media**

Meniere's disease is a disease of cochlea which causes fluctuating sensorineural hearing loss, tinnitus and episodes of vertigo. Atypical meniere's disease may not have all the features of classical meniere's disease.

Similar features may be seen in other disease like acoustic neuroma, CNS diseases, etc.
Suppurative otitis media is a disease of middle ear and causes conductive hearing loss with absence of other features that are seen in Meniere's disease.

6. **c. Low frequency sensorineural deafness is often seen in audiogram**
Meniere's disease is the disease of excess of endolymph in the membranous labyrinth. In this, there is typically low frequency sensorineural deafness; especially in the early stage.
- Carhart's notch and schwartz sign are features of otosclerosis.
- Audiometry is quantity test and hence diagnosis of disease cannot be made with an audiometry.

However; few important types of audiograms are seen in some diseases.
They are given below.

1. Conductive hearing loss
• Conditions that cause increase in the stiffness of tympanic membrane and ossicular chain will lead to upward sloping curve ie more hearing loss at low frequency and less hearing loss at high frequency. Examples of such audiograms is otosclerosis
• Conditions that increases mass of middle ear will give the opposite type curve (downward sloping) ie less hearing loss at low frequency and more hearing loss at high frequency. Examples are: – Fluid in the middle ear as in cases of secretory otitis media.
• A special type of curve is a carhart's notch which is seen in otosclerosis.

2. Sensorineural hearing loss
• Upwards sloping curve is seen in endolymphatic hydrops or meniere's disease
• Downward sloping curve is seen in stiffening of basilar membrane. Examples are: – Ototoxicity, – Noise induced hearing loss
• Flat audiogram is seen in atrophy of stria vascularis. Examples are: – Presbycusis, – Salicylate poisoning
• Trough shaped or "U" shaped curve is seen in congenital hearing loss
• Notch at 4000 Hz is seen in noise induced hearing as well as acoustic neuroma
• Unilateral severe SN loss may be seen in mumps

7. **A. 6**
Meniere's disease is also called ***endolymphatic hydrops.***
Meniere's disease is a complex disease and therefore, the genetic contribution to Meniere's disease is also complex. The single gene/genes mutation may not be sufficient to determine the disease.
It is yet NOT confirmed as to which chromosome is responsible for this disease.
However, from among the above given choices there is a toss between:
- Short arm of chromosome 6, and
- Long arm of chromosome 14.

In case we have to select from these two; go for **chromosome 6**
Depending on the cause of Meniere's disease, it can be divided into two types:

Primary meniere's disease	Meniere's syndrome/ secondary meniere's disease
Is idiopathic in nature May be caused by mutation of gene in short arm of chromosome 6	Caused by other conditions like Syphilis Mumps Cogan's syndrome Hypothyroidism, etc

8. **b. binds to hair cell Na + -K + ATPase channel**
Intratympanic gentamicin is a procedure used in the treatment of Meniere's disease.

THE PROCEDURE OF INTRATYMPANIC GENTAMICIN

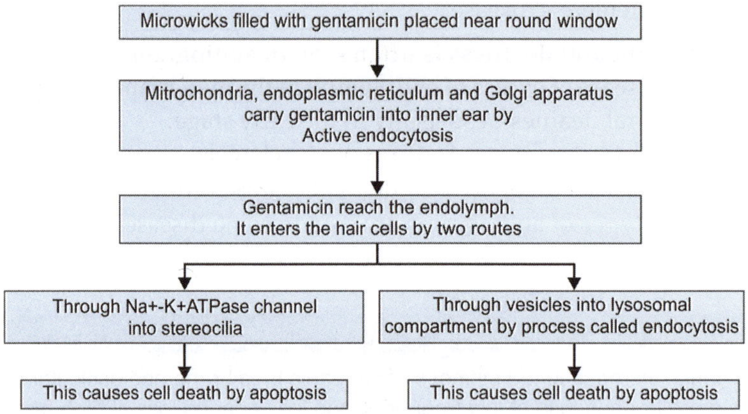

9. **d. Both a and b**

The vasodilator effect in Meniere's disease is seen with both the drugs *i.e*

- Histamine like betadine and
- Nicotinic acid

However, nicotinic acid is NOT used commonly and betadine is a very commonly used drug.
Betadine is histamine analogue.
It has weak agonistic action on H1 and H2 receptors and antagonistic action on H3 receptors.
It causes:

- Vasodilation of stria vascularis and causes improve in microcirculation.
- Decreases asymmetry between the two side vestibular end organ
- Inhibits activity of vestibular nuclei.

10. **b. Electrocochleography is the gold standard investigation for diagnosis**

There is no good investigation for confirming Meniere's disease. That's why Meniere's disease is a clinical diagnosis.
However, few investigations are useful like:

- ***Electrocochleography. This is the most sensitive and most specific investigation and therefore a gold standard investigation.***
- Glycerol test
- Vestibular evoked myogenic potential (VEMP), etc.
  - Medicinal treatment is the main line of treatment. Surgeries are very uncommon done and has unsatisfactory results.
  - Semont's maneuver is done for benign paroxysmal positional vertigo (BPPV)
  - In initial stage of Meniere's disease, the lower frequencies of hearing are affected. The audiogram, therefore, will be ***upwards sloping/right sloping*** and NOT inverted "V".

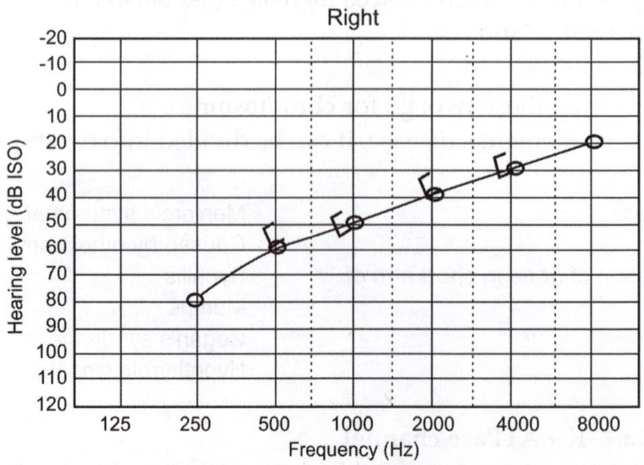

Audiogram showing upward slope

11. **b. Dehiscent superior semicircular canal**

The bony labyrinth has two natural windows on it. They are:

1. Oval window and
2. Round window.

These two windows are necessary for hearing. These two windows must be at ***opposite phase*** of each other during the vibration of the ear caused by sound.

Sometimes there is additional opening on the bony labyrinth. This new window acts as an additional window to the natural two windows. This is the third window. Creation/presence of the third window affects the hearing of the patient. This is called ***third window effect.***

A very important condition causing the third window effect is superior canal dehiscent syndrome.

12. **c. Meniere's diasese**

Endolymphatic sac decompression is one of the earliest surgeries done for Meniere's disease. This surgery was done by Portmann, and therefore is also referred to as ***Portmann's surgery.***

13. **d. Canalith repositioning procedure**

This procedure is also called ***Epley's maneuver.***

During this procedure, the otolith is directed from posterior canal back into the utricle (where it belongs).

IMAGE BASED ANSWER

14. **a. Meniere's disease**

This audiogram shows sensorineural hearing loss in right ear. It also shows more loss at lower frequencies and less loss at higher frequencies. Such an audiogram is described as ***upwards sloping audiogram***.

This finding is seen in **Hydrops or Meniere's diseases**.

Important types or shapes of audiograms and their diagnosis.

For conductive hearing loss:

Types/shapes of graph	Diagnosis
1. Upwards sloping/left sloping (more loss at lower frequency)	• Otosclerosis
2. Downwards sloping/right sloping (loss at higher frequency)	Conditions with increased mass in middle ear • Serous otitis media (SOM) • Ossicular chain damage
3. Dip at 2000Hz/carhart's notch	• Otosclerosis

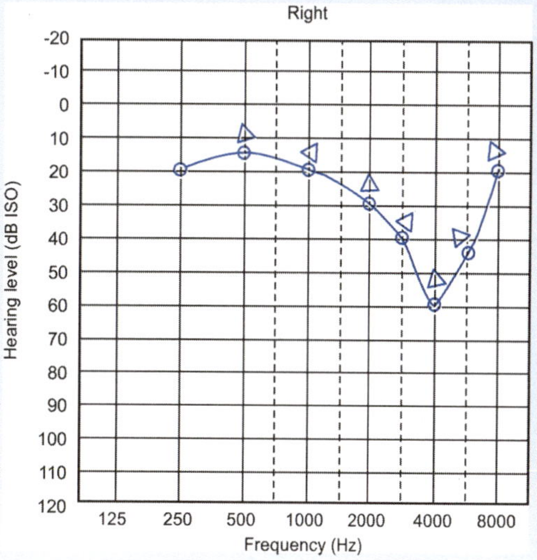

For sensorineural hearing loss

	Types/shapes of graph	Diagnosis
	1. Flat graph	• Striata lesions like presbycusis • Salicylate/Aspirin poisoning
	2. Downwards sloping/right sloping More loss at higher frequencies	**Problems of organ of Corti, e.g.** • Ototoxicity • Noise induced hearing loss (NIHL)
	3. Upwards sloping/left sloping More loss at lower frequency	When membranes stiffens, e.g. • Early stage of Meniere's disease • Other causes of hydrops
	4. Trough shaped or "U" shaped	• Congenital hearing loss
	5. Dip at 4000 Hz	• Acoustic neuroma • Sometimes NIHL

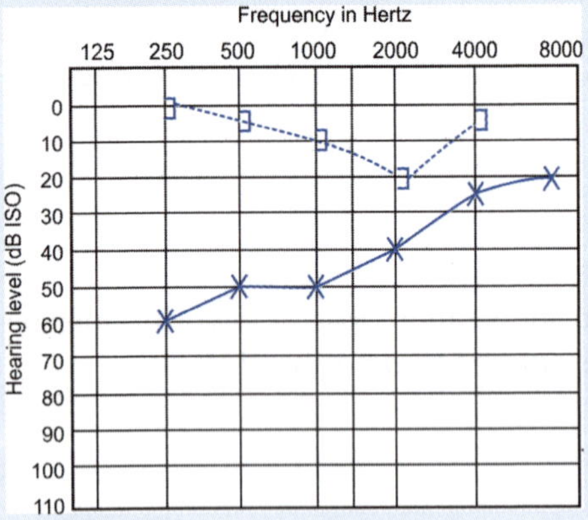

CHAPTER

10 Diseases of the Eighth Nerve/Retrocochlear Diseases

These are diseases of the eighth nerve and central diseases.
Therefore, they have "**retrocochlear features".**
Do you still recall the important **retrocochlear features**

Retrocochlear features seen in neural and central diseases
• Tone decay phenomena will be present
• Roll over curve will be seen
• Speech discrimination score is very poor
• Stapedial reflex will be absent
• The latency between BERA wave I and wave V will increase

ACOUSTIC NEUROMA

More appropriately called **vestibular schwannoma**

Schwannomas
Schwannomas arise most commonly from VIIIth cranial nerve
Second most common having schwannoma is the Vth cranial nerve
Schwannomas cannot arise from Ist and IInd cranial nerves

As the name suggests, it arises from the vestibular branch of VIIIth nerve.

It is a tumor that arises from ***Schwann cells*** of **Superior vestibular nerve more commonly** compared to the inferior vestibular nerve.

Proof of this is below:

The below shown photo is clicked from "Scott-Brown's ORL HNS", Seventh Edition,Page no. 3687, as a proof of the above mentioned fact

> Most tumors (60–80%) arise from the superior division of the vestibular nerve. The tumors seem to arise at somewhat different locations within the meatus.

The most common site of vestibular schwannoma is ***cerebro-pontine angle or C-P angle at the junction of central fibres and peripheral fibres***

This area is known as "**Obersteiner-Redlich zone"**

Two special manifestation which are rare but worth remembering are:

1. Medial vestibular schwannoma	This is a tumour lateral to internal acoustic meatus. It has no extension in the IAM
2. Cystic vestibular schwannoma	There are cyst formation inside the tumour

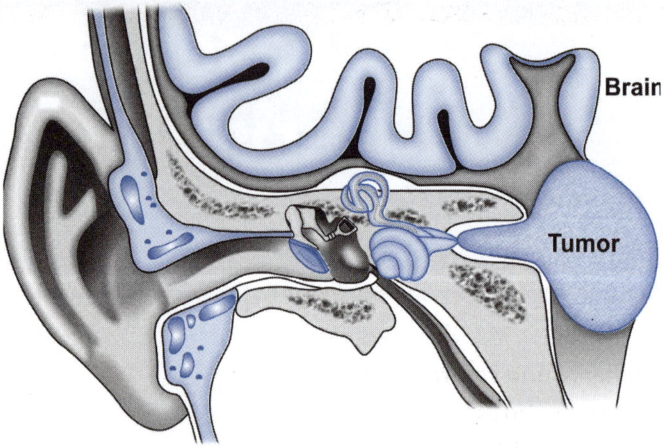

Tumor in the C-P angle and meatus

Three important tumours of C-P Angle in order of frequency are
1. Vestibular schwannoma
2. Meningioma
3. Congenital cholesteatoma

It is a *nonencapsulated slow growing benign tumour of schwann cells of VIIIth cranial nerve.*
It is usually unilateral.
This tumor is common in patient of ***neurofibromatosis type II** (NF2).*
In these patients the tumor is usually bilateral
It has tendency to involve other cranial nerves especially **VIIth nerve and sometimes Vth nerve.**
One of possible causes could be the defect of chromosome 22q. This chromosomal defect is also implicated in NF2.

Common ear Diseases and their Genetic Defects

Diseases	Genetic defects
Otosclerosis	Defective expression of COL1A1 gene
Meniere's disease	Mutation of gene in short arm of chromosome 6
Vestibular schwannoma	Defect of chromosome 22q

The ***most common symptom*** **is unilateral progressive *hearing loss.*** The hearing loss is sensorineural in nature.
NOTE: ***Although, the tumor arises from the vestibular nerve, cochlear symptom (Hearing loss) and not vestibular symptoms, is the first symptom.***
The ***most common manifestation or presentation*** is **loss of corneal reflex.**
This is seen when 5th nerve gets involved.
When Vth nerve gets involved, it indicates that tumor size is > *2.5 cm. in diameter.*
Involvement of 7th nerve leads to *anesthesia/hypoesthesia of posterior-superior canal wall.* This is called **Hitzelberger's sign.**

Important features of vestibular schwannoma	
Hearing loss and tinnitus	Cochlear nerve involved
Vertigo/imbalancing	Vestibular nerve involved
Loss of corneal reflex	Vth nerve involved
Hitzelberger's sign	Facial nerve involved

Some interesting facts about Vestibular schwannoma (Acoustic neuroma)

- It arises from vestibular nerve
- After that, the first nerve it effects is the facial nerve and then may involve the Vth nerve
- Although VIIth nerve gets involved before the Vth nerve, yet Vth nerve symptom (loss of corneal reflex) appears before the VIIth nerve symptom (Hitzelberger's sign.)

Investigation

- Investigation of choice is **MRI (Gadolinium enhanced MRI).**
- This is gold standard investigation.
- X-ray view is *per orbital view* in which we see internal acoustic meatus.
- If different in length of two sides of internal acoustic meatus is **> 2 mm;**
- **Then, it is diagnostic of acoustic neuroma in a suspected patient**.

Other important findings in acoustic neuroma are as given:

- Audiometer
- Audiometry will show sensorineural hearing loss.
- The hearing loss is more **at higher frequencies.**
- Recall that in Meniere's disease, more hearing loss in low frequencies.
- Sometimes, there is **a dip at 4000 Hz frequency.**

  NOTE: In Carhart's notch seen in otosclerosis, the dip is present at 2000 Hz.

  Dip at 4000 Hz may also be present in **noise induced hearing loss (NIHL)**

  Speech discrimination loss is very low

  Stapedial reflex will be absent

  BERA will show increased latency between wave I and wave V

  Special audiometry features like low speech discrimination score, roll over curve, tone decay, etc. may also be present
- **Caloric Test will show reduced response.**
- **Biopsy** may show two types of cells. They are:

Antoni A type (also called Verocay body)	Antoni B type
They are small spindle-shaped cell with densely stained nucleus.	They are aggregation of vacuolated pleomorphic cells.
These cells are tightly/closely packed	They are loosely arranged

- **CT Scan**
- **Gd MRI.** This is the gold standard test for vestibular schwannoma.

Treatment options

There are four options. They are:

1. **Wait and scan**

   This is usually done in very small and slow growing tumour present in elderly person.
2. **Surgery**

   Surgery is the best option for vestibular schwannoma

   The various surgical approaches in acoustic neuroma are as below:

Middle cranial fossa approach	Translabyrinthine approach	Retrosigmoid –sub-arachnoid	Combined approach
Indicated for small tumor of <1.5 cm	Indicated for larger tumor upto 4 cm	For any size tumor	Indicated for larger tumours of >4cm
VIIIth nerve safe or hearing preserved	VIIIth nerve at risk. Hearing destroyed	Hearing preserved	Hearing destroyed
VIIth nerve at risk. Facial palsy	Facial nerve preserved	Facial palsy	Facial palsy

3. **Gamma knife radiosurgery** also called **stereotactic radiosurgery**

   It is a type of radiotherapy.

Gamma knife radiotherapy is useful in many cranial tumors like

- Vestibular schwannoma
- Meningioma, etc.

Not only this, it is also useful option in tumors like

- Glomus jugulare.

During this procedure, the following four stages are to be followed:

Four stages to be followed during gamma knife radiosurgery
1. A rigid stereotactic frame is fitted on the patient's head
2. Radiological images using MRI are taken
3. These images are process and radiosurgery planned
4. Radiation is given in one shot from gamma knife. The source of radiation is the 201 cobalt. NOTE: Unlike radiotherapy where radiation is given in fractions, in gamma knife radiotherapy it is given in a single shot.

Main Advantages of Gamma Knife Radiosurgery are

- It is a non-invasive surgery
- Facial nerve is preserved
- Hearing is preserved in many patients.

4. **Medicines**

   Various drugs are found to be useful for vestibular schwannoma.

   - Tyrosine kinase inhibitors like
     - ***Lapatinib***
     - ***Erlotinib.*** This is ***ErbB inhibitor*** resulting in inhibition of schwann cell proliferation.
   - VEGF inhibitor like
     - Bevacizumab

VESTIBULAR NEURONITIS/ VESTIBULAR NEURITIS

This is infection of vestibular nerve caused by virus usually ***herpes simplex virus type I***.

It infects the **superior vestibular nerve** more commonly as compared inferior vestibular nerve.

In this condition, there is sudden, isolated and total loss of afferent input from unilateral vestibule.

Important features of vestibular neuronitis are given below.

- It is seen in patients > 50-year-old.
- It usually follows URTI.
- It is usually seen 2-3 weeks after URTI
- The main symptoms are vestibular ***nystagmus, vertigo, and nausea***.
- Nystagmus is usually towards the healthy ear/normal side.
- Cochlear symptoms are ***absent***.

Investigations

Vestibular neuritis is usually a clinical diagnosis.

However, most of the vestibular functions like **caloric test, posturography** may have positive findings

The **most important point is that all the hearing test will be normal.** This is because the cochlea is not affected in this condition.

Treatment

It is self-limiting disease, only advice is bed rest for few days.

Corticosteroids and antiviral drugs may be helpful.

However, vestibular symptoms improve due to compensation of the vestibular nucleus.

This compensation may be hastened by **vestibular exercise.**

Therefore, early mobilization from bed rest and vestibular exercise is helpful.

Last minute revision

- Acoustic neuroma is a retrocochlear disease
- It arises from superior vestibular nerve
- C-P angle is the most common site
- It is common in neurofibromatosis type II
- Hearing loss with tinnitus is the commonest symptom
- Loss of corneal reflex is the commonest presentation/sign. This is caused by fifth nerve involvement
- Hitzelberger sign is seen when VIIth nerve gets involved
- Gadolinium MRI is the gold standard investigation
- Surgical excision is the treatment of choice
- Gamma knife radiosurgery can be useful
- Vestibular neuronitis is a very common cause of vertigo. But NO hearing loss is seen
- It is a viral infection of vestibular nerve that follows sore throat in adult males

QUESTIONS

1. **Retrocochlear deafness is seen in:**
   a. Meniere's disease b. CSOM
   c. Acoustic neuroma d. Otosclerosis
2. **Commonly nerve involved in acoustic neuroma is:**
   a. 4th b. 5th
   c. 6th d. 8th
3. **Acoustic neuroma most commonly arises from:**
   a. Superior vestibular nerve
   b. Inferior vestibular nerve
   c. Cochlear nerve d. Facial nerve
4. **In acoustic neuroma cranial nerve to be involved earliest is:**
   a. 5 b. 7
   c. 10 d. 9
5. **Which of the following will cause retrocochlear hearing loss?**
   a. Meniere's disease b. Cochlear otosclerosis
   c. Perilymph fistula d. Acoustic neuroma
6. **Cerebellopontine angle tumor is most commonly:**
   a. Acoustic neuroma b. Cholesteatoma
   c. Meningioma d. All of the above
7. **Loss of sensation in external auditory canal or Histelberger sign is a feature of which of the following:**
   a. Bell's palsy b. Acoustic neuroma
   c. Meniere's disease d. Glomus tumor
8. **Which of the following is not true about 'vestibular neuronitis':**
   a. Probably viral in etiology
   b. There is vertigo and nystagmus
   c. There is sensorineural deafness
   d. Caloric responses are diminished
9. **Retrocochlear deafness is seen in:**
   a. Meniere's disease b. CSOM
   c. Acoustic neuroma d. Otosclerosis
10. **A patient with a developing astroglioma in the primary auditory cortex (Brodmann's area 41) complains of hearing unusual noises. What is the main source of subcortical input to the primary auditory cortex?**
    a. Inferior colliculus
    b. Lateral geniculate nucleus
    c. Medial geniculate nucleus
    d. Superior colliculus
11. **Neurofibromatosis type 2 (NF2) is associated with :**
    a. B/L acoustic neuroma
    b. Café-au-lait spots
    c. Lisch nodules
    d. Posterior subcapsular lenticular cataract
12. **Earliest symptom of acoustic neuroma is:**
    a. Sensorineural hearing loss
    b. Tinnitus
    c. Vertigo
    d. Otorrhea
13. **A patient with suspicion of acoustic neuroma. Investigation of choice is:**
    a. CECT b. Gadolinium MRI
    c. SPECT d. PET Scan
14. **Which of the following would be the most appropriate treatment for rehabilitation of a patient, who has bilateral profound deafness, following surgery for bilateral vestibular schwannoma:**
    a. Bilateral powered digital hearing aid
    b. Bilateral cochlear implant
    c. Unilateral cochlear implant
    d. Brainstem implant

IMAGE BASED QUESTION

15. **A 55 years old gentleman presented with hearing loss and tinnitus. MRI showed a 2 cm mass in the right internal acoustic meatus. The mass was excised and the histopathology slide is shown below.**

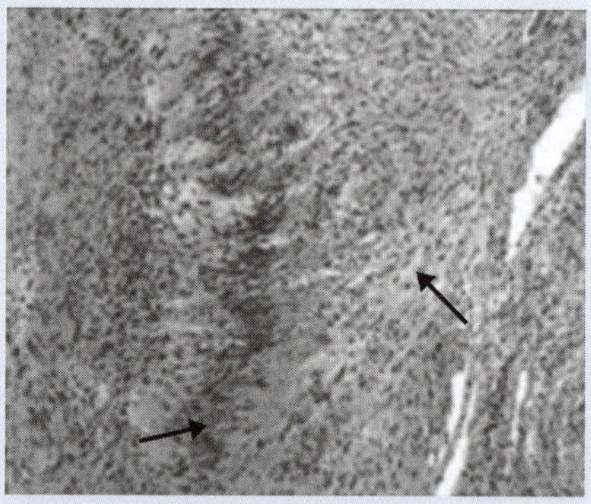

Which is true of this patient?
a. The two arrows point at Antoni A and Antoni B cells
b. This patient has acoustic neuroma
c. This condition is more common in patients with neurofibromatosis type 2
d. All are true

ANSWERS AND EXPLANATIONS

1. **c. Acoustic neuroma**
   Hearing loss can be of the following types:
   1. Conductive, which is caused by diseases in the middle and/or external ear
   2. Sensory/cochlear, which is caused by diseases in the cochlea and

3. Neural/ retrocochlear, which is caused by diseases in the neural pathway.

Acoustic neuroma is most commonly caused in the superior vestibular nerve at the cerebropontine angle and hence will cause retro cochlear deafness.

2. **d. 8th**

Acoustic neuroma also called vestibular schwannoma, most commonly arises from the superior vestibular nerve (a branch of 8th) at the cerebellopontine angle.

This is also the most common tumour of cerebellopontine angle.

However, since the fifth nerve is close to this tumour at the cerebellopontine angle, there is a tendency for it to be involved by the tumour. This leads to `loss of corneal reflex` in patients of acoustic neuroma. In some patient of acoustic neuroma, loss of corneal reflex is the most common presentation.

However, the earliest symptom is hearing loss which is sensorineural in nature.

3. **a Superior vestibular nerve**

Acoustic neuroma arises most commonly from the superior vestibular nerve and the most common site is CP angle. The commonest presentation as loss of corneal reflex.

However, recently a controversy has been created by a publication by a reputed medical institute. According to this publication, the tumor arises from inferior vestibular nerve.

The below shown photo is clicked from "Scott-Brown's ORL HNS", Seventh Edition,Page no. 3687, as a proof of the above mentioned fact

Most tumors (60–80 percent) arise from the superior division of the vestibular nerve. The tumors seem to arise at somewhat different locations within the meatus.

4. **a. 5th nerve.**

Acoustic neuroma is a benign tumor of schwann cells arising most commonly from superior vestibular nerve in the cerebellopontine angle.

As the tumor expands it may involve other cranial nerves.

The earliest nerve it involves is the 5th nerve. This happens when it expands anterosuperiorly.

When this happens patient will have loss of corneal reflex.

Vestibular Schwannoma and Cranial Nerve Involvement

- ***It most commonly arises from superior vestibular nerve***
- ***The first symptoms are hearing loss and tinnitus. These are cochlear symptoms.***
- ***The first nerve involved is V^{th} nerve.***
- ***When V^{th} nerve gets involved, the tumor size is more 2.5 cm.***
- ***Involvement of Vth nerve causes loss of corneal reflex***
- ***Next nerve to get involved is the VIIth nerve***
- ***VIIth nerve involvement may cause Hiztelberger's sign.***

5. **d. Acoustic neuroma**

Retrocochlear hearing loss is caused by diseases affecting the neural pathway of hearing ie diseases beyond the cochlea.

The only disease in the above choices that is in the neural pathway and hence will cause retrocochlear hearing loss is acoustic neuroma.

Rest of the mentioned diseases will cause cochlear hearing loss.

6. **a. Acoustic neuroma**

The common tumours in the cerbellopontine angle are:

- *Acoustic neuroma-most common*
- *Meningioma-second most common*
- *Congenital cholesteatoma*

Acoustic neuroma which is most common tumour in CP angle, arises from vestibular nerve.

7. **b. Acoustic neuroma**

Acoustic neuroma most commonly arises from the superior vestibular nerve but may involve other cranial nerves especially V^{th} and VIIth nerves.

When the VIIth cranial nerve is involved; the sensory fibres are the first to be affected.

Auricular branch of VII th cranial supplies a part of canal wall. Hence in acoustic neuroma, when VII nerve gets involved there is loss of sensation in external auditory canal.

This sign is called Histelberger sign.

8. **c. There is sensorineural deafness**
Vestibular neuronitis is a viral disease which is usually seen in adult males.
It is usually seen 2-3 weeks after a viral upper respiratory tract infection.
It is characterised by vestibular symptom and the ***cochlear symptoms are significantly absent***.
Hence vertigo and nystagmus are present whereas hearing loss is absent.
Caloric responses are diminished.
It is a self limiting disease.

INTERESTING FACT

Vestibular neuronitis is a vestibular nerve disease where cochlear symptoms are absent

Vestibular schwannoma is vestibular nerve disease where cochlear symptoms (hearing loss and tinnitus) are first to appear.

9. c. Acoustic neuroma
Hearing loss can be of the following types:
1. Conductive, which is caused by diseases in the middle and/or external ear
2. Sensory/cochlear, which is caused by diseases in the cochlea and

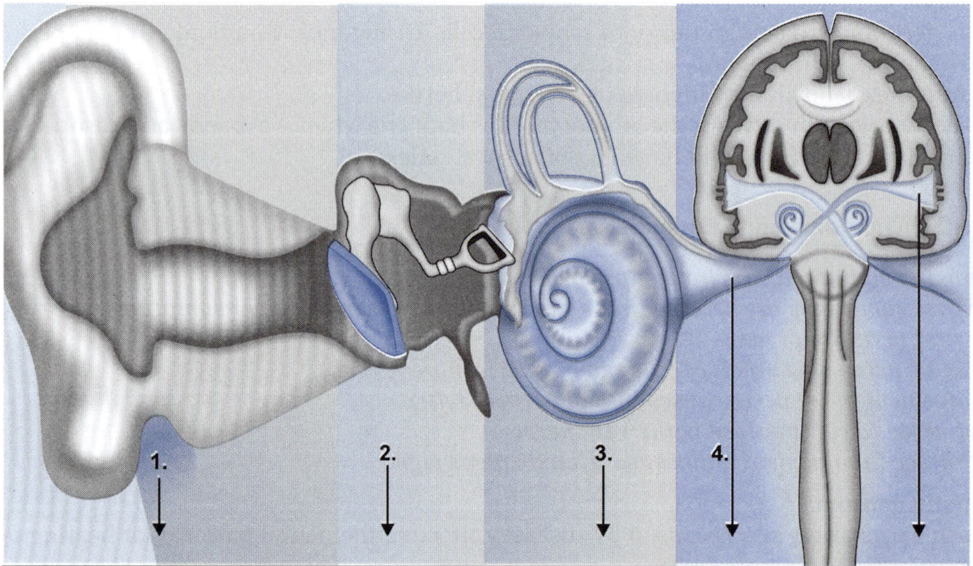

External ear Disease here causes CHL	Middle ear Disease here causes CHL	Inner ear Disease here causes SNHL	Neural ear Disease here causes SNHL	Central auditory part Dieases here causes SNHL
Riennes: BC>AC Weber's lateralizes to same side Audiometry: A-B gap >10-15 dB Otoscopy will show the pathology	Riennes: BC>AC Weber's lateralizes to same side Audiometry: A-B gap > 10 -15 dB **Tympanometry** will clinch the diagnosis Stapedial reflex may be helpful Scan like CT Scan/ MRI may be required	Rienne's: AC>BC Weber's lateraliz to opposite site Audiometry: A-B gap <10-15 dB Recruitment + SISI + Stapedial reflex: present BERA is normal **OAE** is affected **Cochlear microphonics** is affected caloric test may have positive findings	Rienne's: AC>BC Weber's lateralizes to opposite side Audiometry: A-B gap <10-15 dB Stapedial reflex: **Absent** Speech discrimination score is very low Roll over curve: seen **OAE** is normal **Cochlear microphonics:** normal BERA: **Increased latency between wave I & V** Caloric test may have positive findings MRI is helpful	Rienne's:AC>BC Weber's: lareralizes to opposite side Audiometry: A-B gap <10 dB Stapedial reflex: Absent BERA: normal latency CERA: **increased latency** Other central/ neurological features seen Caloric test may have positive findings MRI will clinch the diagnosis

3. Neural/ retrocochlear, which is caused by diseases in the neural pathway.
Acoustic neuroma is most commonly caused in the superior vestibular nerve at the cerebellopontine angle and hence will cause retrocochlear deafness.

10. **c. Medial geniculate nucleus**

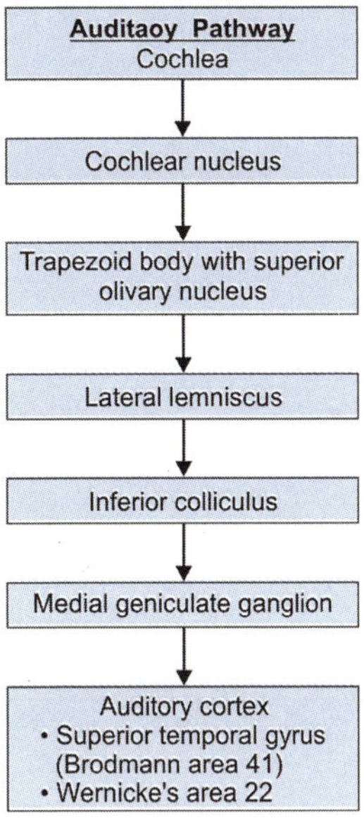

From this auditory pathway, we can see that medial geniculate ganglion is input of auditory input to the auditory cortex.

11. **a. B/L acoustic neuroma**
Both acoustic neuroma and neurofibromatosis type 2 have common genetic defect on chromosome 22q.
Hence, the two may be associated with each other. Usually acoustic neuroma is unilateral but in patient with NF2, it is bilateral.
Rest of the features given in the question are more common features of neurofibromatosis type 1.

12. **a. Sensorineural hearing loss**
- Earliest symptom of acoustic neuroma is a cochlear symptom i.e sensorineural hearing loss, despite the fact that it is a tumour of vestibular nerve.
- Commonest presentation is ***loss of corneal reflex*** due to involvement of trigeminal nerve.
- Otorrhea can never happen due to acoustic neuroma. It is a feature of middle ear disease
- Tinnitus and vertigo may appear later in patient of acoustic neuroma.

13. **b. Gadolinium MRI**
This is gold standard investigation for acoustic neuroma.

14. **d. Brainstem implant**
- Acoustic neuroma is a tumor of the eight nerve.
- A patient had surgery for bilateral acoustic neuroma and had profound hearing loss. This clearly suggests that the eight nerve is damaged during the surgery and hence this patient has ***retrocochlear hearing loss.***
- The best option for retrocochlear hearing loss is ***brainstem implant.***

IMAGE BASED ANSWER

15. **d. All are true**
The picture shows Antoni A and Antoni B cells which is a finding of acoustic neuroma. A person with neurofibromatosis type 2 has almost 80% of having acoustic neuroma.
- Antoni A is highly cellular cells made of palidases of Schwann cell nucleus called ***Verocay bodies.***
- Antoni B is loosely organized with myxomatous and cystic changes.

CHAPTER 11

Hearing Loss—Additional Points You Should Know

Hearing loss could be

- Congenital or genetic, and
- Acquired

Given below are the causes of hearing loss:

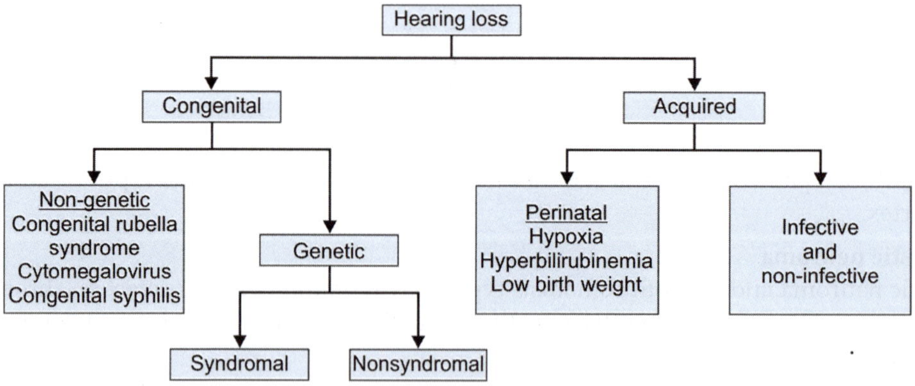

As already discussed in the previous chapters, the hearing pathway can be divided into several parts. Disease to any part will give rise to hearing loss.

These parts can be divided into the following:

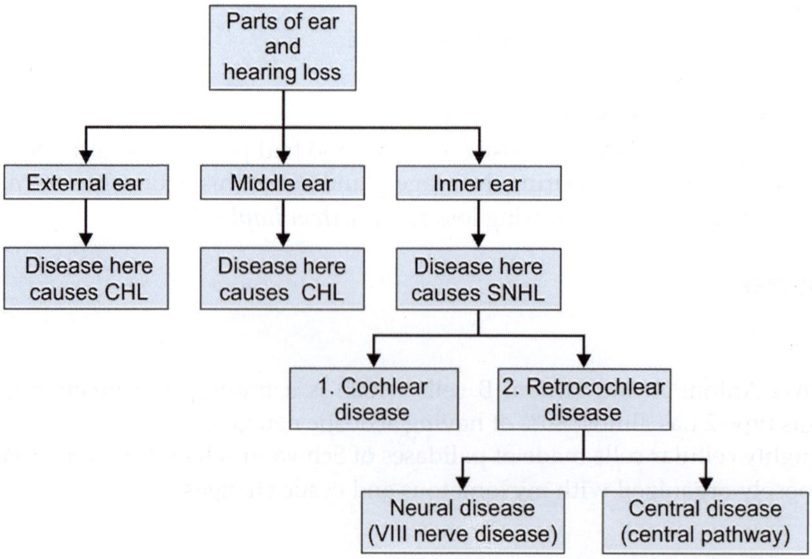

Conductive hearing loss (CHL)	This is caused by disease of 1. External ear 2. Tympanic membrane 3. Middle ear/ossicles
Sensorineural hearing loss (SNHL)	1. Cochlear disease affects inner ear. Their pathology can be three: – Morphogenetic–abnormal development – Cochleosaccular—abnormality in stria vascularis and ionic balance in endolymph – Neuroepithelial—defect in organ of Corti and transduction in hair cells 2. Retrocochlear diseases affect VIIIth nerve and its central pathway

Genetic hearing loss/deafness can be further divided into two types:

1. Genetic syndromal deafness	• *These are less common* • *Usually associated with other features of the syndrome* • *Usually has SNHL*
2. Genetic non-syndromal deafness	• These are more common types • No other symptom • Usually has SNHL, but sometimes can have CHL or mixed loss depending on the syndrome • Divided into three types: 1. Autosomal dominant (DFNA) 2. Autosomal recessive (DFNB) 3. X-linked forms (DFN)

Most of the diseases/conditions leading to the various types of hearing loss are already discussed.
We are now going to discuss the important causes (of hearing loss) from the remaining.

Inner Ear Developmental Anomalies/Aplasia

There are main such conditions. Few important ones are given below.

- **Michel Aplasia**
  The bony and membranous labyrinth is completely absent. In other words, the inner ear fails to develop.
  Therefore, cochlear implant is **NOT** possible in this.
- **Mondini's dysplasia**
  The cochlea has only 1.5 turns instead of 2.5 turns.
  The basal coil is present and the apex part is absent
- **Alexander's dysplasia**
  This is reverse of Mondini's dysplasia.
  In this, the apex is present and the base is absent.
- **Scheibe's dysplasia**
  Only the membranous part of saccule and cochlea are present. Rest of the labyrinth is absent.
  It is also called *cochleosaccular dysplasia.*

FEW IMPORTANT SYNDROMES WITH HEARING LOSS

There are many syndromes having hearing loss. Given below are few important ones.

1. Syndromes causing CHL	2. Syndromes causing SNHL	3. Syndromes causing mixed loss
• Treacher Collins syndrome • Apert's syndrome • Down's syndrome • Pierre Robin syndrome • van der Hoeve syndrome	• Waardenburg's syndrome • Pendred syndrome • Usher syndrome	• Klippel-Feil syndrome • Crouzon syndrome

PRESBYCUSSIS/AGE RELATED HEARING LOSS

This is hearing loss in elderly people.

The hearing loss is usually the **sensorineural type**.

It may be associated with tinnitus.

The hearing loss affects mainly the higher frequency.

Therefore, upward sloping audiogram will be seen.

Depending on the histopathology of these patients, it can be divided into the following:

- ***Sensory type***
  There is loss of hair cells
- ***Neural type***
  In this neurons are degenerated
  This is the **most commom type.**
  Therefore, ***speech discrimination score is very low*** *in these patients*
- ***Metabolic type***
  There is atrophy of the stria vascularis
- ***Mechanical type***
  There is stiffness of the basilar membrane in the cochlea.
- ***Mixed type***
  This one has mixed pathology

Best treatment is hearing aid in both the ears.

NOISE INDUCED HEARING LOSS (NIHL)

Noise induced hearing loss is hearing loss caused either,

1. Single but loud exposure to sound like burst of a cracker near the ear
   This is referred to as ***acoustic trauma***, or
2. Long-term exposure to sound usually seen in patients working in factories.

It is **more common in male.**

Noise induced hearing loss effects mainly the higher frequencies.

The frequency effected most is around 4000 Hz. Similar situation is seen in acoustic neuroma.

Therefore, both these conditions may have ***dip at 4000 Hz in audiogram.***

Conditions which affect mainly the higher frequencies.
In these conditions "downward sloping" audiogram will be seen. (Meniere's has upward sloping audiogram)

- Vestibular schwannoma
- Presbycussis
- Noise induced hearing loss

Note: in addition to downward sloping audiogram, there may be dip at 4000 Hz in the first two.
Otosclerosis has dip at 2000 Hz. It is called "Carhart's notch".

The following could be the causes of noise induced hearing loss.

- Excessive release of **glutamate** in the inner hair cells
- There could be **apoptosis and necrosis** of the outer hair cell.

OTOTOXICITY/DRUG INDUCED HEARING LOSS

There are lots of drugs that can cause ototoxicity. Different books will give different list.

Here is a list of the most important ototoxic drugs.

Common ototoxic drugs	Examples
• Aminoglycosides	Gentamicin Amikacin
• Diuretics	Furosemide Ethacrynic acid
• Analgesics/antipyretics	Aspirin
• Antimalarial	Quinine
• Polypeptide antibiotics	Vancomycin
• Macrolide antibiotics	Erythromycin
• Anti-neoplastics	Cisplatin
• Industrial solvents	Toluene

AMINOGLYCOSIDES

Aminoglycosides are the most popular ototoxic drugs.

This property is also used to treat Meniere's disease as has been discussed already.

In **intratympanic gentamicin,** gentamicin is instilled in th inner ear through the round window of the middle ear. This is done to protect the cochlea and other systemic side effects like nephrotoxicity.

Their main targets of aminoglycosides are the **neuroepithelium of the labyrinth, like**

- Outer hair cells (OHC). This is because OHC are more sensitive than inner hair cell.
- Type I vestibular hair cells
- Crista ampulli

Mechanism of action of aminoglycosides

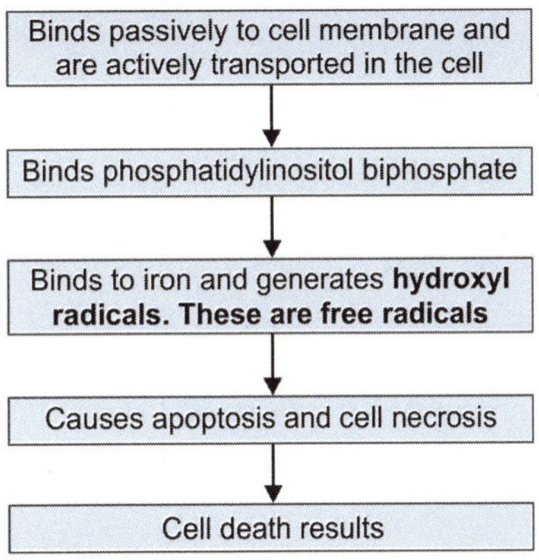

AUDITORY PROCESSING DISORDERS (APD)

This is also called central auditory processing disorder (CAPD).

In this battery of conditions, the external ear, middle ear and the inner ear are normal.

However, patient is unable to process and interpret the sound information which he/she hears.

There are many diseases under this.

One important condition is:

King-Kopetzky Syndrome

King-Kopetzky syndrome is also called **dyslexia of hearing.**

In this, patient is unable to hear properly when there is background noise.

In typical hearing dyslexia, patient can hear the sound but is unable to interpret the sound.

Last minute revision

- *Scheibe's dysplasia is the most common type of dysplasia*
- *Michel's aplasia has complete absence of inner ear*
- *Nonsyndromal congenital hearing loss is caused by viruses like mumps, measles, CMV etc*
- *presbycussis is senile deafness*
- *presbycussis causes sensorineural hearing loss. Weber's test will lateralize to opposite side*
- *Most important ototoxic drugs are the aminoglycosides*
- *They act by binding to phosphatidylinositol and forming free radical and causing cell death by apoptosis.*

QUESTIONS

1. **Conductive hearing loss is seen in all *except:***
   a. CSOM
   b. ASOM
   c. Middle ear effusion
   d. Presbycussis
2. **Which of the following conditions causes the maximum hearing loss:**
   a. Ossicular disruption with intact tympanic membrane
   b. Disruption of malleus and incus as well tympanic membrane
   c. Partial fixation of the stapes footplate
   d. Ottitis media with effusion
3. **Sensorineural deafness may be feature of all, *except*:**
   a. Nail-patella syndrome
   b. Distal renal tubular acidosis
   c. Bartter syndrome
   d. Alport syndrome
4. **Noise induced hearing loss shows dip characteristically at:**
   a. 1000 Hz
   b. 2000 Hz
   c. 3000 Hz
   d. 4000 Hz
5. **Waardenburg's syndrome is characterized by all *except*:**
   a. Heterochromatic iritis
   b. White-forelock
   c. Sensorineural hearing loss
   d. Glomerulonephritis
6. **Hearing loss NOT caused by which of these drugs:**
   a. Kanamycin
   b. Vancomycin
   c. Metronidazole
   d. Quinine
7. **After rupture of tympanic membrane the hearing loss is:**
   a. 10-40 dB
   b. 20 dB
   c. 5-15 dB
   d. 300 dB
8. **Virus causing acute onset sensorineural hearing loss is:**
   a. Corona virus
   b. Adeno virus
   c. Mumps virus
   d. Rota virus
9. **Auditory neurotherapy is an effective modality of treatment for which of the following abnormality of hearing:**
   a. CSOM
   b. Meniere's disease
   c. Malignant otitis externa
   d. Central auditory processing disorder
10. **Dip at 4000 Hz is seen in:**
    a. Otosclerosis
    b. Noise trauma
    c. Meniere's disease
    d. Presbycussis
11. **A patient with kidney disease was repeatedly given high dose of frusemide. After 1 week, this patient started complaining of decreased hearing. All are true about this drug *except*:**
    a. It acts on the cochlea
    b. It acts on inner hair cells
    c. It acts on outer hair cells
    d. It acts on stria vascularis
12. **For drugs causing deafness, true statement is:**
    a. Kanamycin is predominantly vestibulotoxic
    b. Frusemide causes irreversible deafness
    c. Salicylate causes irreversible deafness
    d. Cisplatin causes irreversible deafness

ANSWERS AND EXPLANATIONS

1. **d. Presbycussis**
   Presbycussis is senile hearing loss or hearing loss due to old age. This is due to problems of cochlea or the VIIIth nerve and hence the hearing loss is always sensorineural. Rest of the diseases given in choices are middle ear disease and will cause conductive hearing loss.

Common Diseases Causing Conductive Hearing Loss Are:

1. Wax
2. Tympanic membrane perforation
3. ASOM
4. SOM
5. CSOM

6. Otosclerosis
7. Glomus tumour etc.

Important Diseases Causing Sensorineural Hearing Loss Are:

1. Cochlear otosclerosis
2. Meniere's disease
3. Vestibular schwannoma
4. Presbycussis etc.

2. **a. Ossicular disruption with intact tympanic membrane**
Ossicular disruption with intact tympanic membrane will cause about 54 dB hearing loss.
The only other condition that can cause more than this conductive hearing loss is complete closure of oval window (this causes about 60 dB hearing loss).

3. **d. Alport syndrome**
Nail patella syndrome is an autosomal dominant disease there is dorsal limb structure deformity, nephropathy and glaucoma. SN loss is not a feature of it but has been lately added by some.
Distal renal tubular acidosis is inability to remove acid from the renal tubules. Acidosis resulting from it may very rarely cause SN loss, but this hearing loss is not a part of the disease.
Bartter syndrome is a closely related set of disorders. There are few such related disorders.
It is a disease of kidney tubules resulting in increased aldosterone and reduced serum potassium.
One of the subtypes may have SN loss.
Alport's syndrome is the only one where SN loss is a feature. In this there is loss of kidney function with SN loss.
Hence, the only acceptable answer can be distal renal tubular acidosis.
- I feel there is a mistake in the question. The question should have been, which of the following has SNHL. In that case the answer would have been ***Alport's syndrome.***

4. **d. 4000 Hz**
Noise induced hearing loss (NIHL) is dependent on the intensity and frequency of exposed noise or sound. It is more common when the frequency of exposed noise is between 2000 to
3000 Hz and it increases with the increase in the intensity of noise or sound one is exposed to.
Audiometry typically shows a dip at 4000 Hz. This is also called **"acoustic dip"**

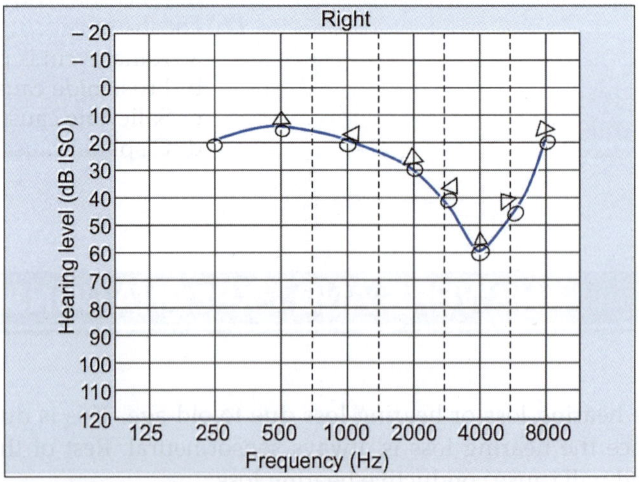

Audiogram of noise induced hearing loss showing dip at 4000 Hz.

There are two more common situations where similar dips are seen. They are:
1. Acoustic neuroma—where a dip is seen at 4000 Hz as in case of NIHL
2. Otosclerosis—where a dip is seen at 2000 Hz and is called ***Carhart's notch.***

5. **d. Glomerulonephritis**
Waardenburg's syndrome is an autosomal dominant disease which have comprises of the following:
- Bilateral sensorineural hearing loss

- Pigmentary anomalies like heterochromatic iritis, white forelock, vitiligo, premature graying etc. and
- Craniofacial features like dystopia canthorum, broad nasal root etc.

It is one of an important syndromal causes of sensorineural hearing loss.
Glomerulonephritis is NOT a feature of Waardenburg's syndrome.

FEW IMPORTANT SYNDROMES WITH HEARING LOSS

1. Syndromes causing CHL	2. Syndromes causing SNHL	3. Syndromes causing mixed loss
• Treacher Collois syndrome • Apert's syndrome • Alport's syndrome • Down's syndrome • Pierre Robin syndrome • van der Hoeve's syndrome	• Waardenberg's syndrome • Pendred syndrome • Usher syndrome	• Klippel Feil syndrome • Crouzon's syndrome

6. **c. Metronidazole**
Here is a list of the most important ototoxic drugs.

Common ototoxic drugs	Examples
• Aminoglycosides	Gentamicin Amikacin
• Diuretics	Furosemide Ethacrynic acid
• Analgesics/antipyretics	Aspirin
• Antimalarial	Quinine
• Polypeptide antibiotics	Vancomycin
• Macrolide antibiotics	Erythromycin
• Anti-neoplastics	Cisplatin
• Industrial solvents	Toluene

From the above mentioned list we understand that metronidazole is NOT ototoxic and therefore will not cause hearing loss.

7. **a. 10-40 dB**
We all know that the tympanic membrane is a very important structure that contributes to hearing. Therefore, perforation of this membrane will lead to hearing loss. The amount of hearing loss caused by tympanic membrane depends on the size of perforation.
Small perforation will cause less hearing loss and large perforation will cause more hearing loss. The range varies from 10-40 dB. Average loss is 38 dB.

8. **c. Mumps virus**
Causes of hearing loss

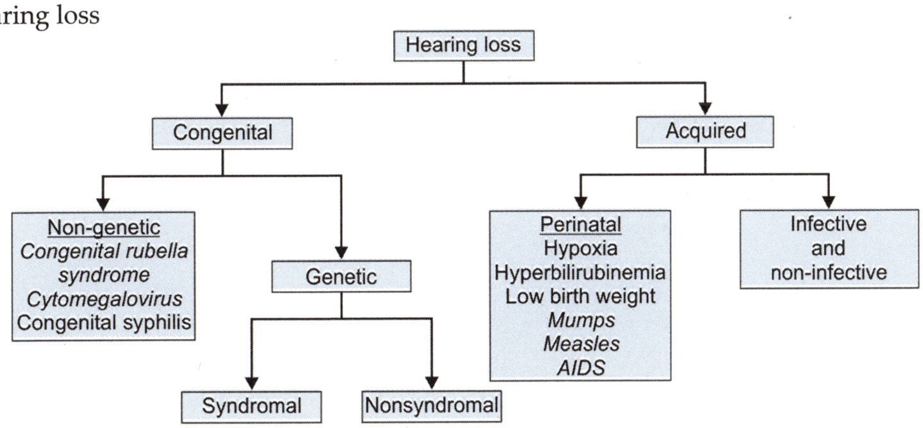

If we look at the ***nonsyndromal non gentic causes of congenital hearing loss***, viruses are some of the major causes of hearing loss.
Same is true of ***perinatal acquired causes*** of hearing loss.

PART 1: EAR

Therefore some of the important virues that can cause hearing oss are:
- Rubella/Measles
- Mumps
- AIDS
- Cytomegalo virus

9. **d. Central auditory processing disorder**
Neurotherapy is a type of treatment modality in which the central neural system is stimulated in oreder to activate it.
It is usually done for central problems.
Auditory neurotherapy is used for central disease of the auditory system.
In the above given choices central auditory processing disorder is the only disease of central origin and there is the correct answer.

10. **b. Noise trauma**
Read explanation in question no. 4

11. **d. It acts on stria vascularis**
The primary action of frusemide is that it causes oedema of stria vascularis and this inturn changes the endolymphatic potential.

Mechanism of frusemide causing hearing loss

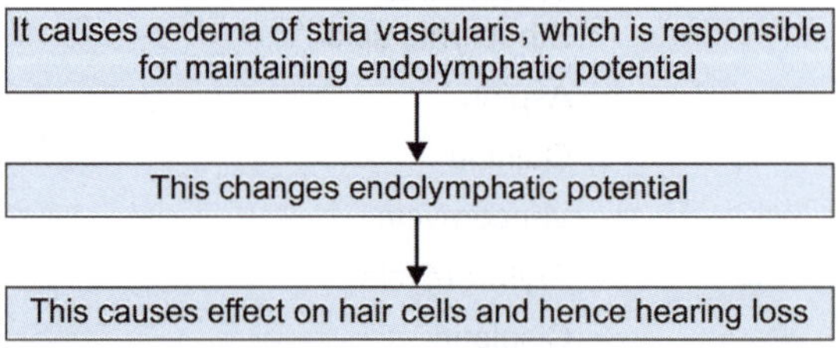

12. **d. Cisplatin causes irreversible deafness**
Most of the aminoglycosides including kanamyin are equally cochleotoxic as well as vestibulotoxic
Drugs like ***loop dieurtics (frusemide), salicylates and erythromycin*** cause **reversible deafness.**
Drugs like ***aminoglycosides, cisplatin and quinine*** causes **irreversible deafness.**

CHAPTER

12 Assistive Devices of Hearing

As we all understand, hearing is the primary function of the ear. Any abnormality of the ear is bound to lead to hearing loss. We treat the abnormalities on its merit. The treatment modality involves various options including different type of surgeries.

In some cases, despite all efforts, the hearing fails to improve. In such patients we have to use one of the hearing devices. Given are few such devices.

HEARING AID

Hearing aid is a device that amplifies sound (same function as middle ear).

It has three parts. They are:

1. Microphone- that picks up sound
2. Amplifier- that amplifies the sound, and
3. Receiver- that finally sends sound in the form of vibrating energy.

Hearing aids come in different models like

- ITE : in the ear
- BTE: behind the ear
- ITC: in the canal
- CIC: completely in canal.

These names are self explanatory.

In patients with bilateral hearing loss, we have option of either unilateral hearing aid or bilateral hearing aid.

These are the advantages of **bilateral hearing over unilateral hearing aid:**

- **It increases range of sound level**
- **Horizontal localization is possible**
- **Has better speech to noise ratio. Patient hears speech better than noise. This property is called *binaural squelch***
- **Suppresses tinnitus and improves sound quality.**

SOME SPECIAL TYPES OF THE HEARING AIDS

BAHA also called ***bone anchoring hearing aid***.

As the name suggests, it is anchored on to the mastoid bone and transmits sound through *bony conduction.*

- **BAHA** has three components:
  1. ***Screw***
  2. ***Abutment***
  3. ***Sound vibrator***
- Some important indications of BAHA are:
  1. External canal damaged beyond repair and
  2. Small child requiring hearing aid

CROS also called ***contralateral routing of signals.***

This is mainly used when the patient has ***unilateral severe hearing loss***.

The most important advantage of CROS is that it gives ***good localization of sound in a patient with unilateral hearing loss.***

ACTIVE MIDDLE EAR IMPLANTS (AMEI)

Active middle ear implants are devices that are implanted inside the middle ear.
They can either be total implantable device or partial implantable device.

Total Implantable Hearing Device

Total implantable hearing device is a type of **middle ear implants.**

In this the implant is attached to the ossicular chain (incus) and the transmission of amplified sound is achieved by what is called ***piezoelectric coupling.***

In simple words, the piezoelectric hearing device is placed between the *head of incus and the head/capitulum of stapes.* The vibration of tympanic membrane and incus is converted into electric energy by this device and is amplified. The amplified sound is converted back to vibrating energy and is transmitted onto the capitulum of stapes. From here it travels to the brain through the normal auditory pathway.

The main advantages of piezoelectric hearing device are:

1. It uses the **natural acoustics** of the external ear, and
2. No cosmetic problem as the implant is beneath the skin.

COCHLEAR IMPLANT

Cochlear implant is a device which is mainly used for **cochlear hearing loss.**

It is usually used when the patient has ***bilateral profound hearing loss with functional VIIIth nerve.***

This device converts vibrating energy into electric energy which then stimulates the ***spiral ganglionic cells of the VIII Nerve.***

For the cochlear implant to function the ***neural pathway has to be intact (there should be NO retrocochlear disease).***

It has five components:

1. **Microphone** – to pick up the sound
2. **Speech processor** – it converts sound energy into electrical energy.
3. **Transmitter** – it transmits this electrical energy onto the receiver which is fitted beneath the skin.
4. **Receiver** – this is fitted beneath the skin and it receives the sound from transmitter and then sends it to the electrodes.
5. **Electrodes/Stimulator** – ***Electrode is the ONLY part of cochlear implant that is inserted inside the cochlea. It is inserted in the scala tympani of the cochlea where it stimulates the VIII nerve.***

Important points to note are:

- It does not have an amplifier like the hearing aid. Instead, it has a speech processor.
- The electrodes have to be inserted into the **scala tympani** of cochlea
- The electrodes pass through the **round window of middle ear.**

Cochlear implant can be inserted into the ear through two routes. They are:

1. Transmastoid, and
2. Middle cranial fossa approach

The more commonly used approach is the transmastoid approach. During this approach, three surgical openings have to be made.

Middle cranial fossa approach is used in cases of CSOM.

1. In mastoid antrum (***cortical mastoidectomy***)
2. In the facial recess on the posterior wall of middle ear (***posterior tympanotomy***)
3. On the anterior lip of round window (***Cochleostomy***).

Most common complication of cochlear implant is **infection of the skin flap.**

The most serious complication is **meningitis caused by *pneumococcus.***

In order to prevent meningitis, patients are vaccinated before the surgery.

BRAINSTEM IMPLANTS

As we have already discussed, the hearing pathway passess through the brainstem.

When this neural pathway or VIIIth nerve (**retrocochlear disease)** is damaged then brainstem implant is the best option.

The implant is placed directly into the brainstem in the ***lateral recess of fourth ventricle.***
Brainstem implant stimulates the ***cochlear nucleus in the pons*** therefore bypasses the VIIIth nerve.

Last minute revision

- *BAHA is bone anchored hearing aid which is used when air conduction cannot be used*
- *CROS is contralateral routing of signals. It is used in unilateral severe hearing loss*
- *Cochlear implant is the best option for profound hearing loss*
- *The electrodes are implanted inside the scala tympani through the round window*
- *For cochlear implant, there should be no retrocochlear disease (VIIIth nerve should be normal)*
- *It stimulates the spiral ganglion of the eight nerve*
- *For retrocochlear diseases, brainstem implants are used.*

QUESTIONS

1. Cochlear implant electrodes are placed at:
 a. Horizontal semicircular canal
 b. Round window
 c. Oval window
 d. Promontory

2. Regarding cochlear implant which of the following is true?
 a. Not contraindicated in cochlear malformation
 b. Contraindicated in < 5 years
 c. Indicated in mild to moderate hearing loss
 d. Implanted through oval window

3. Father of neuro-otology:
 a. Julius Lempert b. John J Shea Jr
 c. William House d. Hayes Martin

4. Cochlear implant is to be done if following is intact?
 a. Outer hair cell b. Inner hair cell
 c. Spiral ganglion cell d. Auditory nerve

5. Cochlear implant:
 a. Stimulate the remaining functional inner hair cells
 b. Today are fully implantable
 c. Are usually indicated in all adult with profound deafness
 d. Give substantial benefit to postlingually deaf adult who usually do not need a long rehabilitation.

6. In a child with hearing aid, the stimulus occurs in the following:
 a. Inner hair cell
 b. Outer hair cell
 c. Cochlear nerve
 d. Spiral ganglion

7. Which is true of hearing aid:
 a. Amplify sound and depend on spiral ganglion cells to stimulate the auditory nerve
 b. Useful in all cases of profound hearing loss
 c. In young profound hearing loss, should be tried for at leasr 6 months.
 d. Should not try in cases where aided threshold exceed 90 db and patient should be referred for cochlear implant.

8. A patient had surgery for bilateral acoustic schwannoma. Following this surgery this patient had bilateral profound hearing loss. Best rehabilitation for this patient would be:
 a. Bilateral high powered digital hearing aid
 b. Bilateral cochlear implant
 c. Brainstem implant
 d. None of the above

9. Which part of the cochlear implant is implanted during the surgery:
 a. Receiver-stimulator b. Transmitting coil
 c. Microphone d. Speech processor

10. A two-year-old child was planned for brainstem implant. All are indications for brainstem implant *except:*
 a. B/L neurofibromatosis
 b. Absent auditory nerve
 c. Absent cochlea
 d. Mondini's deformity

11. During brainstem implant, where is the brainstem implant implanted?
 a. Lateral recess of the 4th ventricle
 b. Floor of 2nd ventricle
 c. CP angle
 d. None of the above

IMAGE BASED QUESTION

12. From the two figures given, which of these is true?

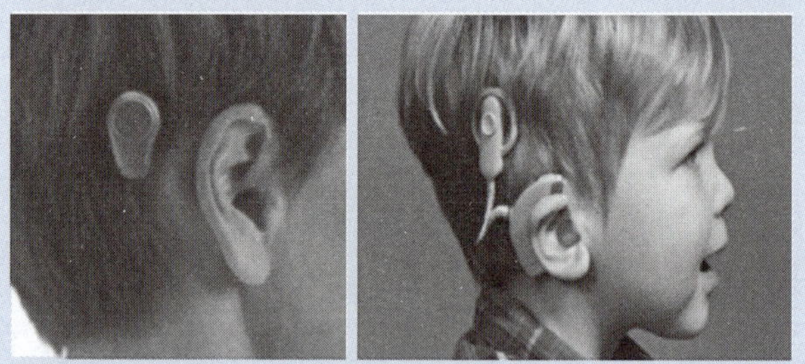

Fig. 1 Fig. 2

 a. Fig. 1 is bone anchored hearing aid and Fig. 2 is cochlear implant
 b. Fig. 2 is bone anchored hearing aid and Fig. 1 is cochlear implant
 c. Both are cochlear implants
 d. Both are bone anchored hearing aid

ANSWERS AND EXPLANATIONS

1. **b. Round window**
The cochlear implant electrodes have to be passed into the scala tympani of the cochlea so as to be closed to the VIII nerve in the cochlea. In order to achieve this, the electrodes should be passed through round window. When electrodes are passed through round window they get inserted into scala tympani.

During the surgery of cochlear implant, three openings are to be made before the electrodes can finally be passed into the cochlea.

Openings created for cochlear implant
1. Mastoid antrum. Cortical mastoidectomy is done
2. Posterior tympanotomy/ facial recess is done
3. Opening is created near the round window

SURGERIES/PROCEDURES WHERE ROUND WINDOW IS USED

- ***Cochlear implant***
- ***Intratympanic gentamicin. A procedure done for Meniere's disease***
- ***Type VI tympanoplasty. The graph is placed over the round window.***

2. **a. Not contraindicated in cochlear malformation**

A cochlear implant is a surgically implanted electronic device that provides a sense of sound to a person who is profoundly deaf or severely hard of hearing. The cochlear implant is often referred to as a **bionic ear.**

- Cochlear implant can be done in patients with certain types of malformations but the number of electrodes which will be inserted is reduced.
- It is not contraindicated in < 5 years patients. In fact, it has been successfully done in patients of 6 month of age.
- Indicated in severe/profound hearing loss. Mild to moderate will respond to hearing aid.
- It is implanted through ROUND window.
- The presence of auditory nerve fibers is essential to the functioning of the device: if these are damaged to such an extent that they cannot receive electrical stimuli, the implant will not work.
- In such a case, brainstem implant is preferred.

Three distinct groups of potential users of cochlear implants with different needs and outcomes.

1. Post-lingually deaf adults
2. Pre-lingually deaf children
3. Post-lingually impaired people (usually children) who have lost hearing due to diseases such as meningitis.

3. **c. William House**

William House has two pioneering work to his credit.

1. He is called ***father of neuro-otology*** because he began surgery for acoustic neuroma and other skull base diseases.
2. He pioneered the cochlear implant and is called ***father of cochlear implant.***

4. **d. Auditory nerve**

Cochlear implant, as the name suggests, is a hearing device that is implanted into the cochlea. The part of the that is implanted into the cochlea are the electrodes. The electrodes are inserted into the scala tympani of the cochlea.

From the scala tympani of the cochlea, the sound from these electrodes has to reach the auditory cortex, where they are perceived. This transmission is done by the auditory nerve.

At least 10% of scala ganglionic cell are also needed for successful hearing from cochlear implant.

5. **d. Give substantial benefit to postlingually deaf adult who usually do not need a long rehabilitation.**

- Cochlear implants stimulate the spiral ganglion cell in the auditory nerve and NOT the hair cells (diagram is shown in the next question).
- Total implantable hearing aids are in the research stage. There are not available in the market yet.
- They are indicated in ***profound hearing loss due to cochlear diseases. They cannot be used in retrocochlear hearing loss.***
- ***Postlingual deaf will always have better outcome and will require less rehabilitation.***

6. **a. Inner hair cell**

Diagram Showing Different Type of Hearing Device Acting at Different Sites of the Hearing Pathway

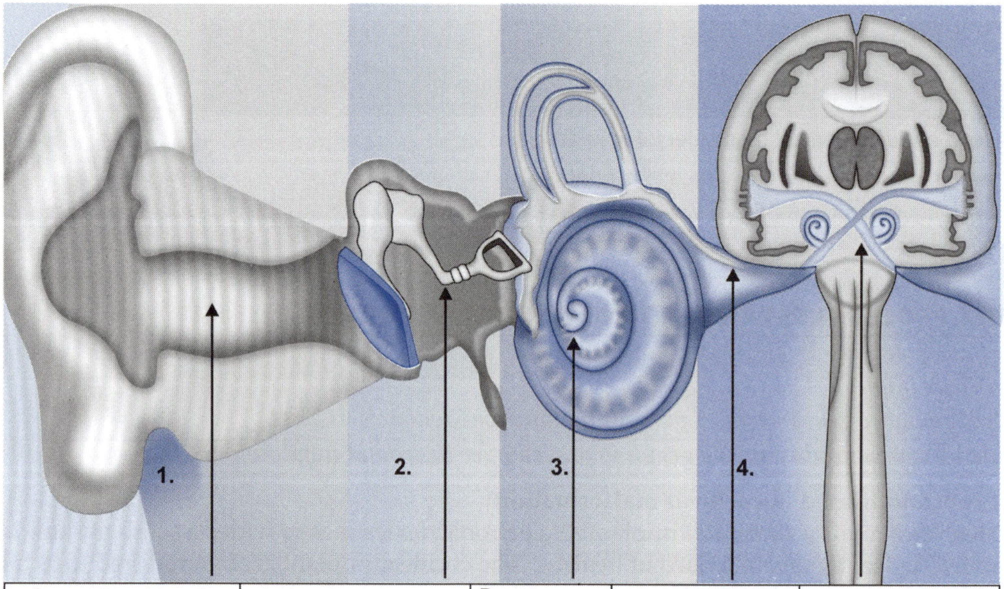

Conventional hearing aid acts here. It uses the entire hearing pathway	Active middle ear implant (AMEI) like ***vibrant soundbridge act on ossicles in middle ear.*** It bypasses external ear.	Bone anchored hearing aid (BAHA) stimulates ***hair cell in the cochlea***. It bypasses external and middle ear.	Cochlear implant stimulates the ***spiral ganglion and VIIIth nerve.*** It bypasses the cochlea	Brainstem implant stimulates the cochlear nucleus. It bypasses the cochlea and VIIIth nerve.

HIGHLIGHTS

- In children a special hearing aid called bone anchored hearing aid (BAHA) is used. It stimulates the inner hair cell in the cochlea
- Active middle ear implants (AMEI) like ***vibrant soundbridge*** acts at ossicle level.
- Cochlear implants stimulate the spiral ganglionic cell in the VIIIth nerve.
- Brainstem implants stimulate the cochlear nucleus in the brainstem (Pons).

7. **d. Should not try in cases where aided threshold exceed 90 db and patient should be referred for cochlear implant.**

Hearing aid is a device which assists in hearing in a person who has impairment of hearing.
It simply amplifies the sound and uses the entire hearing pathway to transmit this amplified sound to the hearing part of the brain. It does not depend on spiral ganglion cells.
It should NOT be used in a patient having profound hearing loss (hearing loss more than 90 dB). In such a patient, cochlear implant should be considered.

Different hearing devices and their indications		
Degree of hearing loss (threshold)	**In adult**	**In children**
Mild loss (26-40 dB)	Convential hearing aid	Bone anchored hearing aid (BAHA)
Moderate till severe loss (41-90 dB)	• Hearing aid • Active middle ear implants	BAHA
Profound loss (>91 dB)	Cochlear implant	Cochlear implant

8. **c. Brainstem implant**
Acoustic neuroma is a tumour of the eighth nerve.
A patient had surgery for bilateral acoustic neuroma and had profound hearing loss. This clearly suggests that the eighth nerve is damaged during the surgery and hence this patient has ***retrocochlear hearing loss.***
The best option for retrocochlear hearing loss is ***brainstem implant.***

9. **a. Receiver-stimulator**
Cochlear implant has five parts which are divided into 2 parts:
External device, and
Internal device

External device	Internal device
• Microphone. Picks up the sound • Speech processor. Converts sound energy into electrical energy. • Transmitter. Transmits this electrical energy onto the receiver which is fitted beneath the skin.	• Receiver. Fitted beneath the skin receives the sound from transmitter and then sends it to the electrodes. • Electrodes/Stimulator. ***Electrode is the ONLY part of cochlear implant that is inserted inside the cochlea. It is inserted in the scala tympani of the cochlea where it stimulates the VIIIth nerve.***

Therefore, receiver-stimulator is implanted.
- Receiver is implanted beneath the skin.
- Stimulator also called electrode is implanted in the ***scala tympani of the cochlea through an opening called COCHLEOSTOME.***

10. **d. Mondini's deformity**
Brainstem implant is indicated in retrocochlear diseases of absent of cochlea.
Mondini's deformity is deformity of cochlea and hence a cochlear disease. In such cases, cochlear implant is a better option.

11. **a. Lateral recess of the 4th ventricle**
As the name suggests, it has to be implanted in the brainstem.
It is implanted in the lateral recess of the 4th ventricle.
And is indicated in retrocochlear diseases.

IMAGE BASED ANSWERS

12 **a. Fig. 1 is bone anchored hearing aid and Fig. 2 is cochlear implant**
In this first figure, the device is attached to the mastoid bone and there is NO implant seen going inside. This is bone anchored hearing aid (BAHA).
In the second figure, an implant can be seen going inside the ear which will finally be implanted inside the cochlea.

PART 2

Nose and Sinuses

CHAPTERS

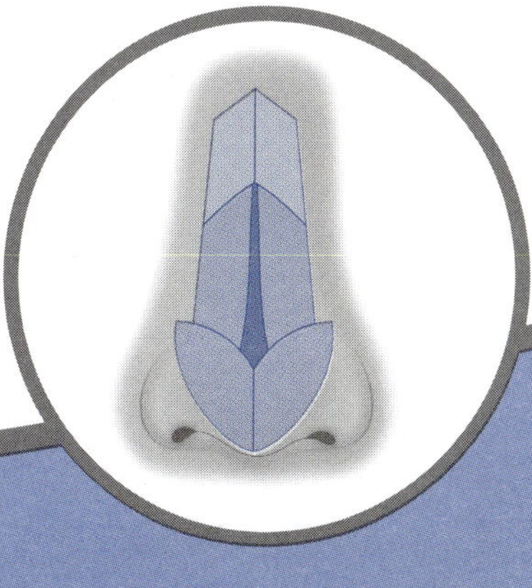

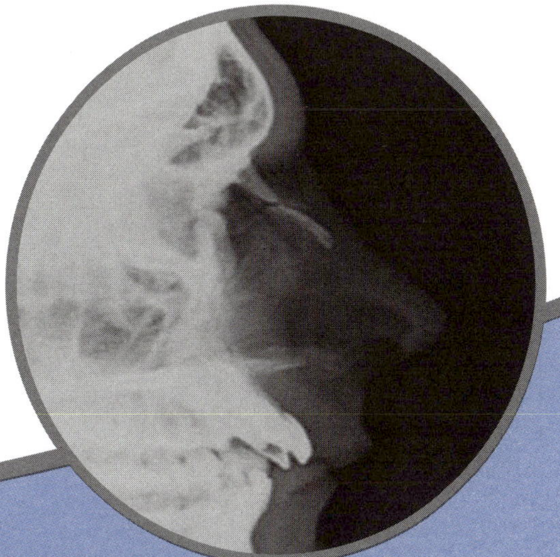

CHAPTER

13 Embryology and Congenital Anomalies of Nose and Sinuses

The first nasal structures are identifiable at 4 week embryo. The process off ossification of the nasal capsule comprises of both endochondral bone formation and membranous bone formations.

During the development of the nasal cavity; few projections appear on its lateral wall. These are:

- One maxilloturbinal
- Followed by five ethmoturbinals, and
- One nasoturbinal.

These turbinals/projections form the various structures.

Turbinals	Structures formed from them
Maxilloturbinal`	Inferior turbinate
1st ethmoturbinal	Middle turbinate
2nd ethmoturbinal	Superior turbinate
3rd ethmoturbinal	Supreme turbinate
4th and 5th ethmoturbinal	No structure
Nasoturbinal	Agger nasi

The middle meatus of the ethmoidal bone has five lamellae/basal lamellae for the attachment of various structures. The various basal lamellae and their attachments are given below:

Basal lamellae	Structure attached
1st basal lamella	Uncinate process
2nd basal lamella	Ethmoid bulla
3rd basal lamella	Middle turbinate
4th basal lamella	Superior turbinate
5th basal lamella	Supreme turbinate

NOTE: Inferior turbinate is NOT attached to the basal lamella because the inferior turbinate is NOT a part of ethmoidal bone. Rather, it is a separate bone, whereas basal lamellae are part of ethmoidal bone.

IMPORTANT POINTS ABOUT THE DEVELOPMENT OF SINUSES

The first sinus that starts to develop in the human embryo is maxillary sinus. It starts to develop at around 7-10 weeks of intrauterine life.

Maxillary Sinus

The maxillary sinus is the first sinus to appear (seven to ten weeks) as a shallow groove expanding from the primitive ethmoidal infundibulum into the mass of the maxilla. Absorption and expansion results.

This is a photo clicked from “Scot Brown ORL andHNS” VIIth edition, page no 1318.

However, maxillary sinus, like most sinuses develop as an out pouching of the **ethmoidal infundibulum.**

The out pouching of the ethmoidal sinus is called *primary pneumaization.*

The last sinus to develop in a human embryo is the **frontal sinus.**

Frontal sinus starts to develop at around **4 months intrauterine life.** It is also the last sinus that completes its development.

Frontal sinuses are **NOT** seen of radiographs in the early human life:

- In a C T scan – till one year
- In an X-ray- till **4-6 years of age**

For this reason, many books say that **frontal sinus is absent during birth** of a child and so starts development **post natally (**this is NOT entirely true).

The sphenoid sinus is different from other sinuses by the following facts:

- It does not develop as an outpouching of ethmoid on the lateral nasal wall.
- It does not have primary pneumatization.

IMPORTANT CONGENITAL ANOMALIES OF NOSE AND SINUSES

Fusion defect	Anomalies
Between maxillary process and premaxilla	Cleft lip
Between palatine process and nasal septum	Cleft palate
Persisting oronasal membrane/bucconasal membrane	Choanal atresia
Epithelial entrapment between maxilla and median nasal elevation	Nasolabial cyst
Entrapment between primitive palate and palatine process	Globulomaxillary cyst

CHOANAL ATRESIA

In the early stage of embryo; the posterior end of the nasal cavity is closed by a membrane. This membrane has various names

- **Oronasal membrane**
- **Bucconasal membrane**
- **Nasobuccal membrane**
- **Hochstetter's membrane/bucconasal membrane of Hochstetter.**

If this is not given in the choices; then **buccopharyngeal fascia is an acceptable answer.**

This membrane normally disappears at around **42–44 days of IUL.** In choanal atresia, this membrane fails to disappear/rupture;

Most common type of choanal atresia is mixed type (partly bony and partly membranous.

2nd most common type is bony. This is the second best answer if mixed is not given in the choices.

It is more common unilateral and in females.

Choanal Atresia

In this rare condition (incidence 1 in 7000 live births), there is complete obstruction of the posterior nasal openings on one or both sides. The blockage has been thought to be either bony or membranous in origin. In reality, a mixed picture is usually seen (70 percent of cases) with the remainder

Scotts Brown's. Page no. 1070

Causes

- Genetic defects
- Hyperthyroid mothers on ***methimazole/carbimazole*** *during pregnancy*
- CHARGE syndrome, etc.

Choanal atresia may be associated with **CHARGE SYNDROME.** This syndrome includes:

C- Coloboma
H- Heart defects
A- Atresia of choana

R- Retardation of growth
G- Genital and urinary anomalies
E- Ear anomalies

Unilateral condition may not cause serious problem.

As a result of this, there is a membrane between the nasal cavity and the nasopharynx.
Hence, the child is unable to breath through the nose.

Bilateral choanal atresia could be life threatening because newborn kids are obligate nasal breather.

Can be diagnosed by the following methods:

- Mucoid nasal discharge
- Absence of air bubbles in the nasal discharge
- Catheter cannot be passed from nose into nasopharynx
- The lateral view of X-ray nasopharynx will show discontinuation of air column of nasal cavity and the air column of the nasopharynx.
- Diagnostic nasal endoscopy will show the membrane.

Management

In case of emergency:

- Intubation
- **McGovern's technique**

Definitive Treatment

- Transpalatal/transnasal surgeries
- Endoscopic surgery (FESS)
- Microdebridement or KTP laser excision
- Use of Mitamicin C.

Is due to bucconasal membrane
Most common is mixed followed by bony and is unilateral
McGovern's technique may be life saving

NASOLABIAL CYST

The other name for this condition is **KLESTADT'S CYST**.

It is a cyst of **nasolacrimal duct and is** non-odontogenic cyst.

CT scan is useful and **surgical treatment** is usually required.

Last minute revision

- *Maxillary sinus is the first sinus to start the development*
- *Frontal sinus is the last to start development. It develops postnatally*
- *Choanal atresia is caused due to bucconasal membrane*
- *McGovern's technique is the life saving technique in this*
- *Nasolabial cyst is a cyst of nasolacrimal duct*

QUESTIONS

1. **Bulla-ethmoidalis is seen in:**
   a. Superior meatus
   b. Middle meatus
   c. Inferior meatus
   d. Sphenoethmoidal recess
2. **Choanal atresia is due to persistence of which of these:**
   a. Buccopharyngeal fascia
   b. Bucconasal membrane
   c. Pharyngobasilar fascia
   d. None of the above
3. **Which of the turbinals may form the agar nasi cell?**
   a. Maxilloturbinal
   b. First ethmoturbinal
   c. Second ethmoturbinal
   d. Nasoturbinal
4. **Sinus NOT present at birth:**
   a. Maxillary sinus b. Ethmoidal sinus
   c. Frontal sinus d. Sphenoidal sinus
5. **Which is the first sinus to start development in an embryo?**
   a. Maxillary sinus b. Ethmoidal sinus
   c. Frontal sinus d. Sphenoidal sinus
6. **All are pneumatization pattern of sphenoid sinus *except*:**
   a. Presellar b. Postsellar
   c. Concha bullosa d. Conchal
7. **Choanal atresia is associated with all *except*:**
   a. Colobomatous blindness
   b. Heart disorder
   c. Renal anomaly
   d. Ear disorder
   e. CNS lesion
8. **All are true of nasolabial cyst *except*:**
   a. They are bilateral
   b. Present in adult
   c. Is derived from odontogenic epithelium
   d. Has female predilection
9. **All of the following procedure is helpful in diagnosis of choanal atresia *except*:**
   a. Anterior rhinoscopy
   b. Passing of red rubber catheter
   c. Breath sound by stethoscope
   d Nasal endoscopy
   e. Acoustic rhinometry
10. **A 2-year-old child is brought to the clinic with a compressible swelling at the root of nose. What is the most likely diagnosis?**
    a. AV malformation
    b. Lacrimal sac cyst
    c. Ethmoid sinus sac
    d. Meningoencephalocele
11. **Which of these syndromes is associated with anosmia?**
    a. Kallmann's syndrome
    b. Turner's syndrome
    c. Down's syndrome
    d. Klinefelter's syndrome
12. **Which of the following is known as the 4th turbinate?**
    a. Superior turbinate b. Agger nasi
    c. Supreme turbinate d. Bullous turbinate

ANSWERS AND EXPLANATIONS

1. **b. Middle meatus**
   Bulla ethmoidalis is the cell of the anterior ethmoidal cell. It is the largest ethmoidal cell. It is also part of the osteomeatal complex.
   Osteomeatal complex is present in the middle meatus and therefore bulla ethmoidalis is also present in the middle meatus.

Important Content of Middle Meatus/Osteomeatal Complex are:

1. *Three ostia i.e*
   a. *Maxillary ostia*
   b. *Frontal sinus ostia*
   c. *Anterior ethmoidal ostia*
2. *Anterior and posterior fontanelles*
3. *Frontal recess*
4. *Uncinate process*
5. *Bulla ethmoidalis*
6. *Infundibulum*
7. *Hiatus semilunaris, etc.*

2. **b. Bucconasal membrane**
Bucconasal membrane usually disappears at around 42 days of intrauterine life.
If it persists after birth, it forms choanal atresia.
In this, the posterior end of nose is blocked. In case of bilateral choanal atresia, the life of the child is a risk.
In such a conditions ***McGovern's technique may be life saving.***

3. **d. Nasoturbinal**
There are various turbinal on the lateral part of nose. They develop in various structures.

The turbinals	Structures formed from them
Maxilloturbinal`	Inferior turbinate
1st ethmoturbinal	Middle turbinate
2nd ethmoturbinal	Superior turbinate
3rd ethmoturbinal	Supreme turbinate
4th and 5th ethmoturbinal	No Structure
Nasoturbinal	Agger nasi

4. **c. Frontal sinus**
This is the best answer, but sometimes sphenoidal sinus is also absent at birth.
Maxillary sinus and ethmoidal sinus are always present during birth of a child

5. **a. Maxillary sinus**
Maxillary sinus is the first sinus that starts to develop in an embryo.

> **Maxillary Sinus**
> The maxillary sinus is the first sinus to appear (seven to ten weeks) as a shallow groove expanding from the primitive ethmoidal infundibulum into the mass of the maxilla. Absorption and expansion results.
> Scot Brown ORL and HNS VIIth edition, page 1318

The sequence of start of development of sinuses is:

Maxillary sinus >> Ethmoidal sinus >> Sphenoidal sinus >> Frontal sinus

Other important points about sinuses are:

Sinuses	Starts development	Status at birth	Age when seen on X-ray
Maxillary sinus	7-10 weeks IUL	Is present at birth	4-5 months
Ethmoidal sinus	9-10 weeks IUL	Is present at birth	12 months
Frontal sinus	3rd month IUL	Is absent at birth	4-6 years
Sphenoidal sinus	4th month IUL	Is absent at birth	4-41/2 years

6. **c. Concha bullosa**
Sphenoid sinus has four general forms of pneumatization. They are:

Pattern of pneumatization	How common is it ?	Other points
Conchal	About 3 %	It is with rudimentary sinus
Presellar	About 10 %	It is till bony wall of pituitary fossa
Postsellar	About 60 %	It is below the pituitary fossa
Mixed	27 %	One or more of above

7. **c. Renal anomaly**
Choanal atresia is associated with a syndrome called **CHARGE SYNDROME.** The features of this syndrome are:
- C- Coloboma of eye
- H- Heart anomaly
- A- Atresia of choanal

- R- Retardation of growth and CNS anomaly
- G- Genital and urinary anomalies
- E- Ear anomalies

From this we can see that CHARGE SYNDROME does not have renal anomalies.

8. **c. Is derived from odontogenic epithelium**
Answer nasolabial cyst is also called ***Klestadt cyst.*** It is formed due to entrapement of epithelial tissue in the line of fusion of medial and lateral nasal process.
It may arise from nasolacrimal duct.
It is **non-odontogenic** and therefore is NOT derived from odontogenic epithelium.
It is more common in adult females and are bilateral.

9. **a. Anterior rhinoscopy**

10. **d. Meningoencephalocele**
In a child less than 3-year-old with any ***compressible swellings inside the nose or on the nasal bridge,* the most likely diagnosis is meningoencephalocele.**
A very important sign in nasal encephalocele is *Furstenberg sign.*

11. **a. Kallmann's syndrome**
The main features of Kallmann's syndrome are ***hypogonadotropic hypogonadism with anosmia/hyposmia.***

12. **c. Supreme turbinate**
Supreme turbinate is present in only 15-20 % of the population. Therefore, the majority of us have only three turbinate. The fourth if present is called the supreme turbinate.
NOTE: The fourth meatus is called *sphenoethmoidal recess.*

CHAPTER

14 Anatomy and Physiology of Nose and Paranasal Sinuses

NOSE

Nose has four walls and two openings. The walls are:

1. Roof
2. Floor
3. Medial wall/ septum
4. Lateral wall

The most important walls from examination point of view are the septum and the lateral wall and to some extend the roof. These walls are made of many bones, it is not necessary to memorise all of them. I am discussing only the relevant points.

ROOF

Nasal roof has four bone but the two that you must remember are:

1. Cribriform plate, and
2. Fovea ethmoidalis

The roof separates the nasal cavity from the anterior cranial fossa and the cribriform plate (which is one of the roof bones) is a very thin bone.

Because of this, this bone gets damaged very easily during endoscopic surgeries of this area.

In fact, **surgical trauma of cribriform plate is the most common cause of CSF rhinorrhea.**

This complication can be avoided if we know the height of the roof **(olfactory fossa).**

The height of olfactory fossa has been divided into three types by **Keros and Kainz.**

Keros and Kainz classification of olfactory fossa/height of nasal roof	
Type I	1-3 mm
Type II	4-7 mm
Type III	> 8 mm

Roof is lined by **olfactory epithelium** which is responsible for olfaction.

The olfactory epithelium has three types of cells. They are:

1. Basal cells
2. Supporting cells, and
3. Receptor cells/olfactory cells.

Receptor cells are main cells for olfaction where transduction for olfaction happens (similar to the hair cells in the cochlea).

The axons of these receptor cells pass through the openings of the cribriform plate in the roof, to form the **olfactory nerve (1st cranial nerve)**. This nerve carries the olfactory signal through the cribriform plate to the **olfactory bulb** which is located in the basal frontal lobe.

In the olfactory bulb, this nerve synapses with the **mitral cell.** About 1000 olfactory nerve fibres synapse with one mitral cell.

The mitral cell, inturn carries this signal to the olfactory cortex where final perception takes place. Therefore:

- The olfactory nerve serves as the **1st order neuron of olfaction and**
- **Mitral cell acts as the 2nd order neuron of olfaction.**

Important Diseases of This Area

Diseases	Features
Esthesioneuroblastoma	Is the tumour of olfactory neuroepithelium
Kallmann syndrome	• Hypogonadotropic hypogonadism • Anosmia
Foster-Kennedy syndrome	• Optic atrophy • Papilloedema • Unilateral anosmia

MEDIAL WALL/NASAL SEPTUM

Nasal septum has three layers.

The central layer is the main layer and is made of:

a. Bones
b. Cartilage, and
c. Membrane

Cartilages in septum	Their numbers
Quadrilateral cartilage	Unpaired cartilage
Upper lateral/alar cartilage	Paired cartilage
Lower lateral/alar cartilage	Paired cartilage
Sesamoid cartilage	Paired cartilage

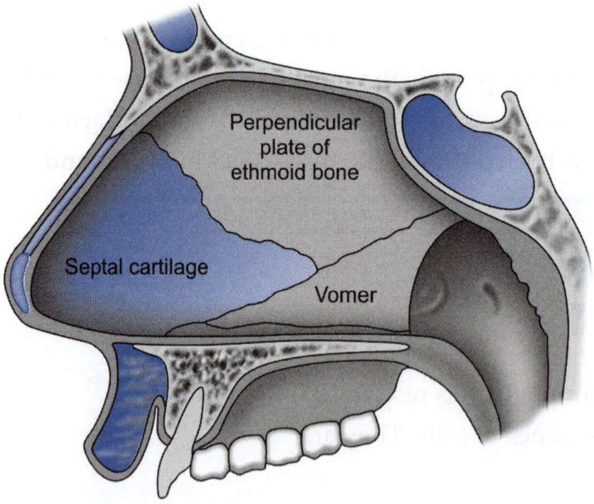

Fig. 1: Nasal septum

This has layers of mucoperichondrium on either side.

Between the mucoperichondrial layer and the central layer, there is a potential space.

This space contains arteries.

Therefore in case of trauma in this layer, these arteries may be traumatized causing bleeding and collection of blood in this potential space. This forms the **septal hematoma.**

The above mentioned cartilages along with the nasal bones form the main framework of the nose.

This nasal frame is important *cosmetic reasons as well as functional properties.*

For this reason nose is divided into three equal parts:

1. Upper third (bony pyramid) is formed of nasal bones
2. Mid-third (nasal vault) is formed by upper lateral cartilages and their fusion with the septal cartilage
3. Lower third is formed by the lower alar cartilage, corresponding septum and superficial musculoaponeurotic system.

The lower third also contains the **nasal tip.**

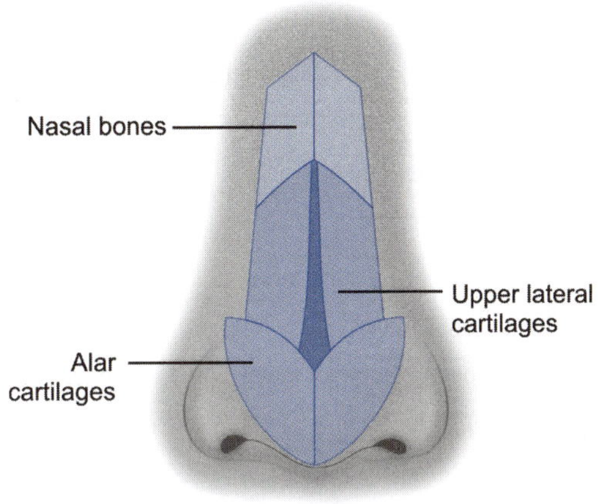

Fig. 2: Nasal bridge

Nasal Tip Supporting Mechanisms are:

- *Lower alar cartilages*
- *Attachment of lower alar cartilages to upper lateral cartilages*
- *Attachments joining the medial crura of lower alar cartilage to the septal cartilage along with intercrural attachments.*

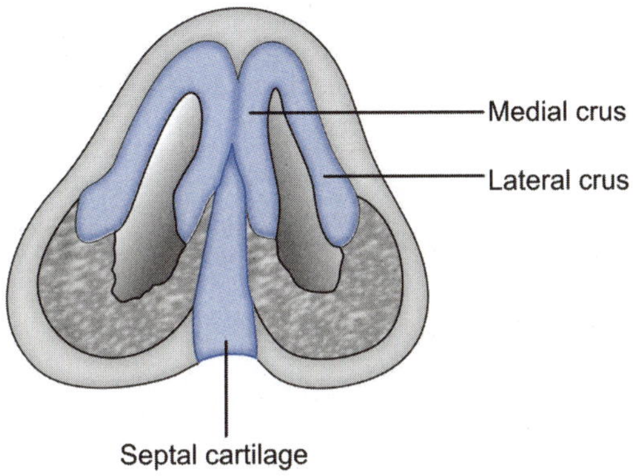

Fig. 3: Nasal tip

Inside the nasal cavity a valve like area exists. This is called ***nasal valve area.***

Nasal valve area is the ***flow limiting area or inflow resistant area.*** This valve controls the nasal air flow. Nasal valve area is formed by the following structures:

- *Caudal/lower margin of the upper lateral cartilage*
- *Corresponding part of nasal septum*
- *Its fibro-adipose attachment to the pyriform aperture, and*
- *The head/anterior end of inferior turbinate.*

The total area of the nasal valve area is **55-65 mm^2** and the angle of internal nasal valve is **10°-50°.**

Any reduction in this area can seriously reduce the nasal air flow. Two important causes that reduce the nasal valve area are:

- **Previous nasal surgeries (this may cause valve collapse), and**
- **Inferior turbinate hypertrophy.**

Inferior turbinate hypertrophy is an important cause inflow resistance in the nose.

Inferior turbinate hypertrophy is common because of its unique blood supply system. This is discussed in relevant topic.

The main artery supplying the nose including the septum is ***sphenopalatine artery*.** This is the terminal branch of maxillary artery and enters the nose through the **sphenopalatine foramen.**

Sphenopalatine fossa is also the site of **juvenile angiofibroma.** Hence, the blood supply of juvenile angiofibroma comes from sphenopalatine artery.

The septal arteries and their sources are:

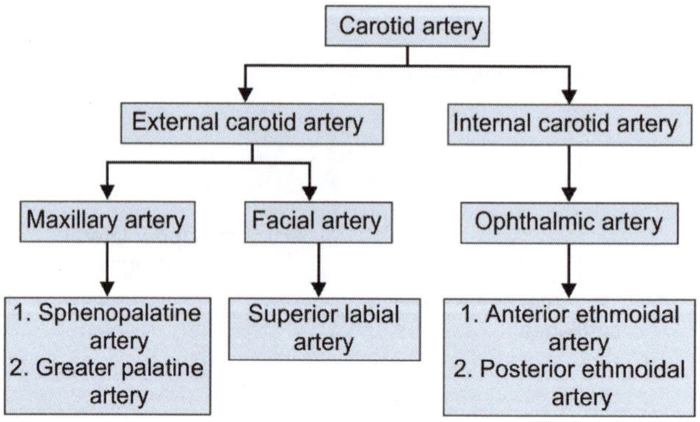

This shows that the septum receives supply from both the carotid arteries.

Out of the five arteries mentioned above, the first four form a plexus on the septum called the **Kiesselback's plexus.**

The area having this plexus is called the **Little's area.**

Little's area is the most common site of epistaxis/nasal bleeding.

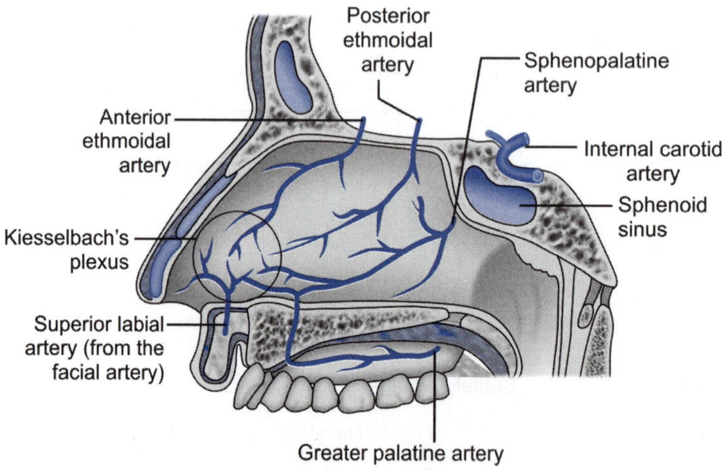

Fig. 4: Septal arteries

The submucosa of nose (especially the inferior turbinate) has a very unique vascular system. It has three types vascular network:

1. ***Subepithelial capillary network***
2. ***Arteriovenous anastomosis, and***
3. ***Sinusoid system.*** This sinusoidal system is controlled by the autonomic system.

This **sinusoid system** is causes the following:

- The cyclical collection of blood into these sinusoids causes normal contraction and expansion of the ***inferior turbinates.***
- This in turn helps in controlling the air flow through the nasal valve of the nose (it acts like a **nasal valve).**
- This expansion and contraction of inferior turbinate is also responsible for the **nasal cycle.**
- Each nasal cycle last for **$2^1/_2$ to 4 hours.**

- When there is ***imbalance in the autonomic control*** of this sinusoid, it leads to a condition called **vasomotor rhinitis.**

LATERAL WALL OF THE NOSE

On the lateral wall of the nose are three turbinates and four meatuses.

The *inferior turbinate* is the **longest turbinate**.

The supreme turbinate is also called **sphenoethmoidal recess**.

Just behind the inferior turbinate is a *plexus of veins* called ***Woodruff's plexus.***

Bleeding from woodruff's plexus is **not** common. However, it may be seen in hypertensives.

Ostia opening in meatuses:

Meatus	Ostia
Sphenoethmoidal recess	Sphenoid sinus ostia
Superior meatus	Post ethmoidal sinus ostia.
Middle meatus	Has three ostias a. Maxillary sinus b. Frontal sinus c. Anterior ethmoidal sinus
Inferior meatus	Does NOT have any ostia. Instead, it has nasolacrimal duct

NASOLACRIMAL DUCT (NLD)

Direction of nasolacrimal duct is **downwards, backwards and outward.**

It has a valve called *Hasner's valve.*

Sometimes a cyst may form in this duct. This cyst is called **nasolabial/Klestadt's cyst.**

When there is blockade of NLD, the patient may have excessive watering of eye (epiphora)

In such a case, a surgical bypass of this duct (NLD) is made between nasolacrimal sac and the nasal cavity. This surgery is called ***dacryocystorhinostomy.***

Some Important Structures in the Middle Meatus are given below

Uncinate process is a sickle shaped or boomerang shaped bone attached onto the lateral wall of nose.

During the functional endoscopic sinus surgery (**FESS**), this is the first bone that is removed. This procedure is called **uncinectomy.**

Bulla ethmoidalis is the *largest ethmoidal air* cell

Agar nasi cell (agger nasi) is the most anterior ethmoidal cell and is often the cause of frontal recess blockade.

Hiatus semilunaris is a half moon shaped two dimensional space between the *uncinate process and bulla ethmoidalis.*

Blockade of this hiatus semilunaris leads to defective drainage from sinuses, causing sinusitis.

Infundibulum is a three dimensional space between the above mentioned structures and the lateral nasal wall.

Osteomeatal complex/picadalli's complex includes all the above mentioned structures along the ostias in the middle meatus. The blockade of this complex is the **most common cause of sinusitis.**

Heller's cell is an ethmoidal cell in the floor of the orbit

Onodi's cell is an ethmoidal cell behind the orbit or lateral to sphenoid sinus.

In few individual, then middle turbinate may get pneumatized. This is called **concha bullosa.**

Given below are the four important ethmoidal cells which every student must remember

Name of cell	Origin	Important point
1. Bulla Ethmoidalis	Anterior ethmoidal cell	Is the largest ethmoidal cell
2. Agar (agger) Nasi	Anterior ethmoidal cell	Most anterior ethmoidal cell
3. Heller Cell	Anterior ethmoidal cell	Is present on the floor of orbit
4. Onodi Cell	Posterior ethmoidal cell	Is present behind the orbit close to optic nerve
NOTE: Some books claim that Heller cell is from posterior ethmoidal cell		

Important Facts about the Mucosal Lining of Nose and Sinuses

The nasal cavity and sinuses are lined by **pseudostratified ciliated columnar epithelium,** which is also called **schneiderans mucosa.**

The submucosa has **seromucinous glands and goblet cells.** They are responsible for nasal secretions.

The nasal secretion composition the following:

Cell type	Secretions	Their composition
• Mucus glands and goblet cells	Mucin	Glycoproteins- 80% Proteins Enzymes and immunoglobulins Cells
• Serous glands and transudation from capillaries	Water and ions	Water and ions

Each columnar cell has microvilli and **50-100 cilia.**

These cilia beat in the **conveyor belt** fashion to propel the nasal secretions backwards.

The speed of beating of nasal cilia is about ***5-10 times***

The speed by which the mucus of the nasal cavity travels backwards is *5-6 mm/min.*

Time taken by the mucus to reach from anterior part of the nose to posterior end of nasal cavity is ***15-20 min.***

NERVE SUPPLY OF NOSE

Nasal cavity is supplied by a number of nerves. You do not have to remember all. The three important points that you need to know are:

1. The main sensory nerve is ***nasopalatine nerve.*** This is branch of maxillary division of trigeminal and enters the nose through the sphenopalatine foramen (along with sphenopalatine artery).

   Therefore when we block this foramen with an anaesthetic agent, it anaesthetizes most of the nasal cavity
2. The gland of the nasal cavity receives **postganglionic sympathetic and parasympathetic from vidian nerve (nerve of pterygoid canal) in the pterygopalatine ganglion.**

   If you remember (while we discussed facial nerve anatomy), vidian nerve is formed by the joining of greater superficial petrosal nerve and deep petrosal nerve.

   The imbalance between these sympathetic and parasympathetic leads to dilation of submucosal sinusoid (discussed above) leading to ***vasomotor rhinitis.***
3. The olfactory neuroepithelium is responsible for olfaction and has the 1st cranial nerve.

Important Functions of Nose and Paranasal Sinuses

Nose is primarily the entry point for air into the body. It also is used for olfaction.

The air that we breathe is NOT conducive for body and therefore, it must undergo a number of changes before it reaches the lower respiratory system.

The nose along with sinuses, bring about these necessary changes. Some of the important changes/functions of nose and sinuses are given below:

- **Breathing/airflow**—Air flow into the lower respiratory system through the nose.

- **Heat exchange**—It brings the temperature of the inspired air close to body temperature.
- **Humidification**—It adds moisture to the inspired air.
- **Protection of airway**—It kills the pathogen in the air and filters the particles from air.
- **Voice**—It adds nasal twang or nasality to voice
- **Olfaction**—It is responsible for the sense of smell.

ANATOMY OF SINUSES

The largest sinus is the **maxillary sinus.**

It is also called the **Antrum of Highmore.**

It is the first sinus that begins to develop in human embryo.

Maxillary Sinus

The maxillary sinus is the first sinus to appear (seven to ten weeks) as a shallow groove expanding from the primitive ethmoidal infundibulum into the mass of the maxilla. Absorption and expansion results.

This is a photo clicked from "Scot Brown ORL and HNS" VIIth edition, page no 1318.

The volume of maxillary sinus is about **15** to **20 cc.**

The floor of maxilla has **alveolus.**

In some people the **2nd pre-molar and the 1st molar** may communicate with maxillary cavity.

If this is not given in the choices, then the acceptable answer is **1st molar.**

This is why the commonest cause of **oro-antral fistula is extraction of the 1st molar.**

The highest sinus in the human body is the **frontal sinus.**

Frontal sinus is the last sinus to start the developing and the last to complete the development.

Ethmoidal sinus is made up of a number of air cells (just like the mastoid in the ear).

The total number of ethmoidal air cell may vary from 3 to 18 cells. On an average a human body has **8-9 ethmoidal air cells.**

These air cells are divided into two groups *i.e.* anterior ethmoidal cells and posterior ethmoidal cells (some books claim that there are three groups)

Few of these ethmoidal cells we have already discussed (bulla ethmoidalis, agger nasi, haller cell, onodi cell, etc.).

Sphenoid sinus is surrounded by important structures. These structures are:

- Internal carotid artery
- Optic nerve
- Maxillary nerve
- Vidian nerve/nerve of pterygoid canal, etc

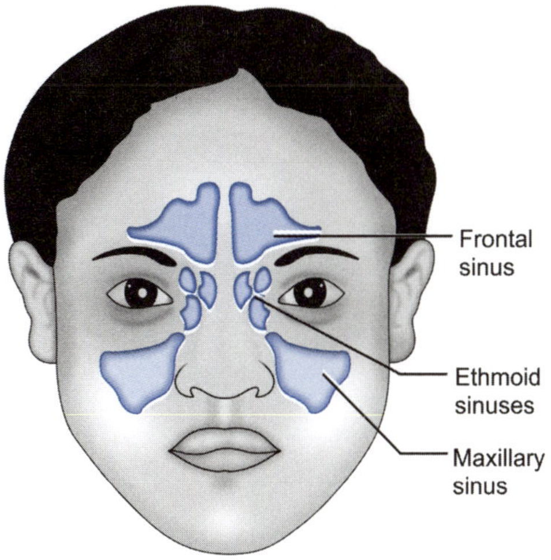

Fig. 5: Relation of sinuses with each other and nose

PART 2: NOSE AND SINUSES

Last minute revision

- Kiesselbach's plexus present on nasal septum is formed of four arteries:
  - Sphenopalatine artery
  - Greater palatine artery
  - Superior labial artery
  - Anterior ethmoidal artery
- This area is called little's area and is the most common site of epistaxis
- Middle meatus has three ostia- maxillary sinus, frontal sinus and anterior ethmoidal sinus
- Inferior turbinate is the largest turbinate
- Nasolacrimal duct opens in the inferior meatus and it runs downward, outward and backward
- Bulla ethmoidalis is the largest ethmoidal cell
- Onodi cell is present behind the orbit near the orbital apex
- Heller cell is present in the floor of orbitfloor of maxilla is formed by alveolus
- Supreme meatus is also called sphenoethmoidal recess
- Maxillary sinus is also called antrum of highmore. It's volume is 15 cc
- 2nd premolar and 1st molar are related with maxillary sinus

QUESTIONS

1. **Maxillary sinus opens in:**
   a. Sphenoethmoidal recess
   b. Superior meatus
   c. Middle meatus
   d. Inferior meatus
2. **All of the following structures open into middle meatus, *except***
   a. Frontal sinus
   b. Anterior ethmoidal sinus
   c. Posterior ethmoidal sinus
   d. Maxillary sinus
3. **Floor of maxillary sinus is related to:**
   a. Incisors and canine
   b. Canine and premolars
   c. Roots of molars
   d. Premolars only
4. **Nasal septum is not contributed by which of these bones.**
   a. Lacrimal
   c. Sphenoid
   c. Ethmoid
   d. Palatine
5. **Direction of nasolacrimal duct is:**
   a. Downwards, backwards and medially
   b. Downwards, backwards and laterally
   c. Downwards, forwards and medially
   d. Downwards, forwards and laterally
6. **Most common site of origin of Nasopharyngeal Angiofibroma is**
   a. Roof of Nasopharynx
   b. At sphenopalatine foramen
   c. Vault of skull
   d. Lateral wall of nose
7. **During inspiration the main current of airflow in a normal nasal cavity is through:**
   a. Middle part of the cavity in middle meatus in a parabolic curve
   b. Lower part of the cavity in the inferior meatus in a parabolic curve
   c. Superior part of the cavity in the superior meatus
   d. Through olfactory area
8. **Commonest sinus involved in infection in infants and young children is:**
   a. Frontal
   b. Maxillary
   c. Ethmoid
   d. Sphenoid
9. **All are component of 'Kiesselbach's plexus' *except*:**
   a. Sphenopalatine artery
   b. Anterior ethmoidal artery
   c. Greater palatine artery
   d. Inferior labial artery
10. **Which of the following innervates the frontal sinus?**
    a. Anterior ethmoidal nerve
    b. Nasociliary nerve
    c. Posterior ethmoidal nerve
    d. Supraorbital nerve
11. **Pain sensations from the ethmoid sinus are carried by:**
    a. Supraorbital nerve
    b. Lacrimal nerve
    c. Nasociliary nerve
    d. Infraorbital nerve
12. **Onodi cells and Haller cells are seen in relation to:**
    a. Optic nerve and floor of orbit
    b. Optic nerve and frontal sinus
    c. Optic nerve and ethmoidal sinus
    d. Optic nerve and nasolacrimal duct
13. **External nose is formed from:**
    a. 3 paired and 3 unpaired cartilages
    b. 3 paired and 1 unpaired cartilages
    c. 3 paired and 4 unpaired cartilages
    d. 1 paired and 1 unpaired cartilages
14. **Osseo-cartilagenous junction of the nasal dorsum is called:**
    a. Nasion
    b. Columella
    c. Rhinion
    d. Glabella
15. **Nasal valve is formed by all except:**
    a. Septum
    b. Middle turbinate
    c. Lower end of upper alar cartilage
    d. Inferior turbinate
16. **Quadrilateral cartilage is attached to all *except*:**
    a. Ethmoid
    b. Vomar
    c. Sphenoid
    d. Maxilla
17. **Maxillary sinus opens in the middle meatus at the level of:**
    a. Hiatus semilunaris
    b. Bulla ethmoidalis
    c. Infundibulum
    d. Agar nasi cell
18. **What is the rate of ciliary movement of nasal mucosa?**
    a. 2-5 mm/min
    b. 5-10 mm/min
    c. 10-20 mm/min
    d. 20-30 mm/min

19. **What is the meaning of parosmia?**
    a. Perversion of smell sensation
    b. Loss of sensation
    c. Reduced smell sensation
    d. Perception of bad smell
20. **Function of mucociliary action of upper respiratory tract is:**
    a. Temperature regulation
    b. Increases velocity of inspired air
    c. Traps particles/pathogens from inspired air
    d. None of the above
21. **Nasal cycle is the cyclical alternate nasal blockade occurring:**
    a. Every 6–12 hours
    b. Every $2^1/_2$ hour–4 hrs
    c. Every 4–6 hrs
    d. Every 8–10 hrs

IMAGE BASED QUESTIONS

22. **Which of the folllowing is NOT true of the picture given:**

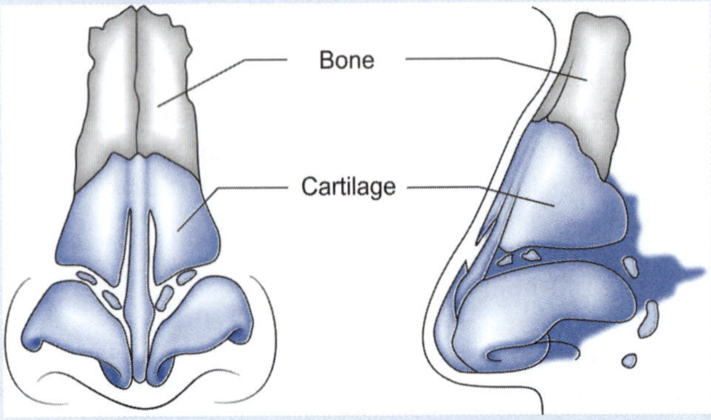

    a. The bone is the nasal bone
    b. The cartilage is upper alar cartilage
    c. This cartilage is a paired cartilage
    d. This cartilage is the most commonly removed cartilage during septoplasty
23. **In the diagram, identify the structure marked with arrow:**

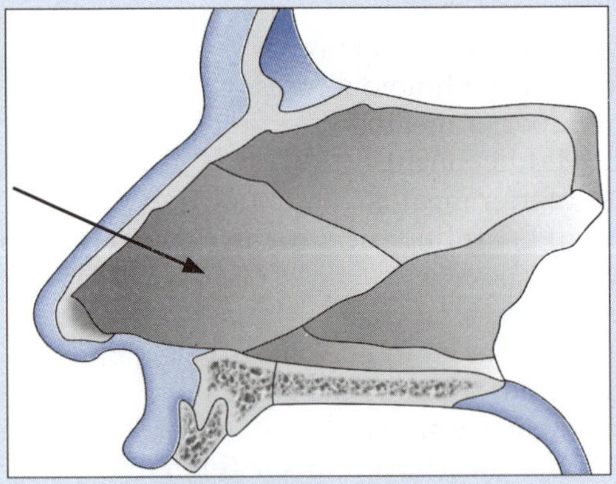

    a. Septal cartilage   b. Vomar bone
    c. Perpendicular plate of ethmoid
    d. Septal membrane
24. **In the CT scan shown below, identify the star (*) marked structure.**

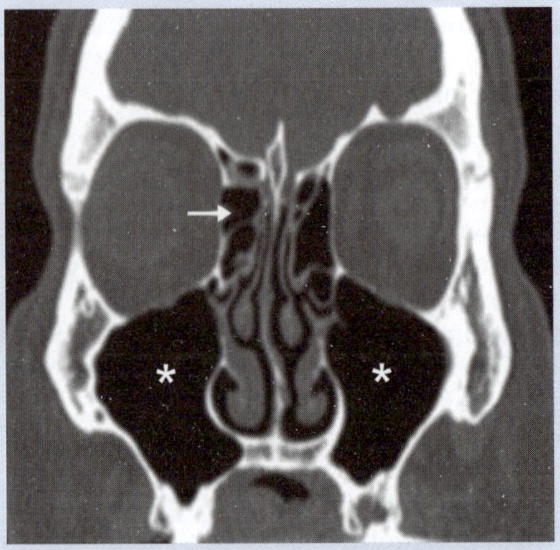

    a. Maxillary sinus   b. Heller cell
    c. Anterior ethmoidal sinus
    d. Inferior turbinate

ANSWERS AND EXPLANATIONS

1. **c. Middle meatus**
2. **c. Posterior ethmoidal sinus**

Lateral wall of the nose has three meatuses. Out of these three meatuses the middle meatus is the most important.

Middle meatus in the nasal cavity is a very important as well as very complex area.

In middle meatus opens the ostia of three sinuses. These sinuses are:

1. *Maxillary sinus*
2. *Frontal sinus and*
3. *Anterior ethmoidal sinus*

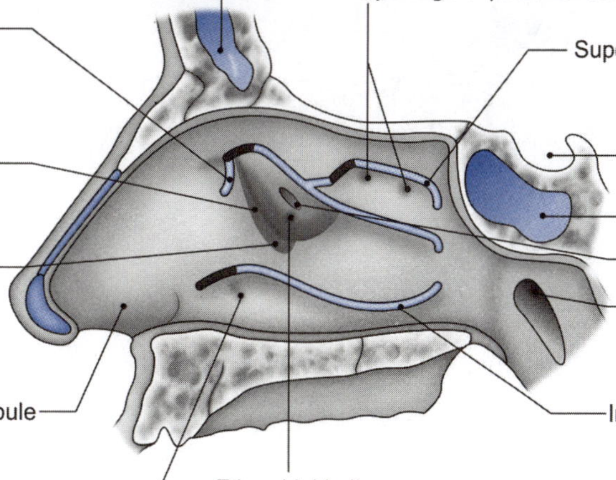

The posterior ethmoidal sinus opens in the superior meatus and the sphenoid sinus opens in the spheno-ethmoidal recess.

NOTE: Inferior meatus is the only meatus that does not have any sinus opening.

It, instead, has opening of the nasolacrimal duct.

Meatus	Ostia
Sphenoethmoidal recess	Sphenoid sinus ostia
Superior meatus	Postethmoidal sinus ostia.
Middle meatus	Has three ostias a. Maxillary sinus b. Frontal sinus c. Anterior ethmoidal sinus
Inferior meatus	Does NOT have any ostia. Instead, it has nasolacrimal duct

3. **c. Roots of molars**

Floor of maxilla is formed by ***alveolus.*** Alveolus has teeth imbedded into it.

Some of these teeth are related to the maxillary cavity. Most common teeth that are related to maxilla are 1st molar and 2nd premolar.

- The best answer to this question is 2nd premolar and 1st molar.
- ***The second best answer is 1st molar and***
- ***The third best answer is molars.***

In the absence of first two options in the choices, the third acceptable answer (in order of Preference) is roots of molars

Note: This question always has controversial choices and so it is very important to remember the order given above.

4. **a. Lacrimal bone**

Lacrimal bone is a part of lateral wall of nasal cavity and not the septum. Bones contributing to septum are:

- Perpendicular plate of ethmoid
- Vomer
- Crest of maxilla
- Crest of palatine bone
- Rostrum of sphenoid

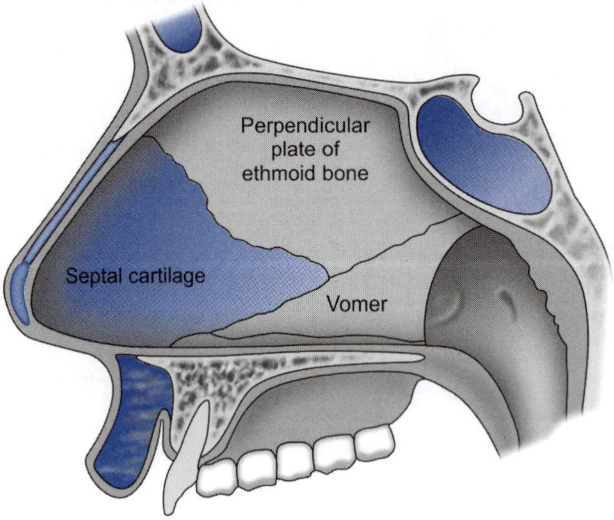

Nasal septum

Note:
- Lacrimal bone separates nose from lacrimal sac
- Lamina papyracea separates nose from orbit
- Fistula is made through this lacrimal bone during dacryocystorhinostomy.

5. **b. Downwards, backwards and laterally**

Nasolacrimal duct is a duct which connects the lacrimal apparatus to nose.
It opens in the inferior meatus of nose and runs:
- Downwards,
- Backwards and
- Laterally.

Nasolacrimal duct has a valve in it. This valve is called ***Hasner's valve.***

6. **b. At sphenopalatine foramen**

Nasopharyngeal Angiofibroma is a very vascular tumour which is very common in juvenile males.
It presents with nasal bleed.
It most commonly arises from the periosteum of sphenopalatine foramen.
Through this sphenopalatine foramen, this tumour easily spreads into pterygopalatine fossa.

7. **a. Middle part of the cavity in middle meatus in a parabolic curve**

This is true for both inspiration as well as expiration.
However during expiration, friction offered at limen nasi converts it into eddies.
This portion of air ventilates the sinuses.
Any obstruction in the nose in the form of growth or disease may disturb this flow.

8. **c. Ethmoid**

Sinus involved in adults is most commonly is the maxillary sinus but in children it is the ethmoid sinus.
In cases of nasal polyps, the reverse is true.
Adults have nasal polyps more commonly in the ethmoid sinus but children have polyps more commonly in the maxillary sinus.

9. **d. Inferior labial artery**

Kiesselbach's plexus is a plexus of arteries present in the little's area of nasal septum.
It is the most common site of epistaxis/nasal bleeding.
Kiesselbach's plexus is formed by four arteries:
1. *Sphenopalatine artery*
2. *Greater palatine artery*
3. *Superior labial artery, and*
4. *Anterior ethmoidal artery*

Inferior labial artery is not a component of Kiesselbach's plexus.
Posterior ethmoidal artey is not a component of Kiesselbach's plexus

10. **d. Supraorbital nerve**
Frontal sinus is located on the upper 1/3 of face and therefore is supplied by branches of ophthalmic division of trigeminal nerve.
Frontal sinus is supplied by ***supraorbital and supratrocheal nerves*** which are branches of frontal nerve. Frontal nerve is a branch of ophthalmic division of trigeminal nerve.

11. **c. Nasociliary nerve**
Nerve supply of various sinuses are:

Maxillary	Ethmoidal	Frontal	Sphenoidal
1. Infraorbital N- V2 2. Alveolar N- V2	1. Nasociliary N- V1 2. Sphenopalatine N- V2	1. Supraorbial B- V1	1. Nasociliary N- V1 2. Sphenopalatine N- V2

12. **a. Optic nerve and floor of orbit**
- Onodi cell arise from posterior ethmoidal cell and is usually present posteriorly near the orbital apex close to optic nerve. If this cell gets pneumatized too much, then it may compress the optic nerve.
- Heller cell arises from the anterior ethmoidal cell and is present in the floor of orbit or roof of maxilla.
- These two cells have NO relation to frontal sinus and nasolacrimal duct.

13. **b. 3 paired and 1 unpaired cartilages**

Cartilages in septum	Their numbers
• Quadrilateral cartilage	Unpaired cartilage
• Upper lateral/alar cartilage	Paired cartilage
• Lower lateral/alar cartilage	Paired cartilage
• Sesamoid cartilage	Paired cartilage

14. **c. Rhinion**
Nasion: Intersection of the nasal bones with frontal bones.
Glabella: The depressed bone between the two superciliary ridges.
Columella: The distal end of the nasal septum that separates the two nasal cavities.

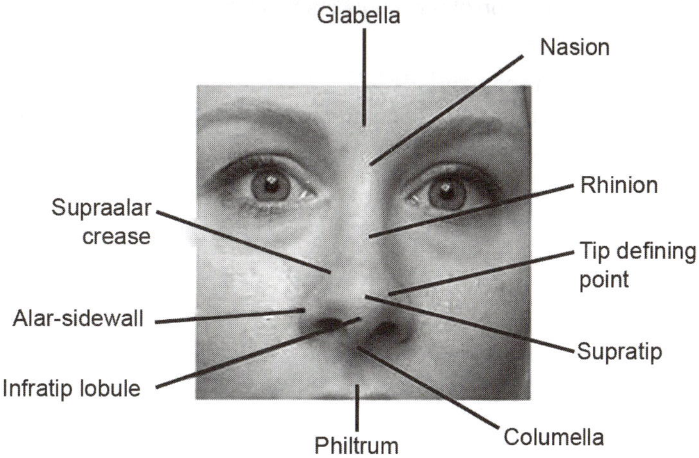

15. **b. Middle turbinate**
Nasal valve area is formed by the following structures:
- *Caudal/lower margin of the upper lateral cartilage*
- *Corresponding part of nasal septum*
- *Its fibro-adipose attachment to the pyriform aperture, and*

The head/anterior end of inferior turbinate.

16. **c. Sphenoid**

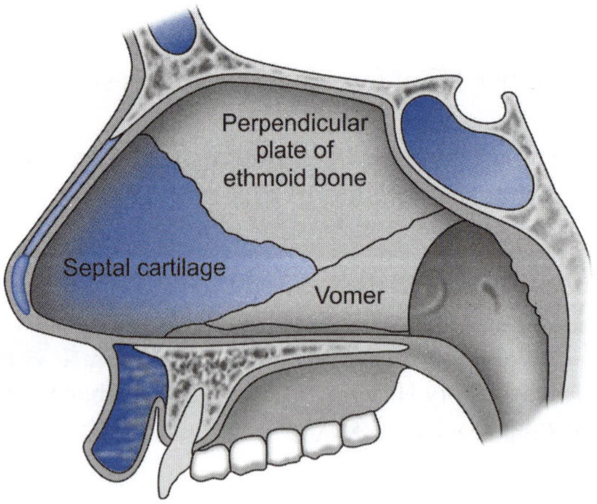

17. **a. Hiatus semilunaris**

Middle meatus has osteomeatal complex which has three ostia opening in it. These ostia are:
- Maxillary sinus ostium
- Frontal sinus ostium
- Anterior ethmoidal sinus ostium.

Maxillary sinus ostium is the most important ostium and it is supposed to drain from the osteomeatal complex through a semilunar shaped opening/door called ***hiatus semilunaris.***

If it opens at the level of hiatus semilunaris, then the drainage will be more effective and so it opens at the level of hiatus semilunaris.

18. **b. 5-10 mm/min.**

Mucosal movement of nasal cilia is 5-10 mm/min and the total time taken for mucus to travel the length of the entire nosal cavity is approx. 15 minutes.

19. **a. Perversion of smell sensation**

1. Anosmia/Hyposmia	Absence of smell/reduced sensation of smell
2. Parosmia	Perversion of smell sensation
3. Cacosmia	Sensation of bad/unpleasant smell

20. **c. Traps particles/pathogens from inspired air**

Mucociliary action has significant innate defence mechanism against inhaled microbes and irritants.

21. **b. Every 21/2-hour–4 hour**

Nasal cycle is alternate blockade of the two nasal cavities. This is produced by the activities of nasal vessels/ venous sinusoids.

Each cycle last for $2^1/_2$-hour–4 hour

IMAGE BASED ANSWERS

22. **d. This cartilage is the most commonly removed cartilage during septoplasty**

Septoplasty is the surgery of nasal septum and NOT the lateral wall of the nose (which is shown in this picture). Septum has the quadrilateral cartilage, which is operated upon during septoplasty.

23. **a. Septal cartilage**

The arrow points at septal cartilage which is also called ***quadrilateral cartilage***.

Nasal septum has one main cartilage (quadrilateral cartilage) and 7 bones.

24. **a. Maxillary sinus. The * marked sinuses are maxillary sinuses and the → marked sinuses are the ethmoidal sinuses.**

CHAPTER

15 Important Tests and Investigations for Nose and Paranasal Sinus

Examination of the anterior part of the nose is simple and easy because one can see through the anterior nasal openings. However, the posterior part and deeper areas of nose and the paranasal sinuses are more difficult to examine.

We shall discuss some of the common examinations and investigations done for nasal diseases.

ANTERIOR RHINOSCOPY

Anterior rhinoscopy is done in almost every patient with nasal complains. Two types of speculum can be used for this.

1. Thudicum Nasal Speculum

This instrument is usually held in the left hand and is used for examination off the anterior part of the nose. The picture is shown below.

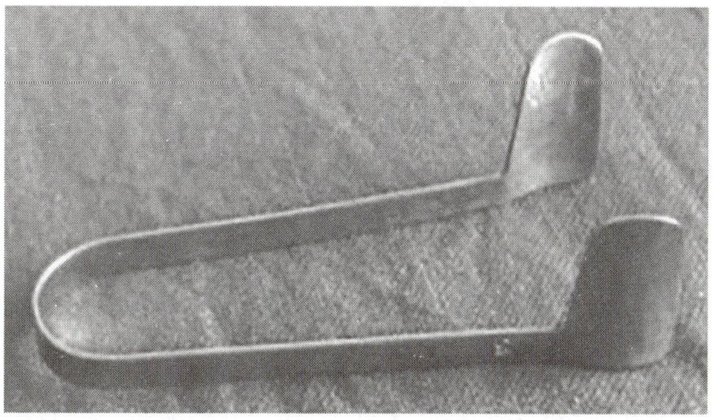

Fig. 1: Thudicum nasal speculum

2. Killian's Nasal Speculum

Killian's nasal speculum is also used for examination of anterior part of the nose. It is much easier to use as compared thudicum's speculum. Killian's speculum is also commonly used during various nasal surgeries. The picture is given below.

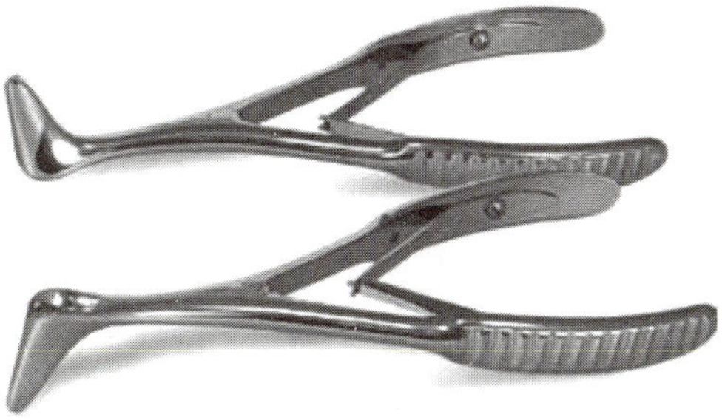

Fig. 2: Killian's nasal speculum

POSTERIOR RHINOSCOPY MIRROR

Posterior rhinoscopy mirror is used for examination of nasopharynx (ADENOIDS) and posterior part of the nose. The picture is given below.

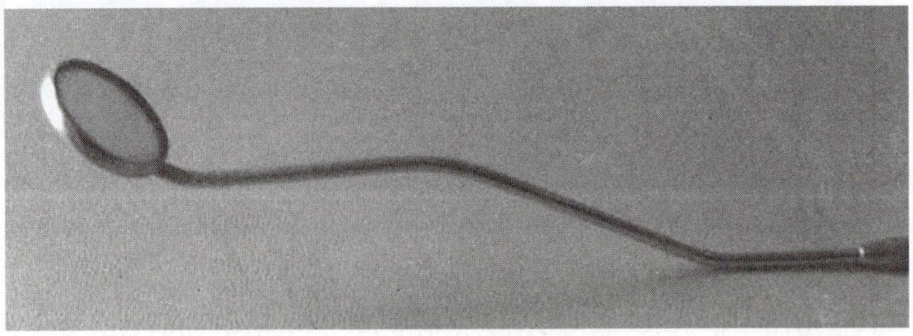

Posterior rhinoscopy mirror procedure is shown in the picture below:

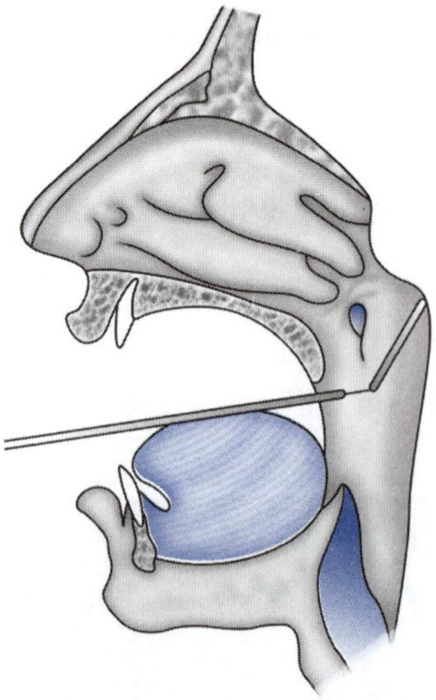

TRANSILLUMINATION TEST

Since sinuses are hollow cavities, transillumination can be done.

It is done in a similar way as in case of cysts. In case of sinusitis, this test can be done only for maxillary sinus and frontal sinus.

DIAGNOSTIC NASAL ENDOSCOPY

For diagnostic nasal endoscopy, the nasal and sinus endoscope is used. The picture is given below.

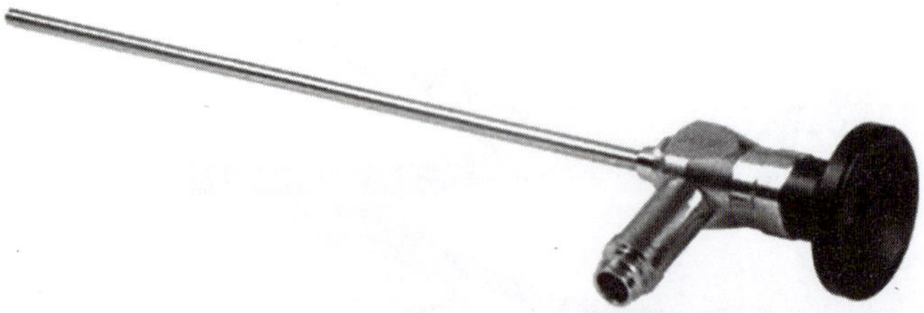

Diagnostic nasal endoscope is an excellent tool for the examination of the entire nasal cavity and the osteomeatal complex (we have already discussed its anatomy).

This procedure is done either:

- From anterior to prosterior direction (this is more commonly done), or
- Posterior to anterior direction (not done commonly)

Anterior to posterior direction is done in three steps or **three passes.**

1. **First pass**—the endoscope is passed below the inferior turbinate. This gives general view of the nose
2. **Second pass**—the endoscope is passed between the inferior and middle turbinate. This shows the middle meatal and the superior meatal areas
3. **Third pass**—in this, the deeper parts and osteomeatal complex are examined.

PROOF PUNCTURE

Proof puncture is an **invasive procedure done to diagnose maxillary sinusitis.**

It is the **most diagnostic** investigation for maxillary sinusitis.

The procedure of proof puncture is similar to a procedure called **antral wash,** which is discussed in a different chapter.

RHINOMANOMETRY

This is used to measure the nasal airflow and its driving pressure. It measures the narrowest part of the nasal cavity.

Acoustic Rhinomanometry

It is used to measure the cross-sectional area along the entire length of nasal cavity.

It gives us a picture of the cross-section of every part of the nasal cavity.

Rhinostereometry

In this investigation, microscopic examination of the inferior turbinate is done to see the changes in the diameter/size of this turbinate. As we have already discussed, this change happens even in a normal situation (**nasal cycle).**

Radiographs

Besides the above mentioned investigations for nasal and paranasal sinus diseases, different types of radiographs are also done.

IMPORTANT X-RAY VIEWS FOR SINUSES

Water's View

The most commonly done X-ray view for sinuses is the *Water's view.*

It is also called ***Occipito-submental with open mouth***

The two main advantages of Water's view are:

- All sinuses seen in one X-ray film.
- The only sinus which is **not** seen very clearly is ***postethmoidal sinus***.
- Water's view is the best view to see the maxilla.

Caldwell's View

It is nearly an A-P view and is the best view for ***frontal sinus***.

Basal View

It is done for sphenoid and ethmoid sinuses.

CT Scan

CT scan is one of the most important investigation for nasal pathologies. You should be able to identify different sinuses on a scan. Given below is a plain CT scan with important areas labelled.

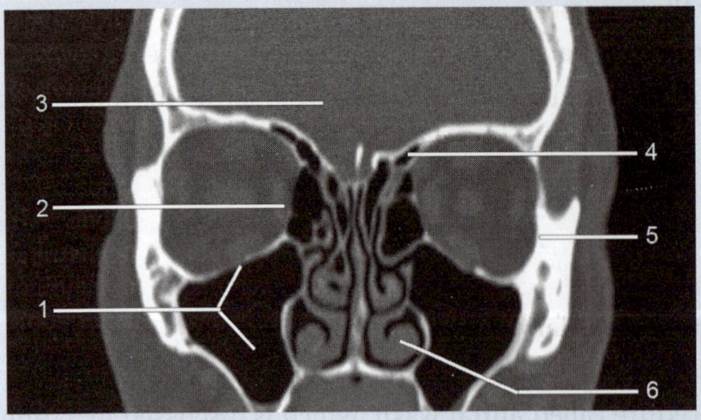

Fig. 6: CT Scan of paranasal sinus

1. Maxilllary sinus
2. Ethmoidal sinus
3. Cribriform plate
4. Frontal sinus
5. Zygoma
6. Inferior turbinate

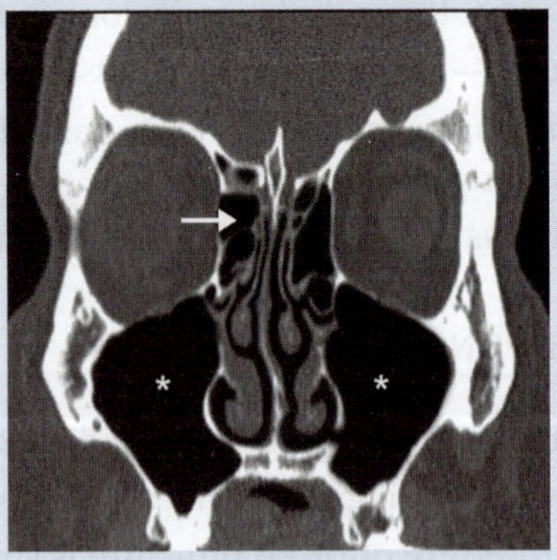

Fig. 7: CT Scan of PNS with: *→

* shows maxillary sinus
→ points at ethmoidal sinus

Last minute revision

- Water's view is the most common X-ray view for sinuses
- Caldwell's view is best for frontal sinus
- Posterior ethmoids are not seen clearly on Water's view
- Posterior rhinoscopy will show the following
  - Choana
  - Posterior end of Vomar
  - Adenoids
  - Eustachian tube opening
  - Fossa of Rosenmüller etc.
- Proof puncture is the best for diagnosing maxillary sinusitis.

QUESTIONS

1. **Which of the following is the most diagnostic method for maxillary sinusitis:**
   a. X-ray of PNS
   b. CT scan of PNS
   c. Proof puncture
   d. Diagnostic nasal endoscopy
2. **In the CT scan shown below, identify the star (*) marked structure.**
   a. Maxillary sinus
   b. Haller cell
   c. Anterior ethmoidal sinus
   d. Inferior turbinate
3. **The instrument shown below is used for:**
   a. Indirect laryngoscopy
   b. Direct laryngoscopy
   c. Posterior rhinoscopy
   d. Anterior rhinoscopy
4. **Best X-ray view for frontal sinus is:**
   a. Caldwell's view b. Towne's view
   c. Water's view d. Lateral view
5. **For viewing superior orbital fissure, which is the best view?**
   a. Lateral view b. Caldwell's view
   c. Towne's view d. Basal view

IMAGE BASED QUESTION

6. **Name the nasal instruments seen in the above diagram:**

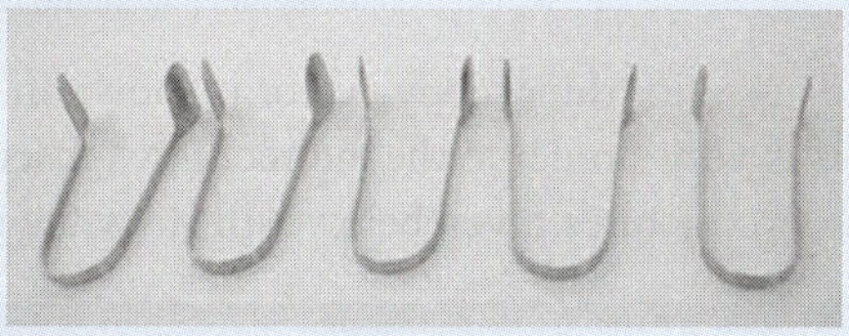

   a. Killian's nasal speculum
   b. Thudicum nasal speculum
   c. Luc's nasal forceps
   d. None of the above

ANSWERS AND EXPLANATIONS

1. **c. Proof puncture**

   Proof puncture is a procedure in which a puncture is made on the medial wall of maxillary sinus through the inferior meatus. If pus begins to flow through this puncture, it is 100% proof of pus in the sinus and hence maxillary sinusitis.

   CT scan and diagnostic nasal endoscopy are also very good a diagnosing maxillary sinusitis but are NOT as specific as a proof puncture.

2. **a. Maxillary sinus**

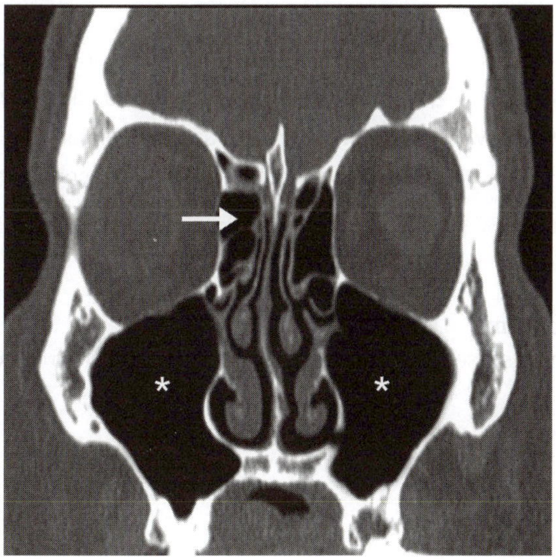

The * marked structure scan show an air filled cavity on both sides on nasal cavity and below the orbits. This → is the location of maxillary sinus.

3. **c. Posterior rhinoscopy**

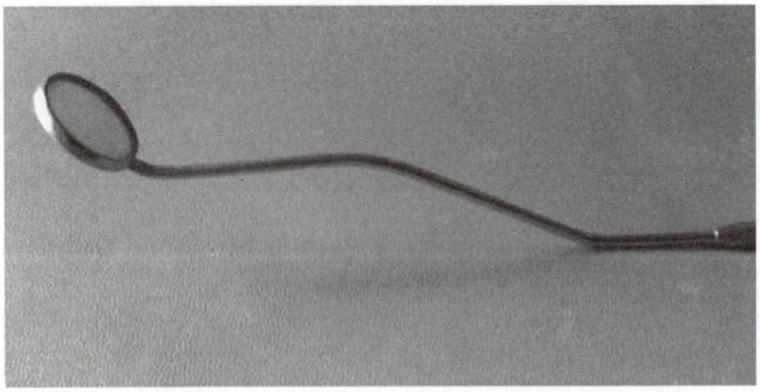

The posterior rhinoscopy mirror is shown in the picture.
This is very similar to the indirect laryngoscopy mirror.
The two pictures given below will show the difference between the two.

Indirect laryngoscopy mirror	Posterior rhinoscopy mirror
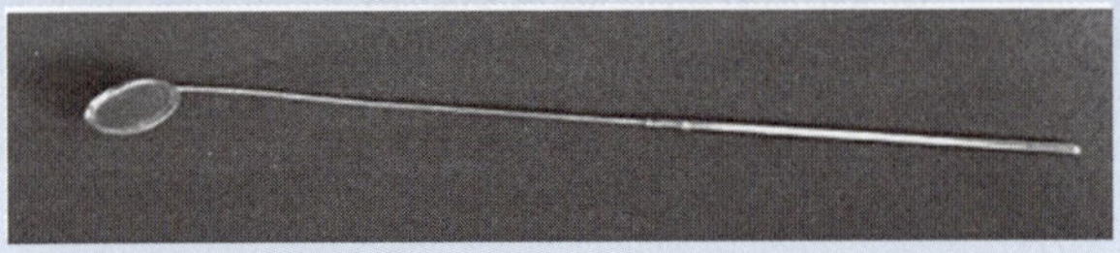	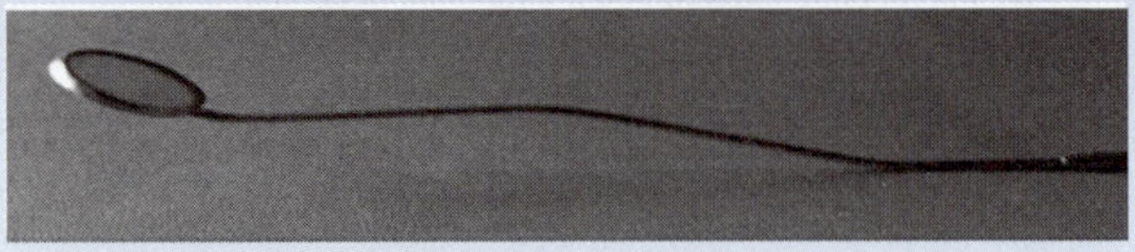
The handle is straight	The handle is "Z" shaped

4. **a. Caldwell's view**
5. **b. Caldwell's view**

IMPORTANT X-RAY VIEWS IN ENT

X-ray view	Structures seen
• Water's view	• All the sinuses EXCEPT posterior ethmoids
• Caldwell's view	• Frontal sinus and superior orbital fissure
• Lateral oblique view	• Posterior ethmoidal sinus
• Basal view	• Sphenoid sinus and posterior ethmoids
• Towne's view	• Comparing the two mastoids and petrous apex
• Schuller's view and Law's view	• Mastoid air cells and mastoid antrum
• Per orbital view	• Comparing the two internal acoustic meatuses

IMAGE BASED ANSWER

6. **b. Thudicum nasal speculum**
Thudicum nasal speculum is used for anterior rhinoscopy. It is also used during nasal surgeries.

CHAPTER 16

Epistaxis

As has been discussed already, nose has blood supply from both the carotid arteries.

- Middle turbinate acts as a boundary between the branches of the two blood major vessels.
- Because of this, there are **internal-external carotid artery anastomoses** in the nose.
- One such important anastomotic site is the **Kiesselbach's plexus** in the **Little's area.**
- For your recollection, I am reproducing the flowchart of nasal blood vessels.

Flowchart 1: Artery supply of septum

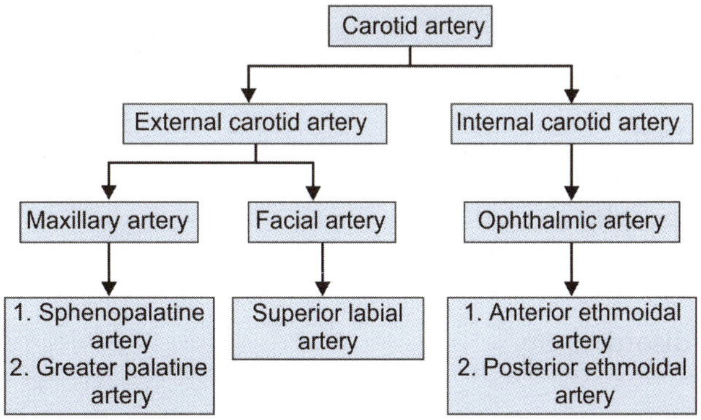

These blood vessels and anastomoses often cause bleeding or epistaxis.

The most **common site** of nasal bleed is the **Little's area**, which has a plexus of four arteries called **Kiesselbach's plexus.**

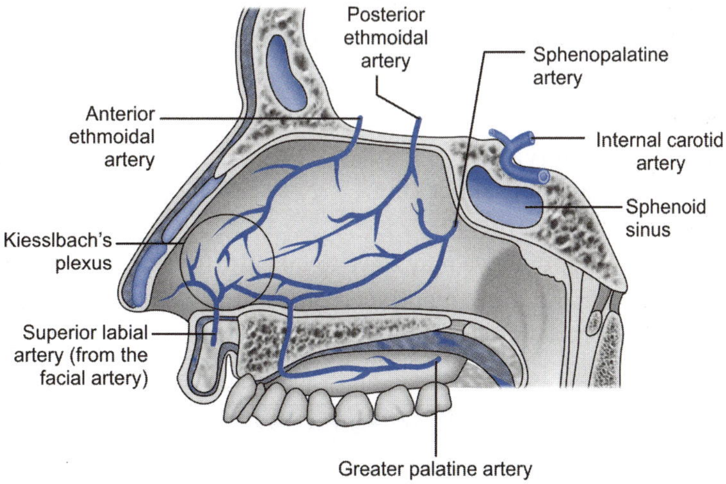

Fig. 1: Little's area 1

The second most common site of nasal bleed is **retrocolumnar vein**.

This usually bleeds due to trauma and therefore more commonly bleeds in *young people*.

Another site of nasal bleed is the **Woodruff's plexus**.

This is a plexus of veins and is present just behind the inferior turbinate on the posterior part of lateral wall of nose.

Woodruff's plexus is NOT an arterial plexus (as suggested in some books), on the contrary it is the ***plexus of veins***.

This area usually bleeds in ***hypertensives and hence may bleed in hypertensive elderly person.***

Note: **Woodruff's plexus is NOT the most common site of epistaxis in elderly people.**
The most common site is Kiesselbach's plexus, but posterior bleed if it happens, is from this plexus.

Important points about epistaxis

Almost any condition of nose can cause epistaxis. So, NO need to memorize all the causes.
The only important disease of nose that CANNOT cause epistaxis is nasal polyps.

The most common cause of epistaxis is idiopathic, but this choice is usually not given.
If this is not given in the choices, nose picking or trauma is the accepted correct answer.

Also in elderly person the cause of epistaxis is idiopathic.

If this is not given, hypertension is the second best answer.

Other Causes of Epistaxis are:

- Foreign body of nose in children
- Angiofibroma, in juvenile age in a male child
- Road side accident in young people
- Nasal growths
- Iatrogenic
- Systemic diseases, bleeding disorders etc.

TREATMENT OF NASAL BLEED

Bleeding is an emergency and hence stopping the bleed is the first priority.

- The first step to stop nasal bleed to **pinch the nose for at least 10 min**.
- This is because the normal clotting time is up to 8 minutes.
- The next thing to be done if the bleeding does not stop is **septal cautery**
- Septal cautery is done using one of the two options:
  - **Silver nitrate (Chemical cautery),** or
  - **Bipolar dithermy (Electrical cautery)**
- The third step to stop nasal bleeding is **nasal packing**.
- Irrigation of nasal cavity with 50° water.
- If all these fail to stop nasal bleeding, then we may have to take drastic measure like **artery ligation.**
- As we attempt to stop bleeding with the above mentioned procedure, we should try to treat the cause of epistaxis like give antihypertensive, anti-fibrinolytics etc.

Important points about nasal packing

- When nasal packing is required for epistaxis, both the cavities should be packed
- The ribbon gauze used for packing should be smeared with petroleum jelly or BIPP
- BIPP is bismuth iodoform paraffin paste. It does not cause adhesions or stenosis.
- The pack should be kept for 24–72 hours
- Posterior nasal packing is done when Woodruff's plexus bleeds
- Foley's catheter can be used for posterior packing.

Important points about artery ligation

- The most commonly ligated artery for epistaxis is the sphenopalatine artery.
- If nasal endoscope is used for this then the name of the procedure is one of the two:
  - Transnasal endoscopic sphenopalatine artery ligation (TESPAL), or
  - Endoscopic sphenopalatine artery ligation (ESPAL)
- If this fails, the second artery ligated is the internal maxillary (IMAL)
- Third artery to be ligated is the external carotid artery
- Finally the anterior and posterior ethmoidal arteries are ligated
  - Anterior ethmoidal artery is 24 mm posterior to lacrimal crest
  - Posterior ethmoidal artery is 12 mm posterior to anterior ethmoidal artery.

Hereditary haemorrhagic telangiectasia (HHT)

- It is also called *Osler-Weber-Rendu syndrome*
- It is autosomal dominant condition affecting blood vessels
- This can cause recurrent epistaxis or persistent epistaxis
- In such situations, we have the following treatment options:

Flowchart 2: Treatment of hereditary haemorrhagic talangiectasia

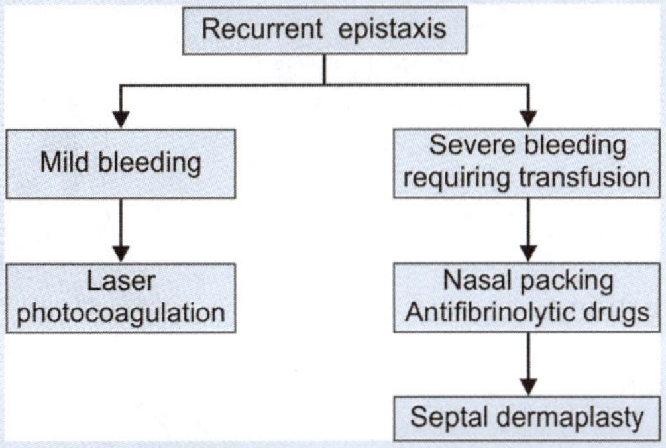

Last minute revision

- *During epistaxis sphenopalatine artery bleeds the most*
- *Nose picking/trauma is the most common cause of epistaxis*
- *Woodruff's plexus may cause posterior bleeding*
- *For epistaxis, pinching should be done for 5–10 minutes*
- *Cautery can be done with silver nitrate*
- *Transnasal endoscopic sphenopalatine artery ligation (TESPAL) is the last resort for epistaxis*
- *Septal dermaplasty may be done in epistaxis due to hereditary hemorrhagic telangiectasia.*

QUESTIONS

1. **Commonest cause of epistaxis in children is:**
   a. Trauma b. Foreign body
   c. Nasal diphtheria d. Enlarged adenoids
2. **Causes of epistaxis are all *except*:**
   a. Allergic rhinitis b. Foreign body
   c. Tumour d. Hypertension
3. **Epistaxis in elderly person is common in:**
   a. Foreign body
   b. Allergic rhinitis
   c. Hypertension
   d. Nasopharyngeal carcinoma
4. **In a 5-year-old child, common cause of unilateral epistaxis is:**
   a. Foreign body
   b. Nasal polyps
   c. Allergic rhinitis
   d. Maggots
5. **Recurrent epistaxis in a 15-year-old female is probably due to:**
   a. Juvenile angiofibroma
   b. Foreign body
   c. Rhinosporidiosis
   d. Hematologial disorders
6. **Treatment of choice in recurrent epistaxis due to hereditary telangiectasia is:**
   a. Anterior ethmoidal artery ligation
   b. Septal dermoplasty
   c. External carotid artery ligation
   d. Any of the above
7. **Regarding bleeding polypus of the nose, which one of the following is true?**
   a. It is an antro-choanal polyp
   b. It is a form of juvenile nasopharyngeal angiofibroma
   c. It is the other name for rhinosporidiasis
   d. It is a capillary haemangioma arising from nasal septum
8. **Source of epistaxis after ligation of external carotid artery is:**
   a. Maxillary artery
   b. Greater palatine artery
   c. Superior labial artery
   d. Ethmoidal artery
9. **Posterior epistaxis occurs from:**
   a. Woodruff's plexus
   b. Kiesselbach's plexus
   c. Atherosclerosis d. Little's area
10. **If posterior epistaxis cannot be controlled, which artery is ligated?**
    a. Posterior ethmoidal artery
    b. Maxillary artery
    c. Sphenopalatine artery
    d. External carotid artery

IMAGE BASED QUESTION

11. **Which is true of the structure that is pointed by arrow?**

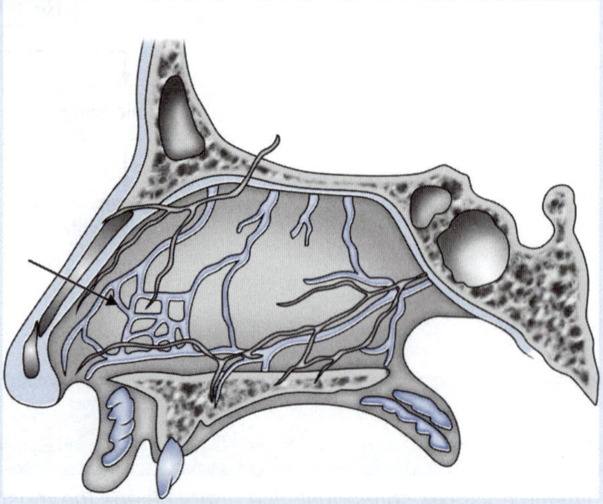

    a. This is Woodruff's plexus
    b. This plexus is formed by four arteries
    c. This is usually present on the vomar bone of the septum
    d. In epistaxis from this site, packing only in the bleeding side is the best treatment

ANSWERS AND EXPLANATIONS

1. **a. Trauma**
   The most common cause of epistaxis is ***nose picking or digital trauma of nose.***
   In elderly, the most common cause of epistaxis is hypertension.
   The most common site of nasal bleed is the Little's area. This is true for both in children as well as elderly
   The second most common site of bleed is retrocollumelar vein.
   Epistaxis may also be seen from Woodruff's plexus.
   This is not a common site of nasal bleed but in hypertensives, Woodruff's plexus may bleed.
   Note: Some books claim that most common site of epistaxis in hypertensives is Woodruff's plexus.

This is not true. Although Woodruff's plexus bleeds very commonly in hypertensives but the most common site remains **Little's area.**

2. **a. Allergic rhinitis**
   Allergic rhinitis usually does not cause epistaxis unless there is supra-added bacterial infection.
3. **c. Hypertension**
   The most common cause of epistaxis is nose picking or digital trauma of nose.
   In elderly the most common cause of epistaxis is hypertension.
   The most common site of nasal bleed is the Little's area. This is true for both in children as well as elderly
   The second most common site of bleed is retrocollumelar vein.
   Epistaxis may also be seen from Woodruff's plexus. This is not a common site of nasal bleed but in hypertensives, woodruff's plexus may bleed.
4. **a. Foreign body**
   In a small child, unilateral nasal bleed with/without foul smell is usually due to foreign body.
5. **d. Hematologial disorders**
   We know that juvenile angiofibroma is seen in juvenile males and NOT in females.
   Foreign body in nose is seen in children and not in adults.
   Rhinosporidiosis (strawberry polyps) has a different presentation.
6. **b. Septal dermoplasty**
   Septal dermoplasty is a procedure in which the ***mucoperichondrium of the nasal septum is replaced with split skin graft***.
   Septal mucoperichondrium has a very rich vascular supply and a plexus called Kiesselbach's plexus.
   Replacing this with split skin graft will reduce recurrent bleeding due to any cause. It is the last resort in patients with recurrent epistaxis due to hereditary telangiectasia and is very effective method of stopping bleeding.

MANAGEMENT OF EPISTAXIS IN HEREDITARY TELANGIECTASIA

- Nasal packing
- Antifibrolytic agents
- ***Laser photocoagulation***
- ***Septal dermoplasty***

7. **d. It is a capillary haemangioma arising from nasal septum**
   Bleeding polypus of septum is haemangioma and is a very important cause on nasal bleed.
   It is an ***inflammatory capillary haemangioma of the septum.***
   It is also called ***pyogenic granuloma.***
   - ***Bleeding polypus is pyogenic granuloma and strawberry polyp is rhinosporidiosis.***
   - Antro-choanal polyp usually does not bleed. In fact, if there is a bleeding mass in nose, it cannot be nasal polyp.
   - Nasopharyngeal angiofibroma and rhinosporidiosis commonly present as bleeding nasal mass but are not septal polypus.
   - Besides angiofibroma and rhinosporidiosis, other common bleeding mass of nose are Ringertz tumour and carcinoma of nose and sinuses.
8. **d. Ethmoidal artery**
   Nose has an extensive and rich blood supply. It is ssupplied from branches of both the:
   1. External carotid artery, and
   2. Internal carotid artery
   1. External carotid artery supplies the nose through three branches. These branches are:
      - Sphenopalatine artery
      - Greater palatine artery
      - Superior labial artery
   2. Internal carotid artery supplies through two arteries. These arteries are:
      - Anterior ethmoidal artery, and
      - Posterior ethmoidal artery

When external carotid artery is ligated, then its three branches cannot cause epistaxis. There bleeding is now only possible through the branches of internal carotid arteries, i.e. ethmoidal arteries.

9. **a. Woodruff's plexus.**
Woodruff's plexus is a venous plexus situated in the lateral wall of nose just behind the inferior turbinate.
It is NOT a very common site of epistaxis. But when it bleeds, it will cause posterior epistaxis.
Kiesselbach's plexus and Little's area are present in the anterior part of nasal septum. This usually causes anterior epistaxis.

10. **c. Sphenopalatine artery**
Posterior part of the nose is mainly supplied by sphenopalatine artery which is a branch of maxillary artery.
    - **The most commonly ligated artery for posterior epistaxis is the sphenopalatine artery.**
    - **If nasal endoscope is used for this then the name of the procedure is one of the two:**
        1. Transnasal endoscopic sphenopalatine artery ligation (TESPAL), or
        2. Endoscopic sphenopalatine artery ligation (ESPAL)
    - If this fails, the second artery ligated is the internal maxillary (IMAL)
    - Third artery to be ligated is the external carotid artery.

IMAGE BASED ANSWER

11. **b. This plexus is formed by four arteries**
This is ***kiesselbach's plexus*** which is present on the quadrilateral cartilage of the septum. Packing in both the nasal cavities is the best treatment.

CHAPTER

17 Rhinitis/Sinusitis (Rhinosinusitis)

Inflammatory conditions of nose and paranasal sinuses (PNS) are common.

Rhinitis is inflammation of the nasal cavity whereas sinusitis is the inflammation of the sinuses. These two are often related and present together. This condition is called **rhinosinusitis.**

Rhinitis and sinusitis are of many types and there are many types of classification given in various books. We are going to talk of rhinosinusitis. You are required to know about the following types:

Types of rhinosinusitis

a. Allergic rhinitis
b. Vasomotor rhinitis
c. Infective rhinitis
d. Irritative rhinitis
   - Simple chronic rhinitis
   - Hypertrophic rhinitis
   - Rhinitis caseosa
   - Rhinitis sicca
   - Atrophic rhinitis

ALLERGIC RHINITIS

The WHO initiative has divided the allergic rhinitis in two ways:

Flowchart 1: WHO classification of allergic rhinitis

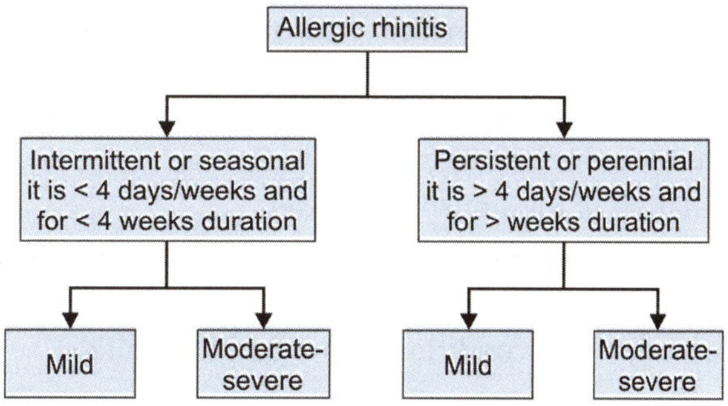

Most common allergen is **house dust.** This has a mite called *dermatophytes,* which is responsible for allergy.

Allergic rhinitis should have two or more of the following symptoms:

- ***Rhinorrhea/running nose***
- ***Nasal blockade***
- ***Itching, and***
- ***Sneezing***

Finding on rhinoscopy examination

- Nasal mucosa is **pale** color with edematous mucosa.
- This is described as **boggy and pale terminates.**
- There is **NO nasal congestion**.

- *Orbital congestion* is often seen with cobble stone appearance of conjunctiva.
- An important investigative finding is presence of ***eosinophils in the nasal discharge.***

Eosinophils in nasal discharge are also seen in other nasal conditions like
• Allergic fungal sinusitis (AFS), • Samter's Triad and • Non-allergic Rhinitis with eosinophilia syndrome (NARES)
Cobblestone conjunctiva is seen in allergic rhinitis whereas cobblestone glottis is seen in tuberculosis of larynx

NOTE:
In a condition called noneosinophilic allergic rhinitis, there is allergic rhinitis. But eosinophils are not raised
In Non-Allergic Rhinitis with Eosinophilia Syndrome (NARES), patient has high eosinophils in the nasal secretion with rhinitis but NO allergy

The main part of treatment is *avoidance* of the allergen and antihistamines.

In severe cases steroids (topical and systemic) may be useful

In chronic cases; **immunotherapy** may be used.

Immunotherapy is a clinical procedure where a controlled amount of allergen is given to the patient, which is gradually increased till a maintenance dose is reached.

Main advantage of immunotherapy is that it gives long-term relief.

The disadvantages are as given below:

- The results are unpredictable
- A very long procedure and hence compliance is not good
- Is a costly procedure
- Patient is often allergic to multiple allergens
- Can cause anaphylaxis and death

VASOMOTOR RHINITIS

This is also called **Non-allergic, non infectious inflammation of nose and PNS**

As we have already discussed, the nasal submucosal has **sinusoidal vascular system.**

This sinusoidal system is controlled by autonomic nervous system. This has both, the sympathetic and parasympathetic control.

In vasomotor rhinitis there is imbalance between the sympathetic and parasympathetic system such that there is increased **parasympathetic/secretomotor** discharge.

This causes vasodilatation or dilation of the sinusoidal vessels.

This in turn leads to **pooling of blood (lakes of blood** are formed) in submucosa and turbinates of nasal cavity.

The nasal turbinates get **engorged, boggy and bluish.**

Therefore, it is difficult to differentiate this condition from allergic rhinitis.

Pathophysiology of vasomotor rhinitis
Defect in the autonomic control ↓ Imbalance between sympathetic and parasympathetic stimulation ↓ Increased parasympathetic stimulation as compared the symapathetic stimulation ↓ Dilation of submucosal sinusoids and venules ↓ Pooling of blood ↓ Watery rhinorrhea and boggy turbinates

A very common presentation is ***early morning bouts or paroxysms of sneezing*** along with nasal blockade and discharge.

Nasal decongestants like oxymetazoline and xylometazoline are usually required.

Isotonic and hypertonic saline may be useful. These ***restore the ciliary motility in the nose.***

Since, the sympathetic and parasympathetic of nose is supplied by the vidian nerve (nerve of pterygoid canal)

Vidian neurectomy may be done in some patients.

Hence, ***vidian neurectomy*** may be indicated in *vasomotor rhinitis.*

INFECTIVE RHINOSINUSITIS

Infective rhinosinusitis can be of the following types:

- Viral
- Fungal
- Bacterial

Infective Rhinitis

Viral Rhinitis

Most common virus causing viral rhinitis is **rhinovirus.**

Fungal Sinusitis

A number of fungal infections can be seen in the nose and PNS.

Overall, the **most common fungus** to infect the nose is ***Aspergillus fumigatus.***

Fungal infections of nose can be divided into the follows:

Flowchart 2: Classification of fungal sinusitis

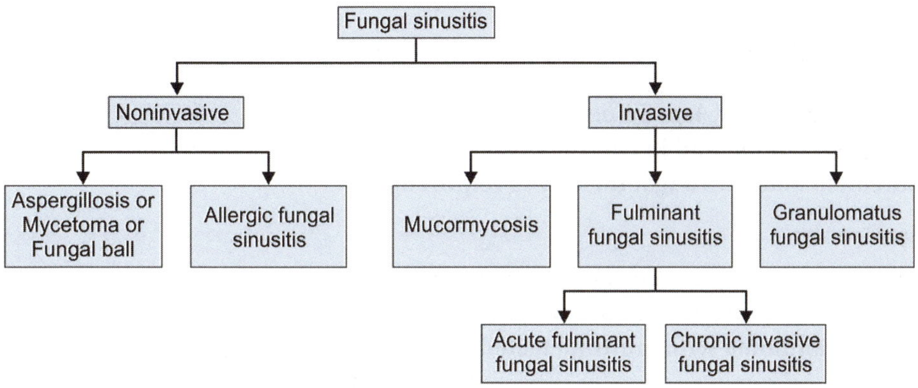

Aspergillosis

Aspergillosis it is the most common type of fungal sinusitis.

- It is caused by ***Aspergillus fumigatus.***
- It presents as ***persistent postnasal discharge and cacosmia (altered smell).***
- It leads to formation of ***aspergilloma or fungal ball*** in the nasal cavity.
- Excision or debridement is the treatment.

Allergic Fungal Sinusitis (AFS)

It is a **type 1 hypersensitivity** reaction to a fungal called **bipolaris.**

AFS is often associated with ***allergic bronchopulmonary aspergillosis (ABPA).***

There are five diagnostic criteria for AFS

1. The patient should be non immunocompromised
2. There should be **no** evidence of tissue invasion
3. Culture should show fungal growth
4. CT Scan shows hypoattenuation , and

5. On microscopic examination, necrotic eosinophilic mucin is seen in the nasal discharge. This nasal discharge called **eosinophilic mucin/allergic mucin** is seen in AFS.

This mucin may look like **peanut butter (peanut buttery mucin).**

This mucin has necrotic eosinophils with scattered fungal hyphae.

Treatment

- The main treatment requires ***corticosteroids and surgery.***
- The surgery of choice is **FESS.**

Some of the other treatment options for allergic fungal sinusitis are:

- Local nasal lavage with Amphotericin B
- Immunotherapy

Mucormycosis/Rhinocerebral Phycomycosis

It is mainly seen in *young immunocompromized patients like diabetics.*

It is an invasive fungal disease which is **angio-invasive.**

It mainly invades arteries and causes necrosis of the involved tissue and may spread to the neighbouring area like **orbital cavity and cranial cavity**.

Presentation

- ***Dark nasal discharge in diabetic person should raise the suspension of mucormycosis.***
- CT scan is done to see extension of the disease.
- Treatment involves *amphotericin B and FESS.*
- In case of evidence orbital spread of mucormycosis, the treatment is more aggressive.
- This includes ***amphotericin B and FESS along with orbital exenteration.***

Acute Fulminant Fungal Sinusitis and Chronic Invasive Fungal Sinusitis

- Acute fulminant fungal sinusitis is for < 4 weeks duration whereas chronic invasive fungal sinusitis is > 4-6 weeks duration.
- These conditions are causes by ***Aspergillus fumigatus.***
- **Pain is the main presentation and in chronic invasive fungal sinusitis, proptosis may be seen.**
- **Surgical debridement and antifungal therapy is required.**

Granulomatous Fungal Sinusitis

- Granulomatous fungal sinusitis is also called indolent fungal sinusitis.
- Granulomatous fungal sinusitis is caused by ***Aspergillus flavus.***
- This condition has **granuloma with multinucleated giant cells and unilateral histiocytes.**

Bacterial Rhinosinusitis

Bacterial rhinosinusitis are of the following types:

Types of bacterial rhinosinusitis	Criteria
1. Acute rhinosinusitis	• Duration < 12 weeks
2. Recurrent rhinosinusitis	• When there are 1-4 episodes of acute rhinosinusitis per year
3. Chronic rhinosinusitis	• Duration > 12 weeks and/or • Radiograph findings for > 4 weeks after starting medication
4. Acute exacerbation of chronic rhinosinusitis	• Worsening of existing symptoms

Acute bacterial sinusitis is mainly caused by three organisms. These three organisms are:

1. Streptococcus pneumonia also called pneumococcus,
2. ***H influenza***
3. ***Morexella catarrhalis***

Chronic bacterial sinusitis is mainly caused by ***Staphylococcus aureau.***

- Most common sinus having sinusitis is the **maxillary sinus**
- But in children the most common sinus involved is **ethmoidal sinus.**

Pathophysiology of rhinosinusitis

Patient has one of the following predisposing factors
- Viral infection (most common predisposing factor)
- Blockade of osteomeatal complex
- Kartagener's syndrome/Cystic fibrosis, etc.

↓

Swelling and occlusion of sinus

↓

Reduced oxygen tension in the sinus

↓

Transudation of fluid and thickening of mucus

↓

Defect in cilia beating in sinus

↓

Stasis of fluid in sinus

↓

Infection of static fluid

The criteria for the diagnosis of rhinosinusitis require:

1. **Two major criteria or**
2. **One major and two minor criteria from the following**

Major criteria/symptoms	Minor criteria/symptoms
• Facial pain/tenderness • Facial congestion • Nasal discharge • Hyposmia/anosmia • Fever • Pus in the nasal cavity	• Headache • Fever • Bad smell/halitosis • Fatigue • Dental pain • Cough • Earache

Tenderness at different site is present for different sinus involvement in rhinosinusitis.

Sinus involved	Site of tenderness
• Maxillary sinusitis	Cheek and alveolus
• Frontal sinus	Below eyebrow This patient also has "office headache"
• Ethmoidal sinusitis	Medial canthus of eye
• Sphenoidal sinusitis	Vertex of skull

IRRITATIVE RHINITIS

Irritative rhinitis can be of the following types:

- Simple chronic rhinitis
- Hypertrophic rhinitis

- Rhinitis caseosa
- Rhinitis sicca
- Atrophic rhinitis

Simple chronic rhinitis and hypertrophic rhinitis are different stages of the same process which occurs due to chronic insult of the nasal mucosa and turbinates.

Simple chronic rhinitis is the early stage of the process in which there is ***hyperaemia and oedema*** of nasal mucosa which **pits** on pressure and is an easily reversible stage.

Whereas, hypertrophic rhinitis has hypertrophy of mucosa that does **not pit** on pressure and is more difficult to reverse.

This hypertrophied turbinates in hypertrophic rhinitis gives **"mulberry like appearance".**

This may cause nasal obstruction and so may require **turbinectomy.**

Two new technologies that are gaining popularity are:

- Co-ablation turbinectomy/radiofrequency turbnectomy, and
- Argon plasma turbinectomy.

RHINITIS CASEOSA

- In this, there is cheesy material in the nasal cavity which looks like cholesteatoma.
- Hence it is also called ***cholesteatoma of nose***.
- Treatment is to clear nasal cavity

RHINITIS SICCA

- In this condition there is dryness in the nasal cavity.
- This is because:
- The normal nasal mucosa which normally is ***pseudostratified ciliated columnar*** epithelium; is replaced by ***squamous epithelium with atrophy of the secretory glands***.
- This occurs when patient works in hot and dry condition like bakeries, glass factories, steel factories, etc.
- The mainly affected area is the **anterior and inferior part of the nose** as this is the part of nose that is mainly exposed to the hot and dry environment.
- Treatment mainly involves prevention of the hot and dry environment.
- The other thing the patient can do is to apply oil based cream/ointment.

ATROPHIC RHINITIS / OZAENAE

In atrophic rhinitis the normal mucosa of the nose, which is pseudostratified *ciliated columnar epithelium also called* ***Schneiderian epithelium,*** is replaced by stratified squamous epithelium. In addition, there is atrophy of the glands with **endarteritis.**

As a result of this, the following are seen:

- Roomy cavity in the nose
- Dry cavity
- **Crust formation (cause of nasal obstruction)**
- Foul smell and
- Bleeding on touch.

Atrophic rhinitis can be two types:

1. primary atrophic rhinitis and
2. secondary atrophic rhinitis

Primary atrophic rhinitis is a condition where the cause is not known. There are many theories. Two main theories are:

a. Infective theory: Mainly caused by ***Klebsiella ozaenae.*** Therefore, this disease is also called **ozaenae**

b. Hormonal theory: It is believed to be due to reduced level of **oestrogen**

Secondary atrophic rhinitis is due to some other disease like syphilis, lupus, etc.

Main complaint in nasal obstruction which is due to crusting in the nose

Some patients have **merciful anosmia also called blissful anosmia.**

The diagnostic finding on rhinoscopic examination is presence of **greenish, dry and foul smelling discharge in widened nasal cavity**.

Sometimes, it may cause secondary infection with maggots.

The most important investigation is MRI. This can show the changes of mucosa and the bones.

Atrophic rhinitis is often confused with empty nose syndrome (ENS).
ENS is iatrogenic conditions, usually caused after "turbinectomy", which is done for turbinate hypertrophy.

Treatment

Medical option

- Alkaline nasal douching
  The content of alkaline nasal solution are:
  1. *Sodium bicarbonate*
  2. *Sodium biborate and*
  3. *Sodium chloride*

  It removes crust and changes the pH of the nasal cavity.
- **25% glucose mixed in glycerin**. This inhibits the growth of proteolytic organisms.
- There are **sprays of estrogen**
- Injections from **placental extract**.
- **Kemicetine solution,** which contains:
  1. Chloramphenicol
  2. Oestradiol
  3. Vitamin D_2
  4. Propylene glycol
- Systemic use of streptomycin
- Potassium iodide

Surgeries

- Young's and modified young's operation.
- Lautenslager's surgery.
  In this the ***lateral nasal wall mucosa is medialized.***
  This is achieved by placing a **silicon block between the lateral wall and its mucosa.**

DIFFERENCE BETWEEN RHINITIS SICCA AND ATROPHIC RHINITIS

In both these conditions there is change of ciliated columnar epithelium to squamous epithelium. The main differences are:

	Rhinitis sicca	Atrophic rhinitis
Cause	Environmental effect	Unknown cause
Area involved	Anteroinferiorly	Entire nose and sinus
Treatment	Avoidance of environment	Medicines and surgeries
Prognosis	Good	Poor/ Bad

Myiasis/maggots

It is the *larva* form of a fly called *chrysomya*.

It mainly presents as pain and bleeding from the nose.

Treatment of Maggots

First kill the larva with

- 10% diluted chloroform, or
- Turpentine oil

And then remove them with forceps.

Last minute revision

- *Allergic rhinitis is most commonly caused by house dust*
- *Vidian neurectomy may be required in vasomotor rhinitis*
- *Aspergillosis is the most common fungal sinusitis*
- *Mucormycosis is also called rhinocerebral phycomycosis. It spreads through blood vessels*
- *It is seen in diabetics and causes dark discharge*
- *Orbital exenteration is done when it spreads into the orbit*
- *Maxillary sinusitis is more common in adult. Ethmoidal sinusitis is moiré common in children*
- *Atrophic rhinitis is also called ozeana*
- *It has merciful anosmia*
- *Alkaline nasal douche contains*
  1. *Sodium bicarbonate*
  2. *Sodium biborate*
  3. *Sodium chloride*
- *Lautenslager surgery may be done in atrophic rhinitis. In this lateral wall is medialized*
- *Maggots are larva of chrysomya.*
- *Chloroform or turpentine oil is the treatment*

QUESTIONS

1. **Alkaline nasal douche contains all of the following *except:***
   a. Sodium chloride
   b. Sodium bicarbonate
   c. Sodium biborate
   d. Glucose
2. **Pathognomonic features of Maxillary sinusitis is:**
   a. Mucopus in the middle meatus
   b. Inferior turbinate hypertrophy
   c. Purulent nasal discharge
   d. Atrophic sinusitis
3. **True about allergic fungal sinusitis are a/e:**
   a. CT shows hyperdense
   b. Orbital penetration
   c. Type 1 hypersensitivity
   d. Corticosteroid is the drug of choice
4. **A 40-year-old diabetic presents with blackish nasal discharge and a mass in the nose likely diagnosis is:**
   a. Mucormycosis
   b. Actinomycosis
   c. Rhinosporidiosis
   d. Histoplasmosis
5. **Which of the following is the most common etiological agent in paranasal sinus mycoses?**
   a. Aspergillus spp.
   b. Histoplasma
   c. Conidiobolus coronatus
   d. Candida albicans
6. **Headache on sunrise and relief at sunset is seen in:**
   a. Maxillary sinusitis
   b. Frontal sinusitis
   c. Anterior ethmoidal sinusitis
   d. Posterior ethmoidal sinusitis
7. **All are true about ozaena *except:***
   a. Common in female
   b. It is usually unilateral
   c. Nasal cavity is filled with greenish crusts
   d. Atrophic pharyngitis
8. **Steroid not given**
   a. Post antrochoanal polyp
   b. Multiple ethmoidal polyp
   c. Postsurgery for chronic rhinosinusitis
   d. Postsurgery for fungal rhinosinusitis
9. **Mulberry like inferior turbinate is seen in:**
   a. Vasomotor rhinitis
   b. Chronic sinusitis
   c. hypertrophic rhinitis
   d. allergic rhinitis
10. **Vidian neurectomy is done in which of these?**
    a. Vasomotor rhinitis
    b. Rhinitis sicca
    c. Atrophic rhinitis
    d. Rhinitis caseosa
11. **Most common cause of nasal obstruction in atrophic rhinitis is?**
    a. Crust formation
    b. Polyps
    c. Synechiae formation
    d. Turbinate hypertrophy
12. **A person uses nasal drops continuously for a long time. Which of the following can be the adverse effect?**
    a. Allergic rhinitis
    b. Vasomotor rhinitis
    c. Mulberry turbinates
    d. Rhinitis medicamentosa
13. **Which of the following is incorrect about atrophic rhinitis?**
    a. Common in females
    b. Seen in 50-60 age groups
    c. Can occur secondary to syphilis
    d. Anosmia
14. **Common organisms causing acute sinusitis are all *except*:**
    a. *Pseudomonas*
    b. *Moraxella catarrhalis*
    c. *Streptococcus pneumoniae*
    d. *H. influenzae*
15. **Most definitive diagnostic of sinusitis is:**
    a. Proof puncture
    b. Diagnostic nasal endoscopy
    c. Transillumination test
    d. X-ray PNS
16. **A 35-year-old male presents with nasal discharge, fever and Facial pain. These symptoms subside with medication. The symptoms recur again after 2 months. On examination, there is mucopurulent discharge in the middle meatus and inflamed sinus opening. Which is the investigation of choice?**
    a. X-ray PNS
    b. CT Scan of PNS
    c. MRI
    d. Inferior meatal puncture

ANSWERS AND EXPLANATIONS

1. **d. Glucose**

Alkaline nasal douche is a solution which is used for treatment of atrophic rhinitis and it contains

- Sodium chloride,
- Sodium bicarbonate and
- Sodium biborate

Glucose is NOT present in the alkaline nasal douche.

The other solution used in atrophic rhinitis is ***Kimecetin solution.***

It contains:

1. Chloramphenicol
2. Oestradiol
3. Vitamin D_2
4. Propylene glycol

2. **a. Mucopus in the middle meatus**

Maxillary sinus ostium opens in the infundibulum in the middle meatus. Hence in cases of maxillary sinusitis, pus from maxilla will come in the middle meatus through the infundibulum. This is pathognomic of maxillary sinusitis

This mucopus can be seen either by:

- Anterior rhinoscopy examination or
- Diagnostic nasal endoscopy,.

Inferior turbinate hypertrophy, purulent nasal discharge and atrophic rhinitis are features of rhinitis and NOT sinusitis.

Other criteria of sinusitis are:

Major criteria/symptoms	Minor criteria/symptoms
• Facial pain/tenderness	• Headache
• Facial congestion	• Fever
• Nasal discharge	• Bad smell/halitosis
• Hyposmia/anosmia	• Fatigue
• Fever	• Dental pain
• Pus in the nasal cavity	• Cough
	• Ear ache

3. **b. Orbital penetration**

Allergic fungal sinusitis is a noninvasive fungal disease of the nose and PNS. In this the patient has hypersensitivity to the fungus. CT Scan shows hyperdensity and steroids are the main drugs given.

Orbital penetration is usually seen in invasive fungal disease like mucormycosis.

There are five diagnostic criteria for allergic fungal sinusitis (AFS).

1. ***The patient should be non immunocompromised***
2. ***There should be no evidence of tissue invasion***
3. ***Culture should show fungal growth***
4. ***CT Scan shows hypoattenuation, and***
5. ***On microscopic examination, necrotic eosinophilic mucin is seen in the nasal discharge.***

4. **a. Mucormycosis**

Mucormycosis is the most dangerous fungal disease of nose and sinuses. It is usually seen in elderly patients who are immunocompromised like diabetics.

Hence, the above mentioned patient is most probably a case of mucormycosis.

Mucormycosis is an angioinvasive fungal disease of the nose and causes necrosis. This causes dark/black nasal discharge.

Fungal Diseases of the Nose and Sinuses

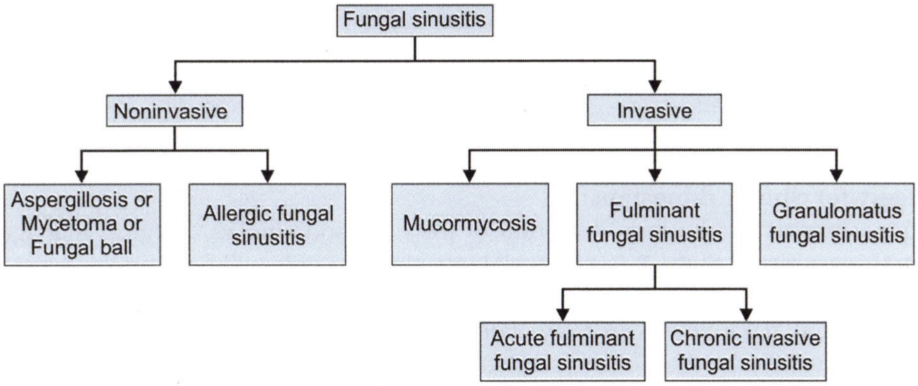

5. **a. Aspergillus spp.**

Fungal Rhinosinusitis

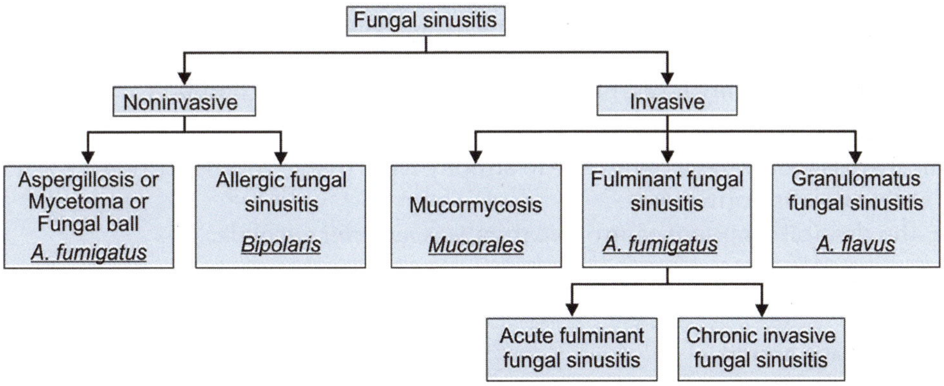

As seen from the above chart, aspergillus is the most common fungi causing fungal rhinosinusitis.

6. **b. Frontal sinusitis**
Headache on sunrise and relief at sunset is called office headache. This is a typical feature of frontal sinusitis. This is also called ***office headache.***

Different Sinusitis and their Tender Site

Sinus involved	Site of tenderness
• Maxillary sinusitis	Cheek and alveolus
• Frontal sinus	Below eyebrow This patient also has **"office headache"**
• Ethmoidal sinusitis	Medial canthus of eye
• Sphenoidal sinusitis	Vertex of skull

7. **b. It is usually unilateral**
Ozaena also called **atrophic rhinitis** is a chronic inflammatory disease of both the nasal cavities.
It is usually a nasal manifestation of some systemic disease and therefore involves both the nasal cavity and may extend to involve other part of upper respirtory pathway lie nasopharynx, sinuses, oropharynx and larynx. Therefore, these patients may have symptoms of pharynx and larynx in addition to nasal symptoms.

Causes of Atrophic Rhinitis (Ozaena)

- Hereditary
- Endocrinal (low estrogen)
- Racial

- Nutritional (Vit D deficiency)
- Infection (***klebsiella ozeana)***, etc.

Ozaena is more common in females as compared to males

The most common symptom is nasal obstruction. Some may have ***merciful anosmia***.

The most significant finding is the presence of greenish crust in both the nasal cavities with atrophy of mucosa and turbinates.

There are lots of medical and surgical options to treat this condition but the results, at best, are average.

8. **c. Postsurgery for chronic rhinosinusitis**

Chronic rhinosinusitis is a bacterial infection of the nose and sinuses. Surgical management is sometimes required in these patients. Since, it is a bacterial infection, steroids will flare up the disease.

Nasal polyps are sometimes caused due to allergy. Therefore, they respond very well to steroids. Postsurgical steroid in cases of all nasal polyps are very effective in preventing recurrence of polyps.

In fungal rhinosinusitis, the drug of choice is steroid. Steroids along with surgery is the main treatment.

9. **c. hypertrophic rhinitis**

In hypertrophic rhinitis the inferior turbinate is described as "***mulberry turbinate***"

The cause of this chronic hypertrophy could be any.

10. **a. Vasomotor rhinitis**

Vasomotor rhinitis is caused due to imbalance between parasympathetic and sympathetic supply from the vidian nerve.

Therefore, vidian neurectomy is one of the treatment options in this condition.

11. **a. Crust formation**

In atrophic there is roomy nasal cavity due to atrophy nasal tissue, yet obstruction is the main symptom. This is due to excessive crust formation.

However, the classical symptom of atrophic rhinitis is ***merciful ansomia.***

12. **d. Rhinitis medicamentosa**

One of the main problems of long-term usage of nasal drops is rhinitis medicamentosa.

13. **b. Seen in 50-60 age groups**

Atrophic rhinitis can be caused due to number of reasons. One of the most common cause of this condition is reduced estrogen levels in **young females** (NOT 50-60 years old).

14. **a. Pseudomonas**

Acute bacterial sinusitis is mainly caused by three organisms. These three organisms are:

1. ***Streptococcus pneumonia also called pneumococcus,***
2. ***H influenza,***
3. ***Morexella catarrhalis***

Chronic bacterial sinusitis is mainly caused by ***Staphylococcus aureus.***

15. **b. Diagnostic nasal endoscopy**

Presence of mucopus in the middle meatus on diagnostic nasal endoscopy is the most diagnostic feature of sinusitis.

16. **b. CT Scan of PNS**

This is most likely a case of chronic sinusitis. CT scan will confirm this condition as well as show the status of osteomeatal complex. This will also help us in deciding the treatment modality.

CHAPTER

18 Complications of Rhinosinusitis

As we have discussed, some of the commonest causes of rhinosinusitis are allergy and viral infections. These types of rhinosinusitis do NOT cause complications. Therefore, complications are uncommon in these patients. Complications are relatively more common in bacterial rhinosinusitis.

One of the **most common complications of rhinosinusitis is osteomyelitis of the frontal bone.**

Osteomyelitits is more commonly seen in patients with maxillary sinusitis.

Some of the important complications of rhinosinusitis are given below.

OSTEOMYELITIS

Osteomyelitis is one of the most common complications of rhinosinusitis.

This complication is more common in maxillary sinusitis.

The most common bony involved in osteomyelitis is the frontal bone.

In children the frontal bone is NOT developed (we have already discussed) and therefore, osteomyelitis in children is seen in maxillary bone.

The osteomyelitis of the frontal bone may lead to subperiosteal abscess. This is called **Pott's puffy tumour.**

MUCOCELE/PYOCELE

Mucocele is a mucus-filled and epithelial lined sac in the sinus.

Mucocele releases lot of bone erosing factors like prostaglandins, leukocytes, cytokines etc. leading to **osteolysis, bone erosion and bone expansion.**

Mucocoele is most commonly seen in frontal sinus or frontoethmoidal complex.

It is most commonly formed as a complication of ***chronic frontal sinusitis***.

When the mucus gets infected it is called **pyocele**

The typical presentation of frontal mucocele is, ***swelling between the medial cantus in the eyeball and the eyebrow***. It pushes the eye and causes ***downward and outward proptosis.***

There are two signs.

1. ***Egg shell crackling sign:*** Walls of sinus ultimately become so thin that they crack into pieces but the pieces of bone are held together by periosteum. Not visible but on touching there is crackling sound.
2. ***Loss of scallops:*** A radiological sign.

Investigation of choice is CT scan.

Treatment is surgical excision of mucocele or FESS.

ORBITAL COMPLICATIONS

Although orbital complications are NOT common, they commonly asked in the examination.

Orbital complications are commonly seen in patients with ***ethmoidal sinusitis.***

Orbital complications are divided into the following types:

- ***Preseptal cellulitis***
- ***Subperiosteal abscess***
- ***Orbital cellulitis***

- *Orbital abscess*
- *Superior orbital fissure syndrome*
- *Orbital apex syndrome*

IMPORTANT FACTS THAT YOU MUST KNOW

Superior Orbital Fissure Syndrome

In superior orbital fissure syndrome there is the involvement of superior orbit fissure by a disease. It can be caused by a number of diseases/conditions.

It can also be seen when the inflammation of rhinosinusitis spreads to involve the superior orbital fissure.

It is also called **Rochon-Duvigneaud's syndrome.**

As the name suggests, the superior orbital fissure is involved and the **nerves passing through this fissure are affected.** These nerves are:

- IIIrd cranial nerve
- IVth cranial nerve
- V1 (ophthalmic division of trigeminal) nerve, and
- VIth cranial nerve. This is the **first nerve that is involved in superior orbital fissure syndrome.**

Orbital Apex Syndrome

Orbital apex syndrome is sometimes WRONGLY called **Jacod's syndrome.**

However, in Jacod's syndrome all the features of orbital apex syndrome are also seen along with few more symptoms.

In this syndrome, the orbital apex is involved and therefore involves the optic nerve (IInd cranial nerve) leading to vision problems.

Tolosa-Hunt Syndrome is similar to superior orbital fissure syndrome, this is idiopathic in nature. Most probably it is caused by granulomatous inflammation of the area.

INTRACRANIAL COMPLICATIONS

Intracranial complications of rhinosinusitis are similar to the ones discussed in CSOM (EAR). One important intracranial complication that you should know is *Cavernous sinus thrombosis.*

Cavernous Sinus Thrombosis/Cavernous Sinus Syndrome

In cavernous sinus thrombosis, the inflammation spreads to the cavernous sinus and involves all the nerves passing through it.

The presentation of cavernous sinus syndrome and orbital cellulitis are very similar.

The important differences are given below.

Orbital cellulitis	Cavernous sinus syndrome/thrombosis
Is unilateral	Is bilateral
Onset is slow	Onset is abrupt/sudden
No chills and rigor	Chills and rigor are very common
Periorbital oedema, chemosis, proptosis and vision problems are common	Along with periorbital oedema, chemosis, proptosis, visoion problems—ophthalmoplegia is also seen.

In case of rhinosinusitis causing orbital complications, these three syndromes (superior orbital fissure syndrome, orbital apex syndrome and cavernous sinus syndrome) happen in a sequential manner.
The sequence is:

Rhinosinusitis (usually ethmoidal)
↓
Superior orbital fissure syndrome
↓
Orbital apex syndrome
↓
Cavernous sinus syndrome

Last minute revision

- Osteomyelitis is the most common complication of sinusitis
- It can also cause potts puffy tumour on the frontal bone
- Mucocele is seen in frontal sinus
- Mucocele has
  - Egg shell crackling sign
  - Loss of scallops
  - FESS is best treatment
- Cavernous sinus thrombophlebitis is the most dangerous complication of sinusitis
- It presents as
  - Sudden fever with chills
  - Chemosis, ophthalmoplegia periorbital oedema, proptosis, diminution of vision etc.

QUESTIONS

1. **Which of the following is a feature of frontal mucocele?**
   a. Straight forward proptosis
   b. Downward and outward proptosis
   c. Downward and inward proptosis
   d. Upward proptosis
2. **Complication of sinusitis include:**
   a. Orbital cellulitis
   b. Cavernous sinus thrombosis
   c. Superior orbital fissure syndrome
   d. All of the above
3. **A patient with sinusitis develops chemosis, B/L proptosis and fever. The diagnosis is:**
   a. Lateral sinus thrombosis
   b. Frontal lobe abscess
   c. Cavernous sinus thrombosis
   d. Meningitis
4. **Most common site of osteoma is:**
   a. Frontal bone b. Ethmoidal bone
   c. Maxillary bone d. Sphenoidal bone
5. **Infection within the right cavernous sinus results in the following *except:***
   a. Constricted pupil to light response
   b. Engorgement of retinal veins
   c. Ptosis of right eyelid
   d. Right ophthalmoplagia
6. **Which of the following statements is true:**
   a. In chronic rhinosinusitis, osteolytic activity is more as compared osteogenesis and sclerosis.
   b. In acute sinusitis, osteogenesis and sclerosis is more than osteolysis.
   c. In mucocoele, osteolysis is mainly due to pressure from the mucocoele.
   d. In mucocoele, the osteolysis is mainly due to release of bone erosion factors like prostaglandins, leukotrines and cytokines.
7. **A young man with a long history of sinusitis presents with frequent episodes of fever, headache with personality changes. Fundus examination reveals papilloedema. Most likely cause is:**
   a. Frontal lobe abscess
   b. Meningitis
   c. Orbital cellulitis
   d. Encephalitis
8. **Orbital cellulitis most commonly occurs after which sinus infection?**
   a. Frontal sinus
   b. Ethmoidal sinus
   c. Maxillary sinus
   d. Sphenoidal sinus

ANSWERS AND EXPLANATIONS

1. **b. Downward and outward proptosis**
   Mucocele is most commonly seen in the frontal sinus and is formed as a complication of chronic frontal sinusitis.
   It usually presents as swelling near the medial end of the eyebrow. Hence, when it enlarges enough, it may push the eyeball forward, downward and outward.
   This is downward and outward proptosis.
   Two important signs seen in mucocele are
   1. Egg shell crackling sign and
   2. Loss of scallops.
   Investigation of choice is CT Scan and treatment of choice is surgical excision of mucocele. The surgery of choice is FESS.
2. **d. All of the above**
   All of the mentioned are orbital complications of sinusitis.
   Orbital complications are divided into the following types:
   - ***Preseptal cellulitis***
   - ***Subperiosteal abscess***
   - ***Orbital cellulitis***
   - ***Orbital abscess***
   - ***Superior orbital fissure syndrome***
   - ***Orbital apex syndrome***
3. **c. Cavernous sinus thrombosis**
   These are features of cavernous sinus thrombosis.

Cavernous sinus thrombosis can happen from any of the five sinuses.
The main features of cavernous sinus thrombosis are:

- Fever with chills and rigor
- Bilateral involvement of nerves running through it (III, IV, V, VI) and ophthalmoplegia.
- Orbital findings like ***chemosis, proptosis, papilloedema, diminution of vision.***
  - Lateral sinus thrombosis has ***picket fence fever***

  It has signs like ***Tobey Ayer sign, crow beck sign, delta sign, Gresinger sign***
  - Frontal lobe abscess and meningitis will have cranial symptoms. Additionally frontal lobe abscess may cause ***papilloedema and personality changes.***

4. **a. Frontal bone**
   Osteomas are benign tumour of the skull. In sinuses it is more common in frontal bone.
5. **a. Constricted pupil to light response**
   Pupils in this case may be non responsive as they are dilated and fixed.
6. **d. In mucocoele, the osteolysis is mainly due to release of bone erosion factors like prostaglandins, leukotrines and cytokines.**
7. **a. Frontal lobe abscess**
   Refer to answer no 3.
8. **b. Ethmoidal sinus**
   Orbital cellulitis is one of the orbital complication of sinusitis.
   Orbital complications can happen from any of the four sinusitis. This is because
   Orbit is surrounded by sinuses from all the sides and all the sinuses have common boundary with orbit.

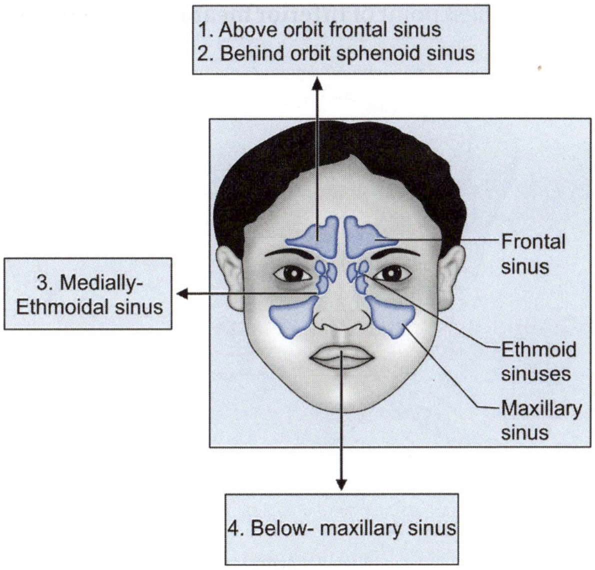

From the above diagram we can see that all the sinuses have common boundary with orbit and therefore infection from all the sinuses can reach the orbit causing orbital complications.
The boundary between ethmoidal sinus with orbit is the ***thinnest and weakes boundaryt.*** This boundary is formed by a ***paper thin bone called lamina papyrecea.*** Therefore ethmoidal sinus can cause orbital cellulitis more commonly as compared to the other sinuses.

CHAPTER

19

Surgery for Sinus

ANTRAL LAVAGE AND INFERIOR MEATAL ANTROSTOMY

These two procedures are very similar with similar principles.

Antral lavage is also called **antral wash.**

If the same procedure is done for **diagnosis of maxillary sinusitis**, the name changes to **proof puncture** (already discussed).

It is done only for maxillary sinusitis.

The two main indications are:

- Chronic maxillary sinusitis
- It is the full proof procedure for conformation of maxillary sinusitis.

A fistula or puncture is made at the highest point of **inferior meatus**. Maxillary lavage is done through this puncture.

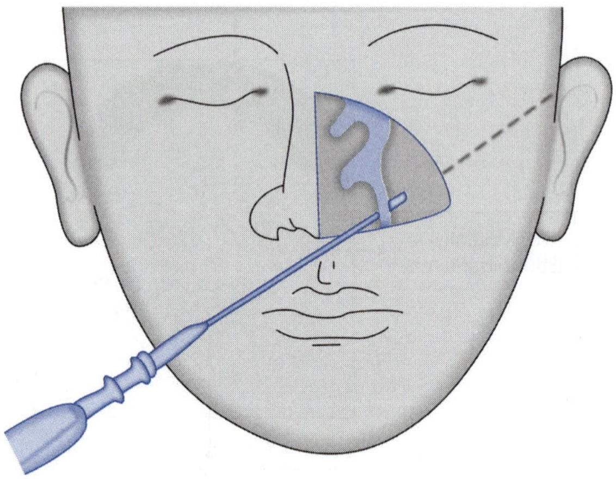

Fig. 1: Antral lavage

The instrument used for creating the fistula in the inferior meatus is called:

- Tilley Lichtwiz trocer and cannula

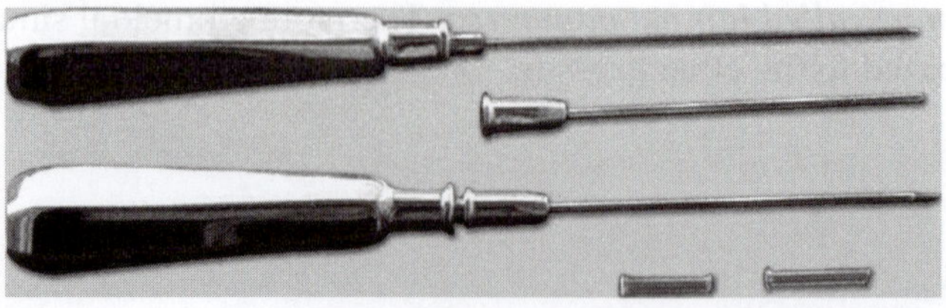

Fig. 2: Tilley Lichtwiz trocar and cannula

The syringe used for lavage is called:

- Higginson's syringe

Complications:

1. Permanent fistula called naso-antral fistula.
2. Osteomyelitis of the medial wall of maxilla
3. Trauma to adjoining structures like nasolacrimal duct (it is near inferior meatus) ***orbital***, cheek etc.
4. Fatal complication like *air embolism.*

CALDWELL LUC'S SURGERY

Caldwell Luc's surgery is another surgery of maxillary sinus.

There are a number of indications:

- Chronic or recurrent maxillary sinusitis. This is the most common indication
- Removal of benign tumors of maxilla like maxillary polyps and cysts
- Removal of foreign body like dentures
- Biopsy for suspicion of malignancy. This is controversial as some believe this will create a pathway for the spread of tumor
- Closure of oro-antral fistula. But this is **not** the primary treatment. In case of oro-antral fistula, conservative treatment is done up to 2 weeks. If this fails to close the fistula, then, surgery is done
- Repair of blow out fracture
- Initial stage of other surgeries like ligation of maxillary artery, approach to nasopharynx and ethmoid.

Incision—***Sub-labial incision is given at the gingivo labial sulcus.***

It extends from **lateral incisor to 2nd premolar.**

After this a puncture is made in **canine fossa** on the anterior wall of maxilla.

Through this opening/window the surgery is done inside the maxillary cavity.

Complications:

- Osteomyelitis
- Fistula called oroantral/gingivo-antral fistula
- Dental trauma
- Damage to ***infra orbital nerve.*** This will lead to cheek, upper lip and ala of nose anesthesia.
- Damage to ***superior alveolar nerve.***

TREPHANING OF FRONTAL SINUS

- This is one of the oldest methods for clearing the disease from the frontal sinus
- During this procedure a 1 cm incision is made ***just above the medial end of the eyebrow***
- The eyebrow will hide the scar mark
- Through this opening, the frontal bone is drilled and opened
- Nowadays, the endoscope is also used in this procedure

OSTEOPLASTIC FLAP SURGERY

- This surgery is done for extensive disease in the frontal sinus
- This gives a complete view of the frontal sinus.

LYNCH AND HOWARTH FRONTO-ETHMOIDECTOMY

- This surgery is also called **external ethmoidectomy**
- In this surgery the frontal sinus is drained via an ethmoidectomy
- ***The Lynch-Howarth incision (curved and concave incision) is given between the medial cantus of eye and the nasal bridge***

  Through this incision the anterior ethmoidal cells are cleared and the drainage pathway for the frontal sinus established.

INTRANASAL ETHMOIDECTOMY

- This procedure is replaced by FESS and so is not done commonly
- As the name suggests, it is used to clear inflammations and polyps from ethmoidal sinus.

TRANSANTRAL ETHMOIDECTOMY (JANSEN-HORGAN SURGERY)

- This procedure is also called **Jansen-Horgan procedure**
- During this procedure the ethmoidectomy is done through the antrum or maxilla.

FESS /ESS (Functional Endoscopic Sinus Surgery)

This has replaced almost all other surgeries.

Advantages:

- Almost all the sinuses can be operated
- Almost all the diseases can be treated with FESS
- FESS can also be done for diseases which are outside the nose and sinuses
- Complications are few
- No external scar etc.

  Almost always the first step during FESS is **uncinectomy and widening of maxillary ostia.**

As mentioned above, FESS can be done for diseases that are outside the nose and sinuses. Some examples are:

- **Repair of CSF rhinorrhea**
- **Choanal atresia**
- **Transnasal endoscopic sphenopalatine artery ligation (TESPAL), in cases of epistaxis**
- **Endoscopic dacryocystorhinostomy (endo DCR)**
- **Orbital decompression**—when there is too much extra-ocular fat
- **Optic nerve decompression**
- **Endoscopic hypophysectomy, etc.**

Complications:

Complications during FESS are not common. The only important and serious ones are:

1. Orbital complications:
   - This happens due to damage of lamina papyracea
   - This may cause collection of blood into the orbit
   - Orbital complication can be prevented by using **Stankiewicz sign** during the surgery.
2. Intracranial complication due to damage of **cribriform plate.**
   - This can cause **CSF rhinorrhea.**
   - ***Surgical fracture (FESS) of the cribriform plate is the most common cause of CSF Rhinorrhea.***

How to Prevent these Complications During FESS

- Using **microdebrider: Microdebrider** is powered instrument which cuts the soft tissue (polyps) very efficiently and quickly and it does not damage the bone. Therefore, bony dehiscence is almost absent. It is used for extensive nasal polyposis/ ethmoidal polyps.
- **Stankiewicz sign:** During the procedure of FESS, we keep pushing the orbit medially. If there is a breach of lamina papyracea, this movement can be seen through the endoscope in the nose.
- Keeping the eye uncovered (do not drape the eye) during the surgery.

BALLOON SINOPLASTY

It is a recent advancement in nasal procedures in which a deflated balloon is inserted in the ostia and then inflated to open it.

It is noninvasive technique for the treatment of sinusitis and holds great promise when done in combination with FESS.

Sinuses	Maxillary	Frontal	Ethmoid	Sphenoid
X-ray view	Water's view	Caldwell's view	Basal view	Basal view
Surgical options	• Antral wash • Inferior antrostomy • Caldwell Luc's Sx • FESS	• Trephaning • Osteoplastic flap • Lynch-Howarth Sx • Rhinofrontal sinuseptotomy or Lothrop Sx • FESS	• Lynch-Howarth Sx • Intranasal ethmoidectomy • Transantral ethmoidectomy or • Jansen-Horgan Sx • FESS	• FESS

Last minute revision

- In antral wash, puncture is made in the inferior meatus
- In Caldwell Luc's surgery, the incision iis given at the gingivo-buccal sulcus and maxilla is entered through canine fossa
- Infraorbital nerve may be damaged in Caldwell Luc's surgery
- FESS is the best surgery for nasal and sinus pathology
- Other surgeries that can be done with FESS are:
  - Endoscopic dacryocystorhinostomy
  - Endoscopic orbital decompression
  - Orbit nerve decompression
  - Endoscopic hypophysectomy etc.

QUESTIONS

1. **Transnasal endoscopic approach is used for surgical access to all of the following organ *except:***
   a. Lacrimal sac b. Cerebellum
   c. Pituitary gland d. Optic nerve
2. **Caldwell Luc operation is done in:**
   a. Maxillary sinusitis b. Ethmoidal sinusitis
   c. Sphenoidal sinusitis d. Frontal sinusitis
3. **Lynch-Howarth surgery is for:**
   a. Nasal septal perforation
   b. Sinonasal tumors
   c. Acoustic neuroma d. Otosclerosis
4. **The current treatment of choice for a large antro-choanal polyp in a 30-year-old man is:**
   a. Intranasal polypectomy
   b. Caldweld Luc operation
   c. ESS (endoscopic sinus surgery)
   d. Lateral rhinotomy and excision
5. **To prevent synachiae formation after nasal surgery, which one of the following packings is the most useful:**
   a. Mitomycin b. Ribbon gauze
   c. Ribbon gauze with liquid paraffin
   d. Ribbon gauze steroids
6. **To prevent synechiae formation after nasal surgery, which one of the following packings is the most useful?**
   a. Mitomycin
   b. Ribbon gauze
   c. Ribbon gauze with liquid paraffin
   d. Ribbon gauze steroids
7. **Child with battery as foreign body in the nose. Which of the following is an important concern?**
   a. Refer to specialist and plan for elective removal
   b. Local release of chemicals from battery and cause tissue destruction
   c. Rhinolith formation
   d. Septal abscess formation

IMAGE BASED QUESTION

8. **What surgery is being performed:**

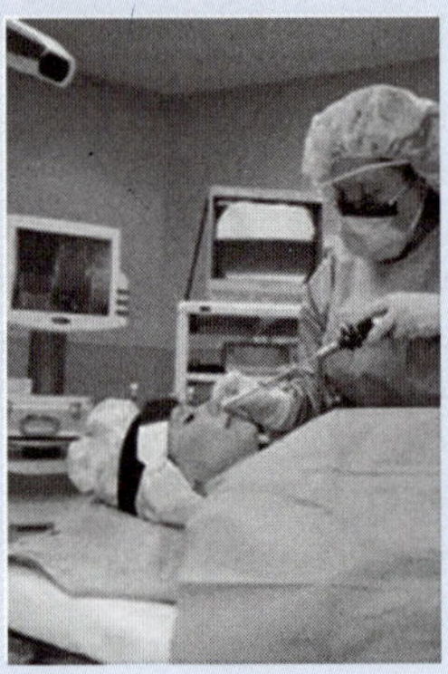

   a. Antral wash
   b. FESS
   c. Tympanoplasty
   d. Mastoidectomy

ANSWERS AND EXPLANATIONS

1. **b. Cerebellum**

Transnasal endoscopic surgeries commonly called **FESS.** This surgery has seen lot of advancement in the last few years. FESS is not only done for nasal and sinus diseases but is also done for diseases outsides the bound of nose and sinuses.

Few such examples are:

- Endoscopic DCR (dacryocystorhinostomy) is done to deal with cases of nasolacrimal duct obstruction in which the medial wall of lacrimal sac is removed via transnasal approach.
- Transnasal hypophysectomy is used for pituitary adenoma.
- Endonasal optic nerve decompression is done when this nerve compresses usually with a hemotoma.
  - Nowadays, FESS is done using powered cutting instruments.
  - Endoscopic nasal surgery is also done in combination with microscopy called ***combined microscopic and endoscopic technique (COMET).***
  - Latest in endoscopic nasal surgery is ***stereotactic surgery.*** For stereotactic nasal surgery a number of technologies are available. Some of them are:
    1. VTI instatrak
    2. Medtronic Xomed LandmarX system
    3. BrainLAB Vectorvision and Kolibri ENT
    4. Stryker navigation system etc.

2. **a. Maxillary sinusitis**
Caldwell Luc operation is done in the maxillary sinus. In this surgery, sublabial incision is given which extends from 2nd incisor to 2nd premolar to expose the maxilla.
Important indications of Caldwell Luc operation are:
- Chronic/recurrent maxillary sinusitis
- Removal of benign growths like antro-choanal polyp, maxillary cyst, etc
- Biopsy from maxilla
- Removal of foreign body from maxilla
- Closure of oroantral fistula, etc.

Important complications of Caldwell surgery are:
- Trauma to infra-orbital nerve leading to anesthesia to teeth and cheek
- Denture trauma
- Sublabial fistula, etc

3. **b. Sinonasal tumors**
Lynch Howarth surgery is done for diseases of frontal sinus and ethmoidal sinus like sinonasal tumors as shown below.

OTHER IMPORTANT SURGERIES OF SINUSES

Sinuses	Maxillary	Frontal	Ethmoid	Sphenoid
X-ray view	Water's view	Caldwell's view	Basal view	Basal view
Surgical options	• Antral wash • Inferior antrostomy • Caldwell Luc's Sx	• Trephaning • Osteoplatic flap • **Lynch-Howarth Sx**	• **Lynch-Howarth Sx** • Intranasal ethmoidectomy	
	• FESS	• Rhinofrontal sinuseptotomy or • Lothrop Sx • FESS	• Transantral ethmoidectomy or • Jansen-Horgan Sx • FESS	• FESS

- Acoustic neuroma is a tumor of vestibular nerve at the cerebellopontine (C-P) angle near the ear. Surgical approaches are:
  - Middle cranial fossa approach
  - Retrosigmoid suboccipital approach
  - Labyrinthine approach
  - Combined approach
- In patients of otosclerosis the surgical options are:
  - ***Stapedectomy***
  - ***Stapedotomy and***
  - ***Fenestration surgery (Type V tympanoplasty)***

4. **c. Endoscopic sinus surgery (ESS)**
Antrochoanal polyp is also called maxillary polyp. It is more common in children and is unilateral.
- The treatment of this is surgical excision. All of the above mentioned surgeries can be done in this case.
- Intranasal polypectomy is the treatment of choice in children whose maxilla is still growing; but this can lead to recurrence.
- The current choice both in children as well as adult would be ESS. This is the least traumatic surgery with equal or better result compared the other mentioned surgeries.
- Caldwell Luc's surgery is preferred for recurrent antrochoanal polyp.
- Rhinotomy and excision is done for extensive polyp and nasopharyngeal tumors.

5. **a. Mitomycin**
Mitamycin-C is an anticancer drug. One of the common complications of nasal packing (specially packing after nasal surgeries) is synechiae formation. A number of methods are being done to prevent this. One of the methods is the application of mitamycin-C in the nasal mucosa.

Methods for Prevention of Synechiae Formation after Nasal Surgeries are

- *Pack the nose with soframycin pack*
- *Place merocele in the nasal cavity*
- *Application of mitomycin-C in the nose, etc.*

Mitomycin-C is also used for treatment of:

- *Laryngeal stenosis, and*
- *Tracheal stenosis*

6. **a. Mitomycin**

Nasal cavity is a very narrow cavity. Moreover, during nasal surgeries like septoplasty, SMR, FESS, etc; the nasal wall gets edematous and traumatized. All this leads to formation of synechiae/adhesions in the nasal cavity.

Knowing this, it is advisable to take steps to prevent postsurgical synechiae formation.

Some of the Common Steps are:

- Application of mitomycin-C in the nasal cavity. This is the best method.
  - About mitomycin-C:
    - The mitomycins are a family of aziridine-containing natural products isolated from *Streptomyces caespitosus* or *Streptomyces lavendulae.*
    - *Application of mitomycin*-C onto the mucosa immediately following dilatation will decrease restenosis by decreasing the production of fibroblasts and scar tissue.
- Nasal packing with **BIPP (bismuth iodide potassium phosphate)**
- Placement of **merocele** in the nasal cavity
- Packing nose with ribbon gauze smeared with soframycin or betadine ointment
- Packing the nose with ribbon gauze smeared with liquid paraffin.
- Steroid is not used

7. **b. Local release of chemicals from battery and cause tissue destruction**

The chemical from battery can cause tissue damage and adhesion formation in the nose.

IMAGE BASED ANSWER

8. **b. FESS**

It is clearly seen at that the surgeon is passing an endoscope into the nasal cavity of the patient. This is functional endoscopic sinus surgery (FESS).

Antral wash is surgery of maxillary sinus, but endoscope is not used.

Tympanometry and mastoidectomy are surgeries of ear and not nose.

CHAPTER

20 Nasal Polyps

Nasal polyps are non-neoplastic pedunculated nasal mass which are **oedematous sacs** lined by pseudostratified ciliated columnar epithelium which sometimes undergo metastatic change into squamous epithelium and has:

- Reduced vascular supply
- Reduced nerve supply
- Reduced secretory glands and goblet cells
- Increased eosinophils

Important points about nasal polyp	
• Has reduced vessels of all three types, i.e. – Submucosal capillaries – Arteriovenous anastomosis – Venous sinusoids	Therefore, polyps are pale in colour and they DO NOT bleed unless infected. Note: Every disease of nose can cause epistaxis **except** nasal polyps
• Has reduced nerve supply	Therefore, they are **insensitive to touch**
• Has reduced glands/goblet cells	Glands undergo cystic degeneration
• Has oedema-filled sacs	Oedema is extracellular Therefore, it is **glistening/shining** white or pale in look

SITE OR ORIGIN

The **most common site of origin is the middle meatus or osteomeatal complex.**

If one has to select a sinus of origin, then most common sinus is ***ethmoidal sinus***.

However, in children, it is more common from the ***maxillary sinus***.

Note: This is reverse in case of sinusitis.

Sinusitis is more common from the maxillary sinus whereas, in children, it is more common from the ethmoidal sinus.

There are five theories for the formation of nasal polyp. They are as given below:

1. Infective theory – due to infection of sinus.
2. Allergic theory
3. Vasomotor theory
4. Bernauli's theory
5. Polysaccharide formation.

IMPORTANT FEATURES OF NASAL POLYP

- Nasal polyps have poor blood supply and so they are ***pale or glistening white in colour***
- On application of vasoconstrictor, there is no significant change/shrinkage in its size.
- It does **not bleed** spontaneously or on pricking. In fact, if nasal mass is bleeding, it CAN'T be polyp.
- However, nasal polyp may bleed when *infected.*
- Nasal polyps are insensitive to touch.

Maxillary Polyp has Various Names Like

- *Antrochoanal polyp*
- *AC polyp*
- *Killians's polyp*

	MAXILLLARY POLYP Antrochoanal polyp (AC polyp) Killian's polyp	ETHMOIDAL POLYP Bunch of grapes
	Grows backward towards the choana	Grows anteriorly
	Children commonly have the maxillary polyp	More common in adults
	Caused by **infection**	Caused by **allergy** or vasomotor rhinitis
	Usually unilateral	Usually bilateral
	Usually single in number	Usually multiple, looks like a *bunch of grapes*
	Not recurrent after treatment	Recurrent after treatment

Important points about nasal polyps

- In case of a polyp-like mass in the nose of a *child less than 2–3 years*; *encephalocele* should be ruled out.
- In child less than 10 years old, *cystic fibrosis* should be ruled out.
- A red polyp-like mass in the nose could have the following differential diagnosis:
  - Malignancy
  - Angiofibroma
  - Ringertz tumour
  - Rhinosporidiosis
  - Infected polyp etc.

Dodd's sign: This is an X-ray finding, in which there is a crescent-shaped space between the antrochoanal polyp and posterior pharyngeal wall.

This is also called the **Crescent sign.**

This sign is absent in case of angiofibroma.

Hence, it is used to differentiate between AC polyp and angiofibroma.

Three important syndromes that can cause nasal polyps (ethmoidal) are:

Samter's triad	Kartagener's syndrome	Young's syndrome
• Ethmoidal polyp • Asthma • Aspirin sensitivity	• Bronchiectasis • Polyp/Sinusitis • Situs inversus/dextrocardia	• Polyp/Sinusitis • Bronchiectasis • Azoospermia/infertility

Treatment

Treatment of the underlying cause with polypectomy

Topical/intranasal steroid sprays are the best medical option.

Sometimes, the combination of systemic and intranasal corticosteroids may completely treat the polyp.

This is called '**medical polypectomy**'.

For polypectomy, there are few surgical options:

- Avulsion of polyp (not done anymore)
- Caldwell Luc's surgery
- FESS
- Ethmoidectomy by either transantral, extranasal or intranasal approach (**outdated**).

Maxillary polyp	Ethmoidal polyp
Corticosteroids + antibiotics Not relieved ↓ FESS (polypectomy) ↓ Recurrence (Recurrence is very uncommon) ↓ Caldwell Luc's surgery	Corticosteroids + antibiotics Not relieved ↓ FESS ↓ Recurrence (Recurrence is very common/almost a rule) ↓ Ethmoidectomy • External ethmoidectomy (Lynch-Howarth) • Transantral (**Jansen-Horgan surgery)** • Intranasal ethmoidectomy

Last minute revision

- *Maxillary polyp is also called antrochoanal polyp and Killian's polyp*
- *Polyps are pale in color, do not bleed and are insensitive to touch*
- *Maxillary polyps are more common in children*
- *Ethmoidal presents as a bunch of grapes and is recurrent in nature*
- *Some important conditions that can cause polyps are:*
  - *Samter's triad*
  - *Kartagener's syndrome*
  - *Young's syndrome*
  - *Cystic fibrosis*
  - *NARES, etc.*
- *Intranasal steroids are the best medicinal treatment for nasal polyps.*
- *Intranasal steroids can treat all symptoms of nasal polyp EXCEPT ANOSMIA.*
- *Anosmia due to polyp is better treated with systemic steroids.*
- *FESS is the best surgical treatment*

QUESTIONS

1. **"Bernoulli's theorem" explains:**
   a. Nasal polyp
   b. Thyroglossal cyst
   c. Zenker's diverticulum
   d. Laryngomalacia
2. **Kartagener's syndrome is characterized by all *except:***
   a. Dextrocardia
   b. Bronchiectasis
   c. Bronchitis
   d. Sinusitis
3. **Killian term is used for which of the following polyp**
   a. Ethmoidal
   b. Antrochoanal
   c. Tonsillar cyst
   d. Tonsillolith
4. **Recurrent polyps are seen in:**
   a. Antrochoanal polyp
   b. Ethmoidal polyp
   c. Nasal polyp
   d. Hypertrophic turbinate
5. **A patient presents with antrochoanal polyp arising from the medial wall of maxilla. Which is the best management option:**
   a. FESS with polypectomy
   b. Medial maxillectomy
   c. Caldwell Luc's surgery
   d. Intranasal polypectomy
6. **Which of the following statements is NOT correct for ethmoidal polyp?**
   a. Allergy is an etiological factor
   b. Occurs in the first decade of life
   c. Are usually bilateral
   d. Are often associated with bronchial asthma
7. **Which of these best differentiates maxillary polyp from ethmoidal polyp?**
   a. Maxillary polyps are multiple
   b. Maxillary polyps are best seen on posterior rhinoscopy
   c. Maxillary polyps are recurrent in nature
   d. Maxillary polyps are bilateral
8. **Most common nasal mass is:**
   a. Polyp
   b. Papilloma
   c. Angiofibroma
   d. Granuloma
9. **A patient presents with multiple nasal polyps. His X-ray shows opacity in the paranasal sinuses. Treatment consists of all *except:***
   a. FESS
   b. Steroids
   c. Amphotericin B
   d. Antihistaminics
10. **Patient with ethmoidal polyp undergoes surgery but presents with a recurrence after 6 months. Which is the correct treatment in this case?**
    a. FESS
    b. External ethmoidectomy
    c. Caldwell Luc's surgery
    d. Intranasal polypectomy
11. **Recurrent epistaxis is NOT a common feature of:**
    a. Nasal polyps b. DNS
    c. Rhinosporidiosis d. Maxillary carcinoma
12. **Treatment of recurrent antrochoanal polyp is:**
    a. Caldwell Luc's surgery
    b. FESS
    c. Intranasal polypectomy
    d. Both a and b
13. **The current treatment of choice for a large antrochoanal polyp in a 10 years old child is:**
    a. Intranasal polypectomy
    b. Caldwell Luc's surgery
    c. FESS
    d. Lateral rhinotomy and excision
14. **Samter's triad include all *except:***
    a. Bronchiectasis b. Asthma
    c. Aspirin sensitivity d. Nasal polyps
15. **Samter's triad is related to:**
    a. Ethmoidal polyp
    b. Nasopharyngeal angiofibroma
    c. Antrochoanal polyp
    d. Nasal glioma
16. **Young's syndrome is:**
    a. Neutrophilia with red papillar rash
    b. Mitral stenosis with atrial septal defect
    c. Infertility with bronchiectasis
    d. Multiple enchondromas with phleboliths
17. **Topical steroids have no role after sinus surgery in:**
    a. Ethmoidal polyp
    b. Antrochoanal polyps
    c. Allergic fungal sinusitis
    d. Chronic allergic sinusitis

IMAGE BASED QUESTIONS

18. **A patient with history of allergic rhinitis, presents with nasal blockade of the left side. On rhinoscopy, the finding is shown in the picture.**

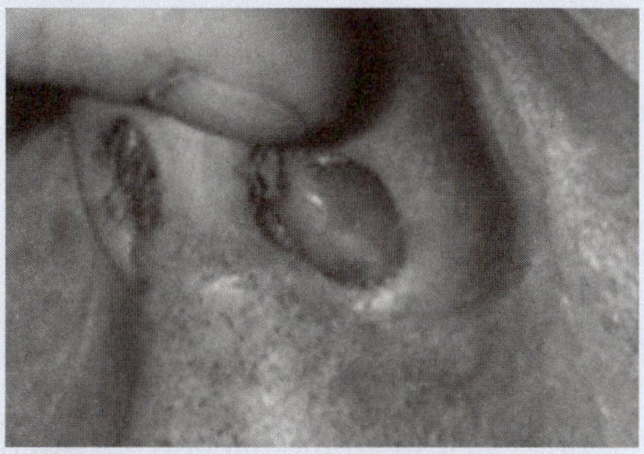

a. This is the case of rhinosporidiosis
b. This is a case of nasal polyp
c. This is a case of inverted papilloma
d. This is a case of rhinophyma

19. **In this CT Scan of PNS of a 16 years old girl; the "*" is most probably:**

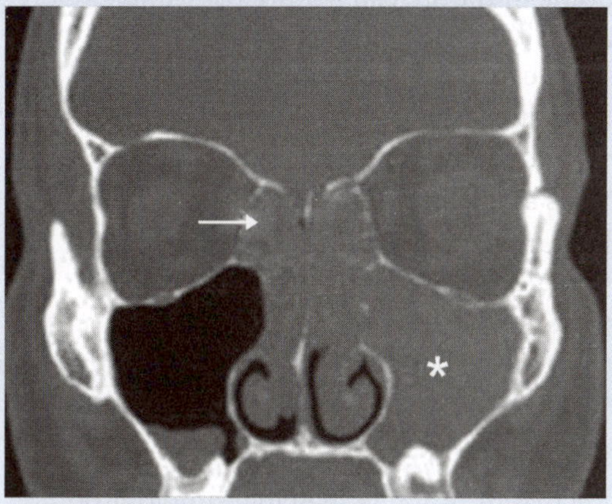

a. Antrochoanal polyp
b. Juvenile angiofibroma
c. Nasopharyngeal carcinoma
d. Sinonasal carcinoma

ANSWERS AND EXPLANATIONS

1. **a. Nasal polyp**

The cause of formation of nasal polyps is not known for sure. There are few theories that explain the formation of nasal polyps. These theories are:

1. **Bernoulli's theorem**
2. **Theory of polysaccharide changes**
3. **Vasomotor rhinitis**
4. **Infective theory and**
5. **Allergic theory**

Few Diseases that can Lead to Formation of Nasal Polyps

- *Samter's triad (aspirin triad)*
- *Kartagener's syndrome (primary ciliary dyskinesis)*
- *Young's syndrome*
- *Cystic fibrosis*
- *Churg-Strauss syndrome, etc.*

2. **c. Bronchitis**

Kartagener's syndrome is also called:

- *Immotile cilia syndrome*
- *Primary ciliary dyskinesia*

This syndrome has absence of ***dynein arm on the peripheral ciliary microtubules and hence the cilia are unable to beat effectively.***

This syndrome has the triad of:

1. **Chronic rhinosinusitis or polyp**
2. **Bronchiectasis and**
3. **Situs inversus**

Bronchitis is not a feature of Kartagener's syndrome.

ENT examination reveals presence of mucus in the nasal cavity.

3. **b. Antrochoanal**
Antrochooanal polyp (short form—AC polyp) is maxillary polyp which is also called **"Killian's polyp"**.
Some of the special features of Killian's polyp by means which it can be differentiated from ethmoidal polyps are:
- Is caused by infection
- Is more commonly seen in younger age group
- Is usually unilateral and
- Is single in number.

Features of nasal polyps are:
- Pale white in color
- Are insensitive to touch
- Do not change in size (shrink) by application of vasoconstrictor and
- Do not bleed

4. **b. Ethmoidal polyp**
Recurrent polyp is seen in ethmoidal polyps because the underlying cause of ethmoidal polyp is **allergy**. We know that allergy cannot be treated but can be controlled and this can lead to recurrence of polyp after the excision.
In patients of ethmoidal polyp (which is caused by allergy), other allergic diseases like asthma may be present.
Presence of ethmoidal polyp, asthma and aspirin sensitivity are seen in **sampter's triads.**

MAXILLLARY POLYP Antrochoanal polyp (AC polyp) Killian's polyp	ETHMOIDAL POLYP Bunch of grapes
Grows backward towards the choana	Grows anteriorly
Children commonly have the maxillary polyp	More common in adults
Caused by **infection**	Caused by **allergy** or vasomotor rhinitis
Usually unilateral	Usually bilateral
Usually single in number	Usually multiple, looks like a *bunch of grapes*
Not recurrent after treatment	**Recurrent** after treatment

Some important points about nasal polyps:
- In a child less than 2 yrs old with nasal polyp, CT scan should be done to rule out encephalocele.
- In a child less than 10 yrs old with nasal polyp, sweat test should be done to rule out cystic fibrosis

5. **a. FESS with polypectomy**
FESS is the best treatment option for all types of nasal polyps. In the modern times, all other surgical options are outdated.
Caldwell Luc's surgery is the second best option for antrochoanal polyp.
Caldwell Luc's procedure is done when polyp arises from areas from where endoscopic removal is difficult (FESS). Two such areas are:
Inferior wall of maxilla and
Lateral wall of maxilla

6. **b. Occurs in the first decade of life**
Refer to the table given in answer no. 4.

7. **b. Maxillary polyps are best seen on posterior rhinoscopy**

MAXILLLARY POLYP Antrochoanal polyp (AC polyp) Killian's polyp	ETHMOIDAL POLYP Bunch of grapes
Grows backward; therefore, can be seen on posterior rhinoscopy	Grows anteriorly; therefore, seen on anterior rhinoscopy.
Children commonly have the maxillary polyp	More common in adults
Caused by **infection**	Caused by **allergy** or vasomotor rhinitis
Usually **unilateral**	Usually bilateral

8. **a. Polyp**
Rest of the mentioned masses are very rare.

9. **c. Amphotericin B**
This is not a fungal disease and so no antifungal drug like amphotericin B is needed.
Rest of the options mentioned are commonly used for nasal polyp.
This appears to be a case of ethmoidal polyp.

10. **a. FESS**
FESS is almost always the best surgical option for all types of nasal polyps. However, if the ethmoidal polyp recurs again and again and that too very frequently, intranasal ethmoidectomy is an option. External ethmoidectomy and intranasal polypectomy are outdated procedures.
Caldwell Luc surgery is done for maxillary problems only.
Surgical options for nasal polyps:
- Avulsion of polyp (not done anymore)
- Caldwell Luc's Surgery
- FESS
- Ethmoidectomy by either transantral, extranasal or intranasal approach (**outdated**).

Maxillary polyp	Ethmoidal polyp
Corticosteroids + antibiotics	Corticosteroids + antibiotics
Not relieved ↓	Not relieved ↓
FESS (polypectomy) ↓	FESS ↓
Recurrence (Recurrence is very uncommon) ↓	Recurrence (Recurrence is very common/almost a rule) ↓
Caldwell Luc's surgery	• Ethmoidectomy (outdated) • External ethmoidectomy (Lynch-Howarth) • Transantral (**Jansen-Horgan surgery)** • Intranasal ethmoidectomy

11. **a. Nasal polyps**

Important points about nasal polyp	
• Has reduced vessels of all three types, i.e. – Submucosal capillaries – Arteriovenous anastomosis – Venous sinusoids	1. Therefore, polyps are pale in color and 2. They DO NOT bleed unless infected.
Note: Most diseases of nose can cause epistaxis except nasal polyps	

12. **d. Both a and b**
In cases of recurrent antrochoanal polyps, we have two surgical options:
1. FESS, and
2. Caldwell Luc's surgery.

13. **c. FESS**
As mentioned before, FESS is almost always the best option for all nasal polyps.

14. **a. Bronchiectasis**

15. **a. Ethmoidal polyp**

Three important syndromes that can cause ethmoidal polyps are:

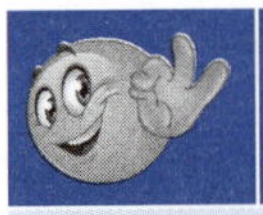 Sampter's triad	Kartagener's syndrome	Young's syndrome
Ethmoidal polyp Asthma Aspirin sensitivity	Bronchiectasis Polyp/Sinusitis Situs inversus/dextrocardia	Polyp/Sinusitis Bronchiectasis Azoospermia/infertility

16. c. **Infertility with bronchiectasis** Refer to the table/box in the previous answer.
17. b. **Antrochoanal polyps** As we know that antrochoanal polyps do not have allergic cause and so steroids are not useful.

IMAGE BASED ANSWERS

18. b. **This is a case of nasal polyp** • Rhinosporidiosis presents as deep red strawberry polyp • Inverted papilloma is again NOT pale as seen in the picture and has no relation to allergy • Rhinophyma is a disease of skin over the nose and has NO growth inside the nasal cavity. It is called potato nose.
19. a. **Antrochoanal polyp** As we can see, it is a homogenous swelling in the maxillary sinus. Therefore, it is most probably a maxillary polyp, which is also called antrochoanal polyp.

CHAPTER

21 Diseases of the Nasal Septum

We all know from our previous discussion the the nasal septum has:

- Bony part
- Cartilaginous part, and
- Membranous part

This is lined with layer of ***mucoperichondrium on both the sides.***

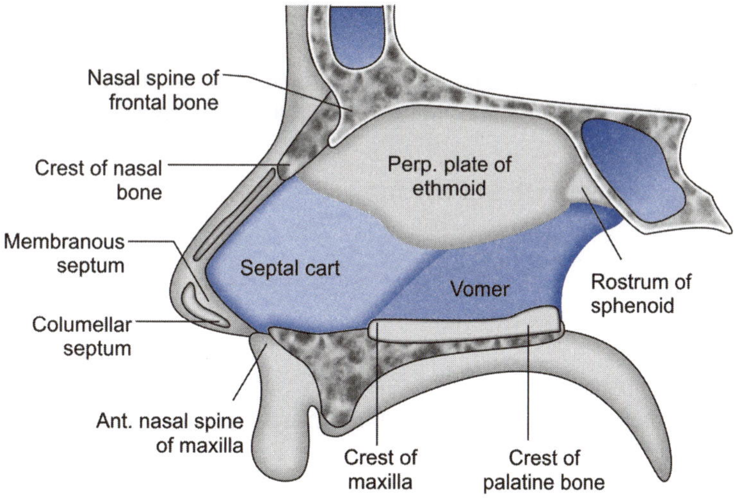

Fig. 1: Nasal septum with parts labelled

We also know that nasal septum has very extensive blood supply and a plexus called **Kiesselbach's plexus.**

We are now going to discuss some important diseases of the nasal septum.

EPISTASXIS

Nasal bleeding most commonly happens from the nasal septum from an area called little's area.
We have already discussed this.

DEVIATED NASAL SEPTUM (DNS) AND SEPTAL SPUR

According to some books up to 20% of children born have DNS/SPUR and by adulthood 60-80% population of world has DNS.

The three most common causes of DNS/spur are:

1. ***Birth trauma or trauma during childhood (most common cause)***
2. Developmental disturbances, and
3. Systemic diseases.

No matter what is cause and what type if DNS, the symptoms are similar.

Spur:

Spur is defined as *sharp or sudden deviation is at the junction of bone and cartilage.*

Presentation

- Most common complaint is ***obstruction/blockade on side of deviation.***
- Sometimes the opposite side also has obstruction.

This happens due to ***compensatory hypertrophy of inferior turbinate.***

The middle and superior turbinates usually do not hypertrophy.

This is because the inferior turbinate has ***erectile tissue and sinusoid vascular system*** which is not present in the other two turbinates.

Middle turbinate may not hypertrophy, but it may be enlarged due to ***pneumatization.*** This condition is called **concha bullosa.**

- The other common complaint is **frontal headache**.

  This is due to the deviated septum impinging onto the **middle turbinate** and hence compresses the **anterior ethmoidal nerve** which supplies this area.

  This causes referred pain to the forehead.

  Since, the nerve involved is ***anterior ethmoidal nerve,*** this headache is called **anterior ethmoidal neuralgia/ anterior ethmoidal syndrome**.

  In some books, this is **wrongly** called ***Sluder's neuralgia.***

  Sluder's neuralgia is actually neuralgia of ***sphenopalatine nerve***.

Common neuralgias of face

- Anterior ethmoidal nerve/*Sluder's neuralgia*
- *Trigeminal neuralgia* is described as sudden lancinating pain (stabbing severe pain) which usually starts near the bridge of nose and travels towards the parietal area.
- *Glossopharyngeal neuralgia* starts near tonsils area and may be referred to middle ear because tympanic plexus derives fibres from glossopharyngeal nerve. Because of the same reason; tumours of the throat may cause referred pain to the middle ear.

- The other less important complains of DNS/SPUR are:
  - Anosmia
  - Bleeding/epistaxis
  - Crooked nose etc.

Complications

- The commonest complication is ***sinusitis.***
- DNS can obstruct the ostia and hence cause of all the sinuses EXCEPT the sphenoid sinus. Hence, *sphenoid sinusitis **cannot** be* caused by DNS.

Cottle's test:s

Cheek on affected side is pulled downwards. If this relieves nasal obstruction, it is positive. This suggests that the nasal obstruction is at the *nasal valve.*

- *Nasal valve* is the narrowest part of nose.
- If obstruction is at nasal valve then Cottle's test will be positive

Treatment

Treatment is mainly surgical.

The two important surgeries are:

1. **SMR or submucosal resection** and
2. **Septoplasty**

Turbinectomy may or may not be required

The difference between SMR and septoplasty are given below:

SMR	Septoplasty
More radical surgery	Conservative surgery
Killian's incision is given on both the sides	**Freer's/Hemitransfixation** incision is given on one side only
Perichondrium flaps are raised from **both sides**	Perichondrium flap is raised from **one** side
Usually the entire middle layer of septum is resected	Repair of the septum is done. There is **no** resection
Two layers of septum are left after the surgery	All the three layers are left after the surgery
Complications are more common, i.e septal perforation	Complications are less common
Less commonly done	More commonly done
Done after the age of 16-17 years	Done after the age of 16-17 years.

As discussed, sometimes there is hypertrophy of the inferior turbinate and has to be treated.
Few treatment options for inferior turbinate hypertrophy are:

Surgical options for inferior turbinate hypertrophy (ITH)

- Thermal coagulation
- Turbinectomy
- Laser excision of turbinate
- Powered instrument (microdebrider)
- Co-ablation turbinectomy/radiofrequency turbinectomy. This is relatively new method and commonly used
- Argon plasma turbinectomy is a new technology

NOTE: Turbinectomy may cause empty nose syndrome (ENS)

Complications of SMR/Septoplasty

- **Nasal bleeding** is the most common complication of SMR/septoplasty.
- ***Septal perforation*** is due to necrosis of septum.
- Large perforation may cause ***saddle nose***.
- **Septal adhesions or synechiae formation**.

NASAL SYNECHIAE/ADHESIONS

- Nasal adhesions are formation of fibrotic tissue between the nasal septum and the lateral wall.
- As a result, the septum gets pulled laterally causing nasal obstruction.
- Nasal synechiae are usually formed due to **nasal surgeries**.
- This can cause all the problems that are caused by DNS.

Treatment of Nasal Synechiae

- Once the synachiae is formed the best treatment is surgical excision of the synechiae.
- It is better to take appropriate steps during the surgery so as to prevent the synechiae.
- On of the recent and effective method is the application of ***Mitomycin-C*** in the nose.
- Packing the nose with **BIPP (bismuth iodide potassium phosphate)** is the other effective method.

SEPTAL HEMATOMA

Septal hematoma is collection of blood between the nasal septum and mucoperichondrial layer.
This causes the bulge on the mucoperichondrium leading to obstruction of the nasal cavities.
The most common cause of septal hematoma is trauma.
In septal hematoma, obstruction/blockage takes place on both the nasal cavities.

COMPLICATION OF SEPTAL HEMATOMA

Flowchart 1: Complication of septal hematoma

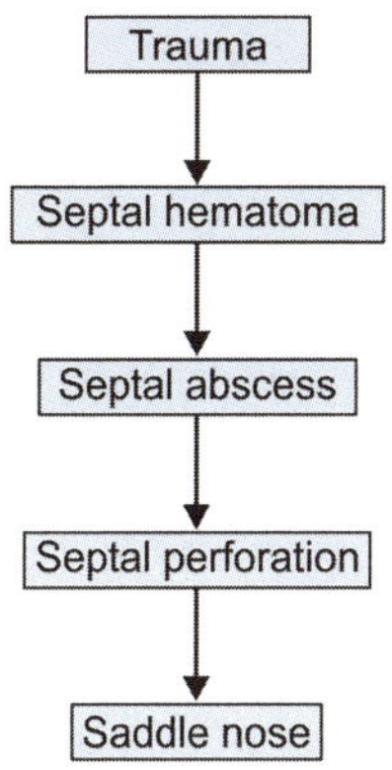

Treatment

Immediate drainage with nasal packing is the treatment of choice.

Antibiotics may be added.

Septal perforation

There are many causes of septal perforation.

The most common cause is surgical trauma (iatrogenic).

Few important causes of septal perforations are:

Important causes of septal perforation

- Nasal surgery- most common cause
- Nose picking
- Alkaline solution released from button battery in the nose (foreign body)
- Cocaine stuffing in the nose
- Malignancies
- Sarcoidosis
- Wegener's granulomatosis. Sometimes septal perforation is the first presentation.
- Tuberculosis/lupus
- Syphilis: Syphilis can cause perforaton of cartilage part as well as *bony part* of the septum. Rest of the infections can cause perforation only in the cartilage part.

Treatment

- Most of the septal perforations are asymptomatic and so does NOT require treatment
- For smaller perforations <2 cm, surgical repair may be helpful.
- For this **ear cartilage or rib cartilage** may be used as graft material.
- For larger perforations > 2 cm, **septal buttons made of silicon can be used.**

Last minute revision

- *Most common cause of DNS is birth trauma*
- *It can cause obstruction due to compensatory hypertrophy of inferior turbinate*
- *It can cause anterior ethmoidal syndrome when the spur touches middle turbinate*
- *Cottle test can be used for diagnosis of DNS*
- *DNS can cause sinusitis of all the sinuses except sphenoid sinus*
- *Incision used for SMR is Killian's incision*
- *Incision for septoplasty is called Freer's incision*
- *Nasal synechiae can be avoided by using BIPP or mitomycin C*
- *Syphilis can septal perforation of the bony septum*

QUESTIONS

1. **Features associated with DNS include all of the following *except:***
   a. Epistaxis
   b. Atrophy of turbinate
   c. Hypertrophy of turbinate
   d. Recurrent sinusitis
2. **Nasal septum perforation occurs in all the following *except:***
   a. Tuberculosis
   b. Nasal surgery
   c. Syphilis
   d. Rhinosporidiosis
3. **DNS may be associated with all *except:***
   a. Recurrent sphenoiditis
   b. Bilateral septal spur
   c. Hypertrophy of inferior turbinate
   d. Epistaxis
4. **The aetiology of anterior ethmoidal neuralgia is:**
   a. Inferior nasal turbinate pressing on the nasal septum
   b. Middle nasal turbinate pressing on the nasal septum
   c. Superior nasal turbinate pressing on the nasal septum
   d. Obstruction of the ethmoidal sinus
5. **Killian's incision is used for:**
   a. SMR operation
   b. Intranasal antrostomy
   c. Caldwell Luc surgery
   d. Septoplasty
6. **Improvement of nasal patency by retracting the cheek laterally and thus testing the valvular component of the nose is called:**
   a. Epley's manoeuvre b. Cottle's test
   c. Schwartz manoeuvre d. Heimlich manoeuvre
7. **After laparoscopic appendectomy, patient has a fall from bed and had swelling on the nose and difficulty in breathing. Next best step in management is:**
   a. I/V antibiotics for 7–10 days
   b. Observation in hospital
   c. Surgical drainage
   d. Discharge after two days and follow up for 8 weeks

ANSWERS AND EXPLANATIONS

1. **b. Atrophy of turbinate**

   In DNS, atrophy is not seen. Atrophy of turbinates are seen in conditions like:
   - Atrophic rhinitis.
   - Rhinitis sicca

   DNS may cause:
   - ***Compensatory hypertrophy of the inferior turbinate and NOT atrophy.***
   - ***Epistaxis. When it comes in contact with the lateral wall of the nose***
   - ***Sinusitis by blocking the ostia of sinuses.***

2. **d. Rhinosporidiosis**

   Nasal septal perforation used to be common problem. The most common cause used to be nasal septal surgeries like sub-mucosal resection. This surgery has now been replaced by septoplasty, yet one of the common causes of septal perforation remains septal surgeries.

   Bacterial infections like ***TB, syphilis, leprosy, lupus and rhinosleroma*** may also cause septal perforations.

   Some of the other conditions causing septal perforation are Wegener's granulomas, sarcoidosis and non-healing midline T-cell lymphoma.

   Rhinosporidiosis is not known to cause septal perforation.

Important causes of septal perforation

- Nasal surgery- most common cause
- Nose picking
- Alkaline solution released from button battery in the nose (foreign body)
- Cocaine stuffing in the nose
- Malignancies
- Sarcoidosis

Important causes of septal perforation

- Wegener's granulomatosis. Sometimes septal perforation is the first presentation.
- Tuberculosis/lupus
- Syphilis. Syphilis can cause perforaton of cartilage part as well as bony part of the septum. Rest of the infections can cause perforation only in the cartilage part.
- Rhinoscleroma

3. **a. Recurrent sphenoiditis**
   Deviated nasal septum (DNS) is of three main types:
   1. Vertical deviation
   2. Horizontal deviation, and
   3. Mixed deviation
   - Horizontal deviation is often associated with septal spur (unilateral or bilateral).
   - The most common complication of DNS is sinusitis. However, DNS can cause sinusitis of all sinuses except sphenoidal sinusitis
   - Compensatory hypertrophy of inferior turbinate is a known presentation of DNS
   - Epistaxis is a known presentation of DNS.

4. **b. Middle nasal turbinate pressing on the nasal septum.**
   This is due to the deviated septum impinging onto the **middle turbinate** and hence compresses the **anterior ethmoidal nerve** which supplies this area.
   This causes referred pain to the forehead.
   Since, the nerve involved is ***anterior ethmoidal nerve,*** this headache is called **anterior ethmoidal neuralgia/ anterior ethmoidal syndrome**.
   In some books, this is **wrongly** called ***Sluder's neuralgia.***
   Sluder's neuralgia is actually neuralgia of ***sphenopalatine nerve***.

5. **a. SMR operation**
   The two important surgeries for DNS are:
   SMR or submucosal resection and
   Septoplasty
   Turbinectomy may or may not be required
   The difference between SMR and Septoplasty are given below:

SMR	Septoplasty
More radical surgery	conservative surgery
Killian's incision is given on both the sides	**Freer's/Hemitransfixation** incision is given on one side only
Perichondrium flaps are raised from **both sides**	Perichondrium flap is raised from **one** side
Usually the entire middle layer of septum is resected	Repair of the septum is done. There is **no** resection
Two layers of septum are left after the surgery	All the three layers are left after the surgery
Complications are more common, i.e. **septal perforation**	Complications are less common
Less commonly done	More commonly done
Done after the age of 16-17 years	Done after the age of 16-17 years.

6. **b. Cottle's test**

Cottle's tests:

Cheek on affected side is pulled downwards. If this relieves nasal obstruction, it is positive. This suggests that the nasal obstruction is at the *nasal valve.*

- *Nasal valve* is the narrowest part of nose.
- If obstruction is at nasal valve then Cottle's test will be positive

7. **c. Surgical drainage**
   This seems to a case of septal hematoma. In septal hematoma, immediate drainage with nasal packing should be done.

CHAPTER

22 Granulomatous Diseases of Nose and PNS and Other Similar Conditions

Granulomatous diseases of the nose and sinuses are of the following types:

Flowchart 1: Granulomatous diseases of nose

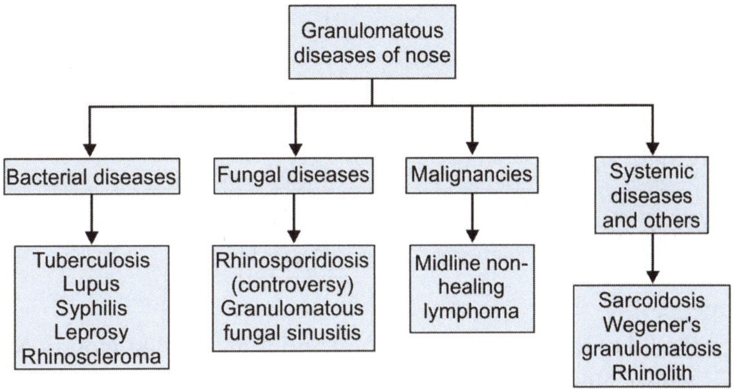

Some important points about some of the above mentioned diseases:

RHINOSPORIDIOSIS

It is a granulomatous disease believed to be caused by ***Rhinosporidium seeberi***.

However, the classification of *rhinosporidiosis seeberi* is not clear. Some consider it to be a water mold.

Molecular biological techniques have recently shown it to be an **aquatic protoctista/protozoa parasite** of a class ***Mesomycetozoea.***

> Unclear whether this organism is a fungus, but sequencing of the 18S small subunit ribosomal DNA sequence from *R. seeberi* has led to its recent reclassification as a member of the protoctista Mesomycetozoea.
> Attempts to isolate: *Scott-Brown's ORL and HNS. 7th edi. pg 2151*

It is seen more commonly in southern India.

The common sites of rhinosporidiosis are:

- Nasal cavity
- Oral cavity
- Eye, and
- Genitalia

It usually presents as **bleeding nasal polyp.**

The polyp often looks like a strawberry and is called **Strawberry polyp or Mulberry polyp. (*Strawberry gums/ gingiva is seen in Wegener's granulomatosis*).**

DIAGNOSTIC INVESTIGATION IS BIOPSY

Diagnosis

> The diagnosis is established by histopathologic examination of tissue sections. These contain large, round or oval sporangia up 350 μm is diameter, with a thick wall and an operculum. The largest sporangia are filled with spores:
> *Scott-Browwn's ORL and HNS. 7th edi. pg 216*

Although, the biopsy may be helpful, it is still diagnosed clinically as a "strawberry polyp". This is partly also because we have NOT been able to culture this pathogen.

CT scan is done to see the extension of the disease.

The drug of choice is **Dapsone** but the treatment of choice is **cautery excision.**

BACTERIAL DISEASES

Bacterial diseases cause granulomatous disease of the nose. They all can cause **perforation** on the nasal septum. They all can cause perforation mainly on the cartilage part of the septum except ***syphilis***, which can cause perforation on the **bony septum** also.

RHINOSCLEROMA

Rhinoscleroma is a bacterial disease caused by gram negative, non-motile enterobacteriaceae called ***Klebsiella rhinoscleromatis***.

This is also called ***Frisch bacillus.***

Sometimes, the entire respiratory tract may be involved.

There is a condition known as laryngoscleroma.

This bacterium is seen in Northern India.

There are three stages:

1. Atrophic stage or catarrhal stage
2. Granulomatous stage
3. Sclerosis/Cicatricial stage

In the granulomatous stage the fill of the nose is like a wood and is also called **woody Nose**.

This condition is also called **Hebra Nose.**

- Most important investigation is biopsy. The findings are:
  - **Mikulicz cell,** which look like the foam cells
  - **Russell bodies,** which looks like the plasma cells.
- CT scan is done to see the extent of disease.

Treatment

- The drug of choice is **streptomycin ± tetracycline.**
- **Rifampicin** can also be used.
- In some cases 2% **acriflavine** may be applied locally.
- The best treatment is **cautery excision**
- **Irradiation with 3000–3500 Gy over 3 weeks is also an option.**

Rhinolith

It is an old foreign body on which calcium and magnesium have deposited.

The calcified foreign bodies look like a stone and hence called rhinolith.

Presentation

A child presents with unilateral nasal discharge with/without foul smell and with/without bleeding.

In children; nasal of body is removed under general anaesthesia.

Non-healing Midline Lymphoma

It is a *T-cell lymphoma,* which affects the midline of the nose. It is a rapidly progressive and destructive disease of the nose and the face.

Wegener's Granulomatosis

The only important fact from ENT point of view is that in this condition; there is granulations on the gums with microabscesses.

This is described as ***strawberry gums or strawberry gingiva.***

Note: *Strawberry polyp is seen in rhinosporidiosis.*

Last minute revision

- *Rhinosporidiosis is caused by rhinosporidium seeberi seen in coastal area of south India*
- *Rhinosporidium seeberi is an aquatic protozoa*
- *It presents as strawberry polyp drug of choice is dapsone*
- *Klebsiella rhinoscleromatis or Frisch bacilli causes rhinoscleroma*
- *It is also called woody nose*
- *Mikulicz cell and Russell bodies are biopsy finding*
- *Cautery excision and streptomycin are used for rhinoscleroma*
- *Rhinolith is old calcified foreign body of nose*
- *Nasal foreign body presents as unilateral foul smelling nasal discharge with bleeding*

QUESTIONS

1. **True statement about Rhinosporidiosis is:**
   a. Most common organism is klebsiella rhinoscleromatis
   b. Seen only in immunocompromised patients
   c. Presents as a nasal polyp
   d. Can be diagnosed by isolation of organism
2. **Rhinosporoidiosis is caused by:**
   a. Protozoan infection
   b. Viral infection
   c. Bacterial infection
   d. Fungal infection
3. **Maggots in nose are best treated by:**
   a. Chloroform diluted with water
   b. Liquid paraffin
   c. Systemic antibiotics
   d. Lignocaine spray
4. **Most common cause of unilateral nasal discharge in a child is:**
   a. Syphilis
   b. Foreign body
   c. Juvenile nasopharyngeal angiofibroma
   d. Rhinolith
5. **Commonest cause of unilateral nasal obstruction and persistent rhinorrhea in 8-year-old child is:**
   a. Foreign body
   b. Choanal atresia
   c. Nasopharyngeal carcinoma
   d. Enlarged adenoids
6. **Rhinophyma is associated with:**
   a. Hypertrophy of the sebaceous glands
   b. Hypertrophy of sweat glands
   c. Hyperplasia of endothelial cells
   d. Hyperplasia of epithelial cells
7. **A child has retained disc battery in the nose. What is the most important consideration in the management?**
   a. Battery substance leaks and causes tissue damage
   b. It can lead to tetanus
   c. Refer the child to the specialist for removal
   d. Instill nasal drop
8. **Rhinoscleroma is due to:**
   a. Spirochetes
   b. Chlamydia
   c. Klebsiella
   d. Autoimmune
9. **Bony nasal septal perforation is characteristically seen in:**
   a. Wegener's granulomatosis
   b. Leprosy
   c. Rhinophyma
   d. Tuberculosis
10. **All are true about T-cell lymphoma except:**
    a. Associated with EBV
    b. Cell express T-cell marker
    c. Is locally invasive
    d. Wide local excision is the treatment of choice
11. **Mikulicz cell and Russel bodies are seen in:**
    a. Rhinosporidiosis
    b. Rhinoscleroma
    c. Lupus vulgaris
    d. T-cell lymphoma
12. **Apple jelly nodules are seen in:**
    a. Rhinosporidiosis b. Rhinoscleroma
    c. Lupus vulgaris d. Syphilis
13. **Nasal polypoidal mass with subcutaneous nodules are seen in:**
    a. Zygomycosis b. Rhinosporidiosis
    c. Sporotrichosis d. Aspergillosis

IMAGE BASED QUESTIONS

14. **A 40 years old patient presents with nasal blockade and epistaxis. Rhinoscopy shows the finding in the 1st picture. This patient was operated and the mass removed is shown in the 2nd picture.**

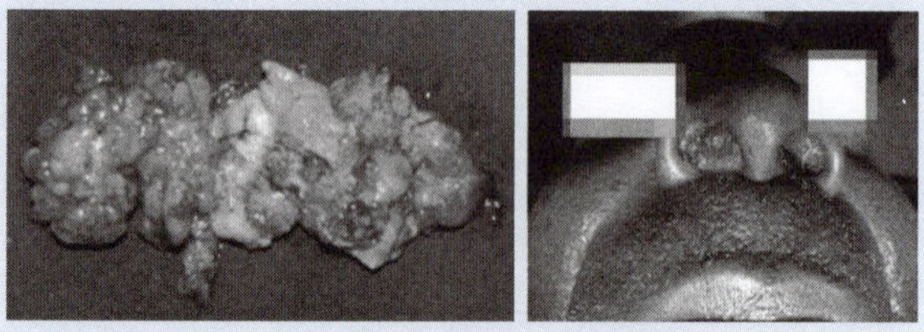

    a. This is a case of nasal carcinoma
    b. This is a case of rhinosporidiosis
    c. This condition is also called woody nose
    d. This condition is seen in northern India
15. **An adult male presented with nasal blockade for few months. On anterior rhinoscopy, both the nasal cavities were partially stenosed/sclerosed. Biopsy was taken and the histopathological slides under high magnification are shown above. Which of this is true?**

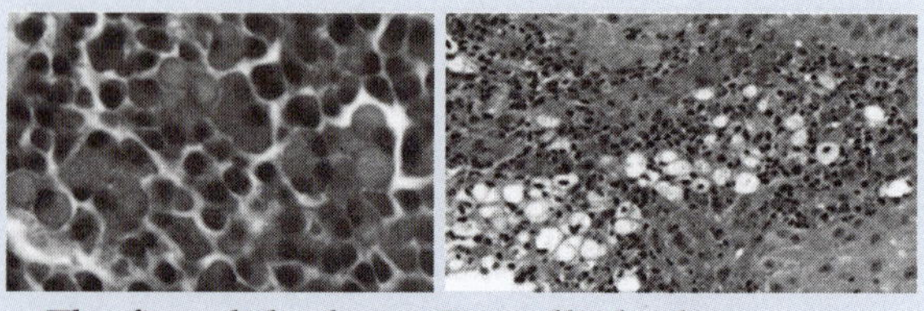

    a. The first slide shows Russell's bodies
    b. The second slide shows Mikulicz cells
    c. This is a case of rhinosporidiosis
    d. All are true

ANSWERS AND EXPLANATIONS

1. **c. Presents as a nasal polyp**
Rhinosporidiosis is caused by *Rhinosporidium seeberi.*
It is not a disease of immunocompromised individuals.
Diagnosis is usually made by isolating spores or "sporangia" and not the organism.
The most common presentation is bleeding nasal polyp. It is also described as ***strawberry polyp***.
   - Klebsiella rhinoscleromatis causes rhinoscleroma
   - It is still NOT clear as to the type of pathogen *Rhinosporidium seeberi* is.
   - This is because isolation and culture of this pathogen is NOT possible.
   - Molecular biological techniques have recently shown it to be an **aquatic protoctista/protozoa parasite** of a class ***Mesomycetozoea.***

Unclear whether this organism is a fungus, but sequencing of the 18S small subunit ribosomal DNA sequence from *R. seeberi* has led to its recent reclassification as a member of the protoctista Mesomycetozoea.[9]
Attempts to isolate: *Scott-Brown's ORL and HNS. 7th edi. pg 215*

   - Because it cannot be cultured, clinical presentation is diagnostic. It presents as ***strawberry polyp.***
   - However, Scott brown has this to say:

Diagnosis

The diagnosis is established by histopathologic examination of tissue sections. These contain large, round or oval sporangia up 350 μm is diameter, with a thick wall and an operculum. The largest sporangia are filled with spores: *Scott-Browwn's ORL and HNS. 7th edi. pg 216*

2. **a. Protozoan infection**
Rhinosporidiosis is caused by Rhinosporidium seeberi, which is an invasive disease seen in coastal areas of Southern India.
However, the classification of rhinosporidiosis seeberi is not clear.
Most consider it to be a water mold. Molecular biological techniques have recently shown it to be an ***aquatic protistan parasite of a class Mesomycetozoea.***

Unclear whether this organism is a fungus, but sequencing of the 18S small subunit ribosomal DNA sequence from *R. seeberi* has led to its recent reclassification as a member of the protoctista Mesomycetozoea.
Attempts to isolate: *Scott-Brown's ORL and HNS. 7th edi. pg 215*

The most important point about rhinosporidiosis is that is presents as ***strawberry/mulberry polyp*** in the nose. It is diagnosed by biopsy which shows inclusion bodies.

Diagnosis

The diagnosis is established by histopathologic examination of tissue sections. These contain large, round or oval sporangia up 350 μm is diameter, with a thick wall and an operculum. The largest sporangia are fulled with spores: *Scott-Browwn's ORL and HNS. 7th edi. pg 216*

Dapsone is the drug given but treatment of choice is diathermy knife excision with cauterization of the base. It is one of the differential diagnosis of bleeding nasal mass/polyp.

3. **a. Chloroform diluted with water**
The other treatment option is turpentine oil. Chloroform and turpentine oil kill the maggots also called myiasis. Maggots is caused by fly chrysomya.

4. **b. Foreign body**
Nasal discharge in most diseases is usually bilateral.
Unilateral nasal discharge in children is typically seen in case of foreign body / rhinolith of nose.
NOTE: In case of unilateral nasal discharge in a child, foreign body nose should be ruled out.
Other presentations of FB nose are:
   - Foul smell from the nose
   - Unilateral nasal bleeding

5. **a. Foreign body**

In cases of a child with unilateral nasal discharge specially persistent rhinorrhea,foreign body of the nose is the most common cause. The other presenting features of foreign body of nose are:

- Unilateral nasal blockade
- Foul smell from nose
- Unilateral nasal bleed.

A nasal foreign body in a child should be ideally be removed under general anaesthesia.

6. **a. Hypertrophy of the sebaceous glands**

Rhinophyma is also called **potato nose** and is due to acne rosacea causing hypertrophy of the sebaceous glands.

The treatment is cosmetic surgery of nose.

7. **a. Battery substance leaks and causes tissue damage**

- If the disc battery remains in the nasal cavity it may lead to leakage of the battery substance.

The battery substance is alkaline in nature and is very damaging to the nasal mucosa followed by fibrosis and stenosis of the nasal cavity.

If the child aspirates the same alkaline substance, this can cause damage of the lungs.

8. **c. Klebsiella**

Rhinoscleroma is a bacterial disease with usually involves nose and upper respiratory tract.

It is caused by ***Klebsiella rhinoscleromatis***.

Klebsiella rhinoscleromatis is also called ***Frisch bacilli***

Rhinoscleroma is more common in Northern India and has three stages. These stages are

1. Atrophic stage
2. Granulomatous stage where it feels like a wood and hence this condition is also called **woody nose.**
3. Cicatricial/sclerotic stage.

The most important diagnostic feature is presence of ***Mikulicz cells and Russell bodies*** in the biopsy.

The drug of choice is streptomycin plus tetracycline.

This is continued till two biopsy reports are negative. However, surgical excision may be required.

9. **a. Wegener's granulomatosis**

Wegener's granulomatosis is necrotizing vasculitis which may affect the nose. In such cases it may cause perforation of **bony as well as cartilaginous septum.**

Granulomatous disease that cause performation on cartilaginous septum only	Granulomatous diseases that cause performation on cartilaginous and bony septum	Granulomatous diseases that do NOT cause performation
• Tuberculosis • Leprosy	• Syphilis • Wegener's granulomatosis • T-cell lymphoma	• Rhinoscheroma • Lupus valgaris • Rhinosporidiosis • Rhinophyma • Sarcoidosis • Fungal infections

Granulomatous diseases of nose and their important presentations

Granulomatous diseases of nose	Their presentations
Tuberculosis	Cartilaginous perforation
Leprosy	Cartilaginous perforation
Lupus valgaris	Appel jelly nodule
Rhinoscleroma	Woody nose/Hebra nose/Taper nose
Syphilis	Snuffles/gummas/Bony & cartilaginous perforation
Rhinosporidiosis	Strawberry/mulberry polyp
Rhinophyma	Potato nose
Sarcoidosis	Lupus pernio/strawberry gingival

10. **d. Wide local excision is the treatment of choice**
T-cell lymphoma is a very aggressive nasal disease that needs an aggressive treatment.
It required chemotherapy + radiotherapy.

11. **b. Rhinoscleroma**
Most important investigation in rhinoscleroma is biopsy. The histopathology findings are:
Mikulicz cell, which look like the foam cells
Russell bodies, which looks like the plasma cells.

12. **c. Lupus vulgaris**
Apple jelly nodules are brown coloured nodules that do not blanch on pressure and is seen in lupus vulgaris.

13. **b. Rhinosporidiosis**
In rhinosporidiosis, the most important presentation is strawberry nasal polyp or nasal polypoidal mass which may bleed on touch.
The fingers of the patient may get contaminated and may then inoculate in the skin leading to subcutaneous nodules.

IMAGE BASED ANSWERS

14. **b. This is a case of rhinosporidiosis**
This is a case of rhinosporidiosis which is also called strawberry polyp and is seen in coastal area of southern India.

15. **d. All are true**
The history and finding are suggestive of rhinosporidiosis. The slides are that of **Russell bodies and Mikulicz cells** respectively. This further proves that it is **rhinosporidiosis**.
    - **Russell bodies** are plasma like cells. They are eosinophilic, large homogenous immunoglobulin containing inclusions. **Mikulicz cells** are foamy vacuolated histiocytes.

CHAPTER

23 Fractures of Facial Bones

Facial bones are some of the most commonly fractured bone and so this topic becomes very important from the point view of examination.

Important points about fractures of facial bones are given below:

FRACTURE NASAL BONE AND NASAL SEPTUM

Nasal bones fractures are often accompanied with fractures of the septum.

They are the **most commonly** fractured bone on the face.

Nasal bone fractures are of three types:

Class I fracture	Class II fracture	Class III fracture
• The force of blow is low • No gross displacement seen • Nasal bridge may be depressed • May be accompanied with Chevallet fracture of septum • No reduction required	• The force of blow is moderate • Deformity is usually seen • May lead to "Open Book fracture" • May be accompanied with Jarajaway fracture of septum • Closed reduction is required	• It is also called naso-orbito-ethmiodal fracture • The force is severe • Severe deformity seen • "Telescopy" of nose into ethmoid may happen • This may lead to CSF rhinorrhea, telecanthus, etc • "Pig like/pig snout" may be seen • Open reduction is required

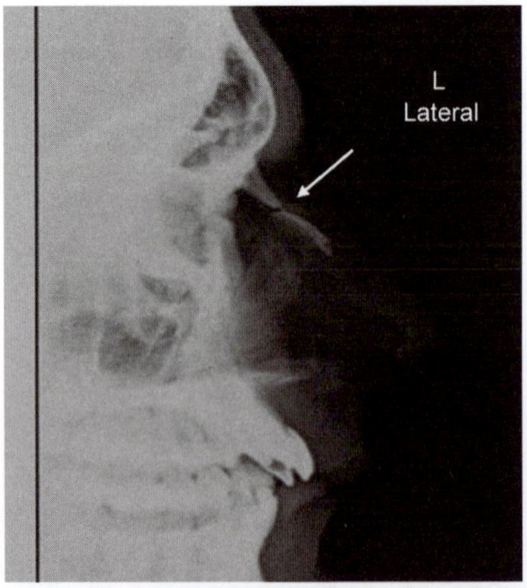

Fig. 1: X-ray showing nasal bone fracture

SEPTAL FRACTURES

As mentioned above, nasal bone fractures are often accompanied with fractures of septum.

Septal fractures are of two main types:

Chevallet fracture	Jarajavay fracture
Blow is from below upwards When septal fracture line is vertical	The blow if from side of nose when the fracture line is **horizontal**

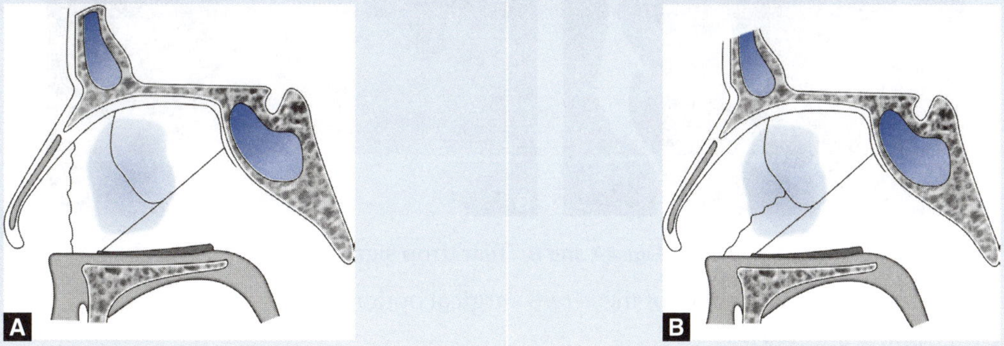

Figs 2A and B: Showing differences between two fractures

TREATMENT OF NASAL BONE AND SEPTUM FRACTURES

- If reduction of fractures is required, then it must be done as soon as possible **(immediately)**.
- After few hours, assessment will be difficult due to oedema.
- If the patient comes after few hour and oedema has taken place; we should wait for 5-7 days for oedema to settle and then reduction should be undertaken.
- If the patient present very late and the fractures will heal and osteotomies will be required.
- The forceps required for these reductions are shown below:

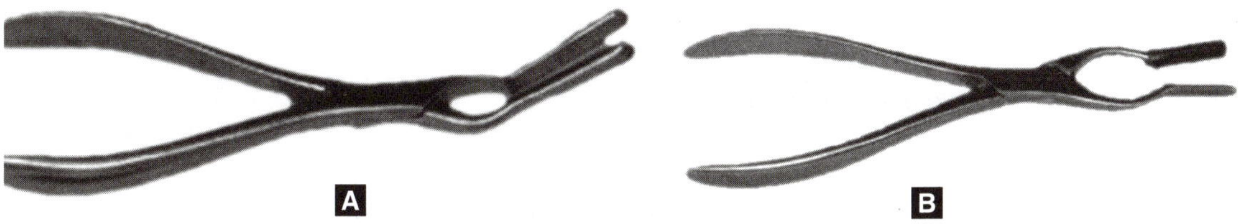

Figs 3A and B: (A) Asche's forcep used for septum; (B) Walsam's forcep used for nasal bone

FRACTURES OF MAXILLA

Fractures of maxilla are classified as Le Fort fractures.

They are three types as given below:

Le Fort I fracture	Le Fort II fracture	Le Fort III fracture
• This is also called longitudinal fractures • Is also called Guerin fractures	• This is called pyramidal fractures	• This is called craniofacial disjunction
• Fracture passes through floor of nose and maxilla	• Fracture passes from maxilla to floor of orbit to root of nose. • "Panda facies" may be seen	• Facial bones separate from cranial bones
• Fixation may be required	• Fixation may be required	• Fixation may be required

BLOW OUT FRACTURE

This is an **isolated** fracture of **floor of orbit**.

Some books say that in this fracture, the medial wall of orbit (lamina papyracea) is also fractured along with orbital floor.

X-ray finding in this fracture is ***Tear drop sign/hanging drop sign.***

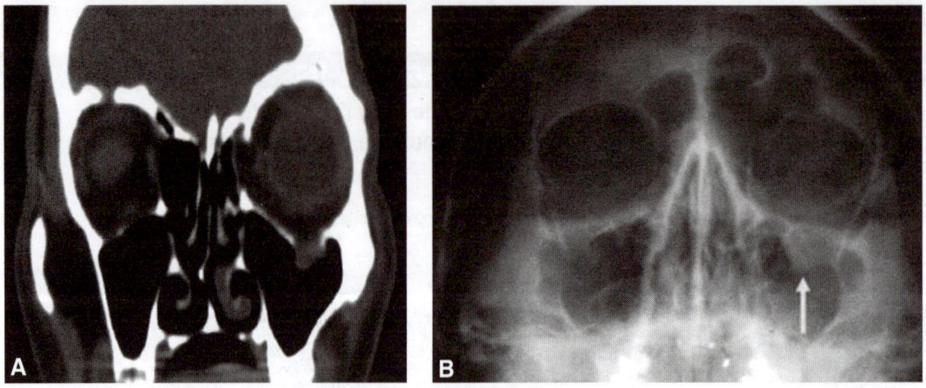

Figs 4A and B: Tear drop sign

Treatment is surgical repair with either of these two surgical options:

- Endoscopic transantral approach
- Caldwell Luc's surgery

Zygoma/Zygomaticomaxillary Complex Fracture

This fracture is also called **Tripod fracture** because

Three articulations are disrupted

- Fronto-zygomatic
- Infraorbital rim
- Zygomatico-maxillary butress

  The main finding is ***loss of malar eminence.***

  In most cases no treatment is required.

Open reduction and wiring is needed in the following situation:

- Patient wants it for cosmetic reasons
- Entrapment of vessel or nerve like infraorbital nerve

Mandibular Fracture

The most common site of fracture on the mandible is the **neck of condyle or subcondyle.**

Guardsman Fracture

It is seen when somebody falls down with chin hitting the ground.

The fracture involves ***symphysis and condyles (usually both the condyles).***

CSF Rhinorrhea (Most Important Topic in this Chapter)

CSF rhinorrhoea is flow of CSF through the nasal cavity due to fracture of the roof of nose.

The most common cause of CSF Rhinorrhea is the **surgical trauma of cribriform plate of the ethmoid bone**.

Some books claim that fovea ethmoidalis fracture is the most common cause. This is NOT true.

Flowchart 1: Causes of CSF rhinorrhea

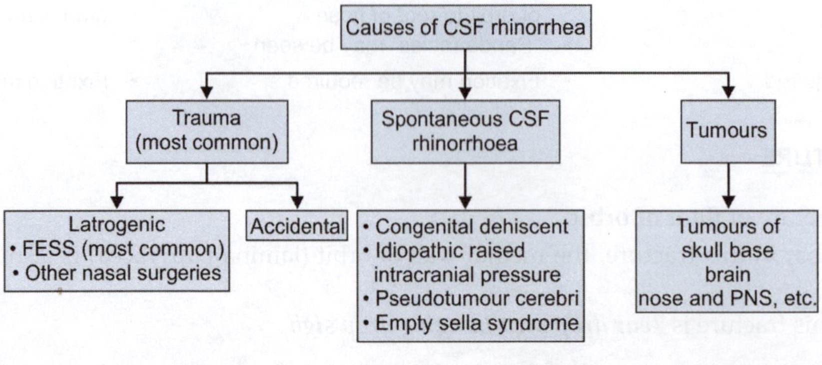

Few Features Are

- The nasal discharge cannot be sniffed back
- There is a clear fluid with **no** sedimentation
- **Handkerchief sign**: No stiffening on drying the handkerchief after wiping the discharge
- **Halo sign**: If we take a drop of nasal discharge on blotting paper, there is blood stain in centre surrounded by region of clear fluid and hence looks like a halo.
- **Target sign:** same as halo sign
- **β_2 transferrin:** This is ***most specific and most sensitive*** indicator of CSF rhinorrhea. It is seen on immunoelectrophoresis.
- **Glucose** content of the discharge is more than **30 mg/dL**.
- **Diagnostic nasal endoscopy**: We can see fracture site.

Investigation

HRCT used to be standard investigation for CSF Rhinorrhea.

But it has been seen that **CT cisternography and MR cisternography** are alternate investigations. Both of these have some advantages and some disadvantages. Hence, one cannot be better than the other. The best results are seen when both are done together.

Flowchart 2: Investigation for CSF rhinorrhea

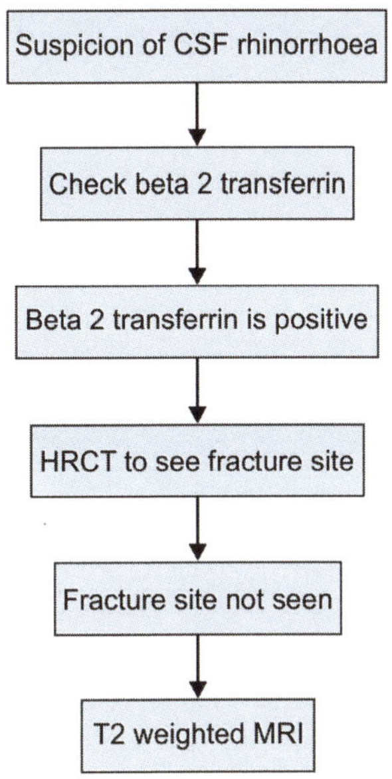

Treatment

- Conservative treatment is given for 1-2 weeks. First line of treatment
- Surgical repair when this fails to heal the defect.
- For surgical repair FESS is one of the good options.

Oroantral Fistula

Oroantral fistula is a fistula between the oral cavity and antrum of highmore (Maxilla).

The **most common cause of oroantral fistula is tooth extraction.**

As we have discussed, 2nd premolar and 1st molar teeth are closely related to the maxillary cavity.

Extraction of these teeth may result in oroantral fistula.

Treatment

The primary treatment is conservative management. We should wait for about 2 weeks for spontaneous repair.

If it fails to repair within 2 weeks, then surgical repair should be done.

Caldwell Luc's surgery is a good option.

Last minute revision

- *Most common fractured bone on the face is the nasal bone*
- *Chevallet fracture is vertical fracture of septum*
- *Jarjavay fracture is horizontal fracture of septum*
- *Le Fort fractures are fractures of maxilla*
- *Le Fort fracture is also called craniofacial dysjunction*
- *Blow out fracture is fracture of orbital floor*
- *Tear drop sign is diagnostic finding*
- *Tripod fracture is fracture of zygoma*
- *Most common site of fracture of mandible is the subcondyle/condyle*
- *CSF rhinorrhea is caused by traumatic fracture of cribriform plate*
- *Beta transferring is diagnostic of CSF rhinorrhea*
- *Conservative management is the first line of treatment*
- *Oroantral fistula is caused by tooth extraction*
- *Conservative management is the treatment of choice.*

QUESTIONS

1. **The most common site of leak in CSF rhinorrhoea is:**
   a. Sphenoid sinus. b. Frontal sinus.
   c. Cribriform plate. d. Tegmen tympani
2. **Common site for CSF Rhinorrhoea is:**
   a. Ethmoidal sinus b. Frontal sinus
   c. Petrous d. Cribriform plate
3. **CSF rhinorrhea is leak of CSF into the nasal cavity through:**
   a. Cribriform plate b. Ethmoidal air cell
   c. Frontal sinus
4. **CSF rhinorrhoea is diagnosed by:**
   a. Beta 2 microglobulin
   b. Beta 2 transferrin
   c. Thyroglobulin
   d. Transthyretin
5. **All of the following about CSF rhinorrhea is true *except:***
   a. MC site is fovea ethmoidalis
   b. B2 lactoferrin specific
   c. Investigation of choice is MRI
   d. Trauma is the most common cause
6. **A person present with cribriform plate fracture with CSF rhinorrhea. What will be immediate treatment?**
   a. Frequent blowing of nose
   b. Plugging of nose with paraffin
   c. Craniotomy
   d. Antibiotics with wait for 7 days.
7. **In Chevallet fracture of nasal bone, mechanism of trauma is:**
   a. Blow from side b. Blow from below
   c. Blow from front d. Blow from above
8. **CSF otorrhea (ear CSF discharge) occurs due to:**
   a. Trauma of tympanic membrane
   b. Trauma of petrous temporal bone
   c. Trauma of cribriform plate
   d. Trauma of parietal bone
9. **Immediate action to be taken in CSF rhinorrhea is:**
   a. Nasal packing
   b. Prophylactic antibiotic and X-ray
   c. Head low position and vasoconstrictors
   d. Exploration
10. **Management of undisplaced fracture of Zygoma is:**
    a. Wiring to frontal bone
    b. No-specific treatment
    c. Open reduction
    d. Closed reduction
11. **Not seen in fracture of maxilla is:**
    a. Anesthesia of upper lip
    b. CSF rhinorrhea
    c. Mobility of maxilla
    d. Malocclusion
12. **A patient of head injury is brought to hospital. Patient is conscious and is having clear discharge from the nose. NCCT head was done which showed nonoperable injury of frontobasal area. What is the most appropriate management:**
    a. Wait and watch
    b. Do a MRI to localize the leak and control the discharge endoscopically
    c. Put a dural catheter to control CSF leak
    d. Approach transcranial to repair the damage frontobasal region.
13. **Most important primary care in faciomaxillary trauma is to:**
    a. Assess the level of consciousness
    b. Ensure adequate airway
    c. Look for CNS injury
    d. Immediate fracture reduction
14. **Ideal time for correction of nasal bone fracture:**
    a. Immediately
    b. After 1 week
    c. After 4 weeks
    d. After 6 weeks
15. **While playing a young boy was hit on the nose and developed DNS. However, the septum was not deviated. The following of the patient is true:**
    a. He should be taken for open reduction after 1 week
    b. He should be taken for closed reduction as soon as oedema subsides
    c. Septoplasty should be done along with nasal bone reduction
    d. He is having Jarjavay fracture
16. **A patient presents with enophthalmos after trauma to face by a blunt object. This could be due to all *except:***
    a. Fracture maxilla
    b. Fracture zygoma
    c. Fracture nasal bone
    d. Fracture ethmoid
17. **Nerve damaged during zygomatic fracture:**
    a. Supraorbital nerve b. Infraorbital nerve
    c. Facial nerve d. Lingual\nerve
18. **Guardsman's fracture involves:**
    a. Symphysis with condyles
    b. Angle and body
    c. Ramus and body
    d. None
19. **Le Fort fracture does not involve:**
    a. Zygoma b. Maxilla
    c. Nasal bone d. Mandible

ANSWERS AND EXPLANATIONS

1. **c. Cribriform plate**
2. **d. Cribriform plate**
3. **CSF rhinorrhea is leak of CSF into the nasal cavity through:**
   - Cribriform plate
   - Ethmoidal air cell or
   - Frontal sinus

   The most common site is cribriform plate and fovea ethmoidalis .
   Leak from petrous bone will lead to CSF otorrhea and not rhinorrhea.
4. **b. Beta 2 transferrin**
   Beta 2 transferrin is present in CSF and not in nasal discharge and hence is used for the diagnosis of CSF rhinorrhea.
   It is the most specific investigation for this condition.
   - Beta-2 transferrin is a carbohydrate-free (desialated) isoform of transferrin, which is almost only found in the cerebrospinal fluid. It is not found in blood, mucus or tears, thus making it a specific marker of cerebrospinal fluid, applied as an assay in cases where cerebrospinal fluid leakage is suspected.
   - Beta-2 transferrin would also be positive in patients with perilymph fluid leaks, as it is also present in inner ear perilymph. Thus, beta-2 transferrin in otorrhea would be suggestive of either a CSF leak or a perilymph leak
5. **d. Trauma is the most common cause**
   The most common cause of CSF rhinorrhea is ***surgical trauma of the nasal roof mainly the cribriform plate.***
   The incident of surgical trauma has increased with the advent of functional endoscopic sinus surgery (FESS).
   In fact, CSF rhinorrhea is one of the most serious complications of FESS.

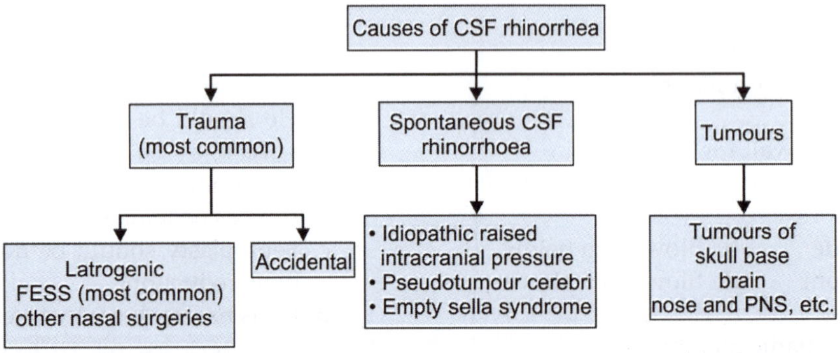

Differences between CSF and Nasal Secretions

CSF fluid	Nasal secretion
• History of sinus surgery, head injury or intracranial tumour	• Sneezing, nasal stuffiness, itching in the nose or lacrimation.
• A few drops or a stream of fluid gushes down when bending forward or straining	• Continuous flow of discharge, No effect of bending forward or straining.
• Cannot be sniffed back	• Can be sniffed back
• Character of discharge is thin, watery and clear slimy (mucus) or clear (tear)	• Discharge is sweet and salty
• Sugar content More than 30 mg/dL	• Less than 10 mg/dL
• Beta 2 transferrin is present (It is most specific for CSF)	• Always absent
• CSF and blood are mixed, double ring sign (or target sign) also called halo sign is seen	• No target sign/halo sign

Treatment

Early cases of post traumatic CSF rhinorrhoea are managed:
- Conservatively by placing the patient in the semi-sitting position, avoiding blowing of nose, sneezing and straining.
- Prophylactic antibiotics are also administered to prevent meningitis.
- Persistent cases of CSF rhinorrhoea are treated surgically by:
  - Nasal endoscopic (FESS) or
  - Intracranial approach.

6. **d. Antibiotics with wait for 7 days.**

CSF rhinorrhea refers to the drainage of cerebrospinal fluid through the nose. It is characterized by
- Unilateral nasal discharge,
- Test positive for glucose and,
- Beta-2 transferrin. It is a sign of basal skull fracture.

Management includes watchful waiting about 90 percent patients respond to conservative management
- Leaks often stop spontaneously. If this does not occur then neurosurgical closure is necessary to prevent the spread of infection to the meninges.
- Packing the nose by inserting a foreign body will increase the risk of infection. It can have devastating complications in some patients, as the communication between the nasal cavity and the cerebrospinal fluid and CNS can result in bacterial infections of the CNS that can have catastrophic effects on the patient
- Blowing of nose will lead to pneumatic cavity in brain which can lead to raised ICT.

7. **b. Blow from below**

Chevallet fracture is the fracture of nasal septum. Septal fractures are often accompanied with fractures of nasal bones.

Septal fractures are of two main types:

Chevallet fracture	Jarjavay fracture
Blow is from below upwards When septal fracture line is vertical	The blow if from side of nose when the fracture line is **horizontal**
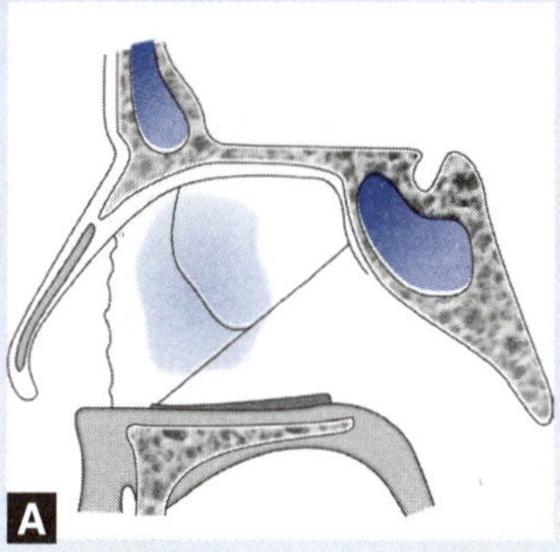 A	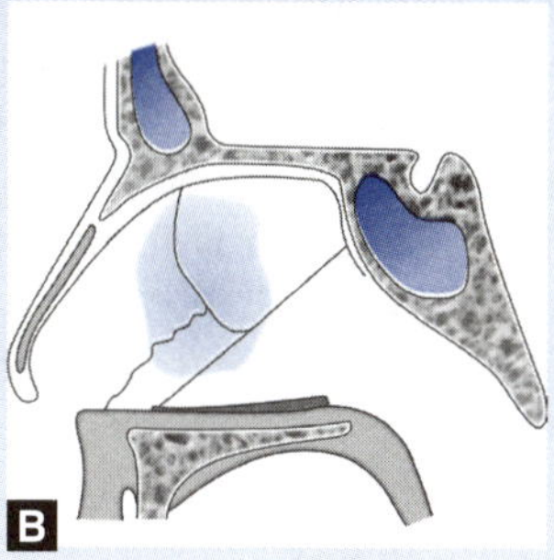 B

8. **b. Trauma of petrous temporal bone**

Ear is located inside the petrous part of the temporal bone. The roof of the ear is called ***tegmen tympani.*** Tegmen tympani separates ear from middle cranial fossa.

Fracture of temporal bone are of three types:

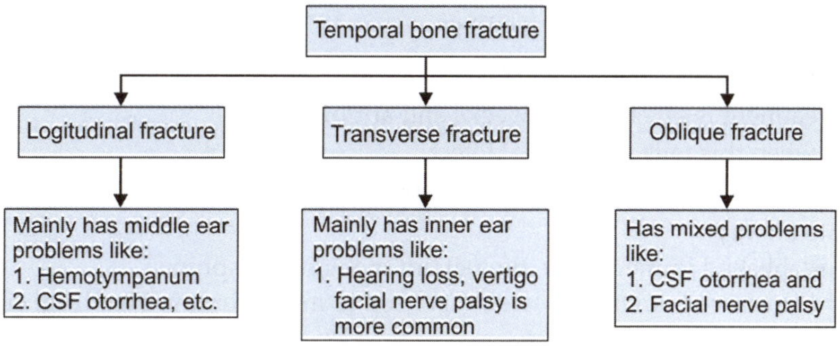

9. **b. Prophylactic antibiotic and X-ray**
In case of CSF rhinorrhea, it is clear that there is fracture in the roof of the nose. The site and size of the fracture has to be identified. For this we can either do
- ***CT Scan or***
- ***X-ray*** (when scan is not possible)

Fracture of the nasal roof also creates direct connection between the nose and cranial cavity. To prevent the nasal pathogens from infecting the cranial cavity, antibiotics should be added.
- Nasal packing cannot stop CSF rhinorrhea. Moreover it is increase the chance of infection.
- Head low position will increase the CSF flow.
- Exploration is the second line of management

10. **b. No-specific treatment**
Zygoma is also called the ***cheek bone.*** It has no function. It only has cosmetic importance.
It is made of three bones and therefore the fracture is called ***tripod fracture.***
This leads to cosmetic deformity and NO functional problem.
Therefore, no treatment is required in most cases.
The only surgical option is open reduction. Indications for this surgery are:
- Patient wants cosmetic correction.
- Comminuted fracture of the bone
- Intrapment of blood vessel or nerve in the fracture site
- Nonhealing of primary fracture, etc.

11. **b. CSF rhinorrhea**
Face is divided into three parts:
1. Upper third
2. Mid third, and
3. Lower third

Maxilla is the part of mid third of face.
Maxillary fractures are divided into three types:
1. Le Fort I fracture
2. Le Fort II fracture and
3. Le Fort III fracture

- Upper lip is supplied by infraorbital branch of maxillary nerve. This nerve runs through infraorbital groove and foramen in the roof of maxilla. This may get damaged in Le Fort II and III fractures leading to anaesthesia of the upper lip.
- The floor of maxilla is formed by alveolus. Alveolus harbers the upper teeth. Therefore, open bite and malocclusion almost always happen in maxillary fractures.
- In Le Fort III fracture (craniofacial dysjuncion), the maxilla is free from rest of the skull leading mobility of maxilla.
- CSF rhinorrhea is seen in fracture of upper third of face and is NOT seen in fractures of mid third and lower third of face
- In a pure maxillary fracture (mid third of face), the base of the skull is NOT fractured. Therefore, CSF rhinorrhea is NOT seen in purely maxillary fracture.
- However, Le Fort III is often associated with fracture of other bones like ethmoidal, nasal roof (upper third of face), etc. These may cause CSF rhinorrhea. Please note that this rhinorrhea is not caused by the maxilla

12. **a. Wait and watch**
This is a case of CSF rhinorrhea following trauma.

TREATMENT OF TRAUMATIC CSF RHINORRHEA

- **Conservative** treatment is given for 1-2 weeks and antibiotics.
- **Surgical** repair when this fails to heal the defect.
- For surgical repair **FESS** is one of the good options.

13. **b. Ensure adequate airway**
If airway is NOT established immediately, the patient may die of asphyxia.
It is well known that in case of emergency we must keep in mind **airway, bleeding, circulation (ABC).**

14. **a. Immediately**

Treatment of Nasal Bone and Septum Fractures

- If reduction of fractures is required, then it must be done as soon as possible **(immediately)**.
- After few hours, assessment will be difficult due to oedema.
- If the patient comes after few hour and oedema has taken place; we should wait for 5-7 days for oedema to settle and then reduction should be undertaken.
- If the patient present very late and the fractures has heal and osteotomies will be required.

15. **b. He should be taken for closed reduction as soon as oedema subsides**
As we have seen in the previous question; reduction should be done immediately. This choice is NOT given in the question. From the question it is assumed that the oedema has already taken place when the child comes to the doctor.

16. **a. Fracture maxilla**
Most common traumatic cause of enophthalmos is **blow out fracture.**
Blow out fracture is the fracture of floor of orbit. Floor of orbit is also the roof of maxilla. Hence, maxillary fracture (roof) can cause enophthalmos.
Fracture of zygoma can cause enophthalmos.
Severe ethmoidal fractures may, in rare cases, cause enophthalmos.
Nasal bone fractures cannot cause enophthalmos.

17. **b. Infraorbital nerve**
In fracture of zygoma, the infraorbital area may get involved damaging the infraorbital nerve.

18. **a. Symphysis with condyles**
This is also called **parade ground fracture** because it is seen in guards during parade.
The guards fall on the ground hitting the mid-chin on the ground, fracturing the ***symphysis with both condyles.***

19. **d. Mandible**

Le Fort I fracture	Le Fort II fracture	Le Fort III fracture
• This is also called longitudinal fracture • Is also called Guerin fracture	• This is called pyramidal fracture	• This is called craniofacial disjunction
• Fracture passes through floor of nose and maxilla	• Fracture passes from maxilla to floor of orbit to root of nose. • "Panda facies" may be seen	• Facial bones separate from cranial bones
• Fixation may be required	• Fixation may be required	• Fixation may be required

CHAPTER

24 Growth and Tumour of Nose and PNS

RHINOPHYMA

Rhinophyma is a disease of the skin overlying the nose.

In this condition, the sebaceous glands of this undergo hypertrophy leading to large looking nose.

Because of the look, this condition is also called **potato nose.**

This condition is more commonly seen in patients suffering from rosacea.

Rhinophyma is a cosmetic problem and so cosmetic treatment is required.

Some treatment options are:

- Oral tetracycline and topical metronidazole
- Removal using Silver's knife
- Removal with electrocoagulation
- Removal with laser

FIBROUS DYSPLASIA

Fibrous dysplasia is a bony disease where the normal bone is replaced by irregular trabecles of immature, nonlamellar and metaplastic bone.

It is a benign condition of the bone.

Fibrous dysplasia **most commonly affects the maxillary and the mandible.**

It has two types:

1. Monostotic: This is the more common type.

2. Polyostotic: This is less common type.
Polyostotic type of may be associated with McCune-Albright syndrome.

Presentation

Fibrous dysplasia presents as ***diffuse, gradually progressive and painless swelling in the cheek (maxilla) or forehead (frontal bone) in a young child.***

NOTE: Any young child with slow growing painless swelling which may cause cosmetic distortion of the face should raise the suspicion of fibrous dysplasia.

X-ray finding.

In X-ray and CT Scan give **ground glass appearance.**

Treatment

- In most cases, NO treatment is needed.
- If it causes cosmetic deformity then chiseling or saving may be needed.
- If it encroaches on vital structures, then craniofacial resection may be required.

MUCOSAL MALIGNANT MELANOMA

Mucosal malignant melanoma is an extremely rare condition.

When it happens, **nasal mucosa is the most common site.**

This tumour is seen in adult males.

Like the skin melanomas, the mucosal melanomas are also very aggressive tumours.

The best treatment is ***radical excision of the tumour with adjuvant postoperative radiotherapy.***

Prognosis is very poor.

INVERTED PAPILLOMA

Inverted papilloma is a benign epithelial tumour of the nose.

This has various names

Names of tumours

- *Inverted papilloma*
- *Ringertz tumour*
- *Transitional cell tumour*
- *Schneiderian's tumour.*

It may be benign but has malignant potential

It arises most commonly from the ***lateral wall of nose (from meatal meatus).***

It is usually seen in males more than 50 years old.

The most common presentation of this tumor is ***nasal obstruction with bleeding mass in the nasal cavity.***

NOTE: It is one of the differential diagnoses of *bleeding nasal mass.*

Histopathology

Inverted papilloma has inversion of neoplastic epithelium into the underlying stroma.

Treatment

- Radical excision with a wide margin.
- The surgery of choice is **Medial Maxillectomy**.
- **FESS** may be done for smaller tumour.

Olfactory Neuroblastoma

Olfactory neuroblastoma is a neuroendocrine tumour

Olfactory neuroblastoma is also called **aesthesioneuroblastoma.**

It is tumour of **basal cells of the olfactory neuroepithelium.**

It has bimodal distribution (20 years and 50 years) and is more common in females.

Treatment

- Total excision followed by radiotherapy.

Carcinoma of the Sinuses

Among the sinuses; carcinoma most commonly arises from the **maxillary sinus.**

Ethmoidal sinus carcinoma is seen more commonly in *wood workers.*

Most common type of carcinoma in PNS is the squamous cell carcinoma, but in wood workers the most common is adenocarcinoma

It is seen in the age group of 40-60 years.

Presentation

The most common presentation is ***bleeding from nose or bleeding nasal polyp.***

NOTE: this is a differential diagnosis of ***bleeding nasal mass.***

The usually involved lymph nodes are:

- Submandibular lymph nodes, and
- Jugulodigastric lymph nodes

Classification

- **Ohngren's Classification**
  In this, an Ohngren's line is drawn from the angle of mandible to medial canthus of eye.
  The area above this line is called *suprastructure* and the area below this line is called *infrastructure,*
  Growth inferior to this line has better prognosis as compared to growth above the line.
- **Lederman's classification**
  In this; two lines are drawn called ***Sebileau's line.***
- **AJCC Classification is also an option**.
  This is based on TNM classification.

Treatment

- Is combination of surgery and radiotherapy

Last minute revision

- *Rhinophyma is also called potato nose*
- *Rhinophyma is hypertrophy of sebaceous glands*
- *Fibrous dysplasia presents as gradual swelling on the cheek of young children*
- *CT Scan shows ground glass appearance*
- *Inverted papilloma is also called ringertz tumour*
- *It arises from lateral wall of nose in adult males and presents as nasal bleeding*
- *Olfactory neuroblastoma also called esthesioneuroblastoma is tumour of olfactory epithelium*
- *Sinonasal carcinoma is seen in woodworkers and is adenocarcinoma*
- *Ohngren's line is used in maxillary carcinoma*
- *Sinonasal carcinomas are treated with surgery + radiotherapy*

QUESTIONS

1. **Which of these is also called potato nose?**
   a. Rhinophyma
   b. Rhinoscleroma
   c. Calcified foreign body in the nose
   d. None of the above
2. **True about inverted papilloma is:**
   a. Arises from nasal septum
   b. Common in children
   c. Risk of malignancy
   d. Postoperative radiotherapy is useful
3. **Woodworkers are associated with which of these sinonasal carcinoma?**
   a. Adenocarcinoma
   b. Squamous cell carcinoma
   c. Anaplastic carcinoma
   d. Melanoma
4. **Maxillary carcinoma stage III (T3N0M0), treatment of choice is:**
   a. Radiotherapy
   b. Surgery plus Radiotherapy
   c. Chemotherapy
   d. Chemotherapy plus surgery
5. **Commonest site of ivory osteoma**
   a. Frontoethmoidal region
   b. Mandible
   c. Maxilla
   d. Sphenoid
6. **Ohngren's line classification is based on:**
   a. Imaginary line between medial canthus and angle of mandible
   b. Imaginary line between lateral canthus and angle of mandible
   c. Horizontal lines passing through floor of orbit and floor of maxillary sinus
   d. Horizontal line passing from tragus of pinna to the lateral cantus of eye
7. **A 15-year-old child has a slow growing swelling in the right cheek for the past few months. The swelling is not painful and non-tender. What could be the diagnosis?**
   a. Maxillary carcinoma
   b. Fibrous dysplasia of maxilla
   c. Juvenile angiofibroma
   d. Inverted papilloma
8. **Tumour arising from olfactory nasal mucosa is:**
   a. Adenoid cystic carcinoma
   b. Inverted papilloma
   c. Nasal gloma
   d. Aesthesioneuroblastoma
9. **Which of these is true of head and neck mucosal malignant melanoma?**
   a. Most common site is head and neck is nasal mucosa
   b. Head and neck mucosa is the most common site overall
   c. Prognosis is very good
   d. All are true
10. **Inverted papilloma is characterized by all *except:***
    a. Is called schneiderian papilloma
    b. More common in females
    c. Presents with epistaxis and nasal obstruction
    d. Arises from lateral nasal wall
11. **Ground glass appearance of maxilla is seen in:**
    a. Maxillary sinusitis
    b. Maxillary carcinoma
    c. Maxillary polyps
    d. Maxillary fibrous dysplasia
12. **First lymph node involved in maxillary carcinoma:**
    a. Submental b. Submandibular
    c. Clavicular d. Lower jugular

IMAGE BASED QUESTION

13. **Study the CT Scans of PNS given below. Which of the statements given is false?**

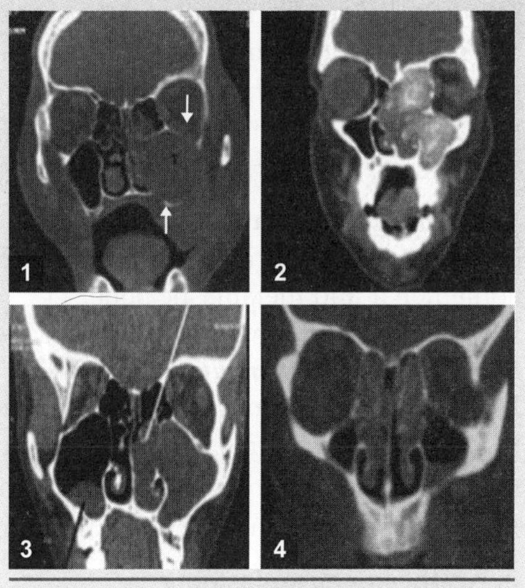

    a. Figure 1 shows maxillary carcinoma
    b. Figure 2 shows fungal sinusitis
    c. Figure 3 shows antrochoanal polyp
    d. Figure 4 shows ethmoid carcinoma

ANSWERS AND EXPLANATIONS

1. **a. Rhinophyma**
Rinophyma is a disease of sebaceous glands which undergo hypertrophy leading to large nose.
Because of the look, this condition is also called **potato nose.**
Rhinoscleroma is called **woody nose.**

2. **c. Risk of malignancy**
Inverted papilloma is a ***benign tumour with malignant potential.***
It is usually seen in adult males and arises from lateral nasal wall.
Excision with wide margin should be done.
Radiotherapy may cause malignant changes.

3. **a. Adenocarcinoma**
Although, the most common type of sinonasal carcinoma is the squamous cell carcinoma; in ***woodworkers adenocarcinoma is more common.***
Sinonasal carcinoma is seen in the following professionals:
   - ***Woodworkers***- adenocarcinoma is more common
   - ***Leather workers***
   - ***Nickel workers.***

4. **b. Surgery plus Radiotherapy**
Almost in stages of maxillary carcinoma, the treatment of choice is surgery plus radiotherapy.

5. **a. Frontoethmoidal region**
Ivory osteoma is a dense and compact tumour of the mature lamellar bone with little medulary space and deficient haversian canals.
The most common site is frontoethmoidal area.

6. **a. Imaginary line between medial canthus and angle of mandible**
Ohngren's line is an imaginary line between medial canthus and angle of mandible.
This line divides the maxillary sinus into two parts:
   - ***Supero-lateral part, and***
   - ***Inferomedial part.***

   It is believed that inferomedial carcinomas of maxilla have better prognosis compared to the superolateral carcinomas.

7. **b. Fibrous dysplasia of maxilla**
Fibrous dysplasia is a bony disease where the normal bone is replaced by irregular trabecles of immature, nonlamellar and metaplastic bone.
Fibrous dysplasia presents as ***diffuse, gradually progressive and painless swelling in the cheek (maxilla) or forehead (frontal bone) in a young child.***
X-ray/scan shows **ground glass appearance.**
   - Maxillary carcinoma is usually seen in adult males and presents with nasal bleeding.
   - Juvenile angiofibroma is seen in juvenile males and presents with severe epistaxis.
   - Inverted papilloma is ringertz tumour. It presents as nasal growth with bleeding.

8. **d. Aesthesioneuroblastoma**
Olfactory neuroblastoma is also called **aesthesioneuroblastoma.**
It is tumour of **basal cells of the olfactory neuroepithelium.**

9. **a. Most common site is head and neck is nasal mucosa**
Malignant mucosal melanoma is a very uncommon tumour in the head and neck region.
When present, it is most common in the nasal mucosa.
It is a very aggressive tumour with very poor prognosis.

10. **b. More common in females**
Inverted papilloma is more common in males.

11. **d. Maxillary fibrous dysplasia**
Fibrous dysplasia presents as ***diffuse, gradually progressive and painless swelling in the cheek (maxilla) or forehead (frontal bone) in a young child.***
NOTE: any young child with slow growing painless swelling which may cause cosmetic distortion of the face should raise the suspicion of fibrous dysplasia.

X-RAY FINDINGS

X-ray and CT Scan give **ground glass appearance.**

12. **b. Submandibular lymph nodes.**

IMAGE BASED ANSWER

13. **d. Figure 4 shows ethmoid carcinoma**
    - Figure 1 shows a mass in the maxillary sinus and there is bony destruction as a result of which the mass has spread into the cheek. This is maxillary carcinoma.
    - Figure 2 shows a destructive mass occupying the entire nose and sinuses of one side. The important point is that there are hyperdense areas in the mass which are ***calcified areas***. This is finding of fungal sinusitis.
    - Figure 3 shows a nondestructive mass in the maxilla. This is maxillary/antrochoanal polyp.
    - Figure 4 shows non destructive mass in both the ethmoids. These are ethmoidal polyps. Carcinomas are usually unilateral which may spread to the other side and will also show bony destruction.

PART 3

Throat

CHAPTERS

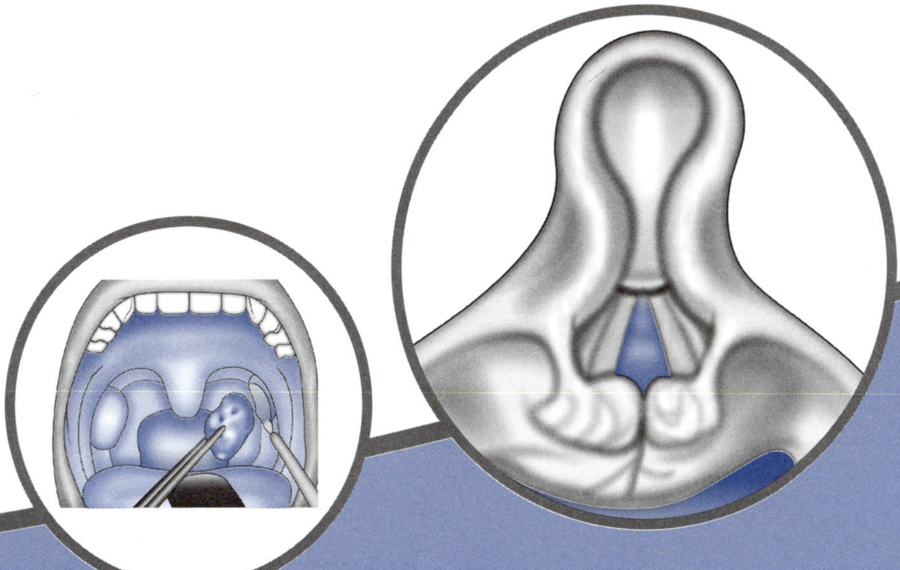

CHAPTER

25 Embryology of Throat

Most of the important facts about embryology of throat are already discussed along with ear embryology in 1st chapter.

This chapter is mostly repeatation of that.

The embryology of throat is related with the pharyngeal arches.

The pharyngeal arches appear in the **4–5 weeks of intrauterine life (IUL).**

Given below are important related to pharyngeal arches:

Arches	Important structure from cleft and arch	Important structure from pouch	Nerve and artery of the arch
First	• Maxilla • Malleus and Incus • **Meckel's cartilage** • Muscles of mastication	• Middle ear cleft with Eustachian tube	• Mandibular nerve • Maxillary artery
Second	• **Reichert's cartilage** • Stapes • Muscles of facial expression	• Bed of tonsil	• Facial nerve
Third	• Part of hyoid bone • Stylopharyngeus muscle	• Thymus • **Inferior parathyroid**	• Glossopharyngeal nerve
Fourth and Sixth	• Laryngeal cartilages **except epiglottis** • Laryngeal muscles	• **Ultimobranchial body (from V arch)** • **Superior parathyroid**	• Vagus nerve

Note: All The Laryngeal Cartilages Develop From IVth And Vth Pharyngeal Arches Except Epiglottis Which Develops From Hypobranchial Eminence (IIIrd Arch)

Few important arch anomlies	Syndromes from these anomalies
• 1st arch anomalies	• Treacher Collins syndrome • Goldenhar syndrome • Pierre Robin syndrome • Branchio-Oto-Renal syndrome
• IIIrd and IVth pouch anomaly	• DiGeorge syndrome

DEVELOPMENT OF LARYNX

The cephalic end of the ventral outgrowth of developing foregut **develops into the glottis and infraglottis.** The supraglottis develops from the compression of foregut by the pharyngeal mesoderm.

Difference between Infantile Laryx and Adult Larynx

Infant larynx	Adult larynx
• Is higher up at $C_{2\text{-}3}$ vertebrae • As a result; epiglottis is close to soft palate and the two appose against each other during suckling. Therefore, an infant can swallow as well as breathe simultaneously.	• Is lower down between C3 to C6-7 vertebrae
• It is cone shaped	• It is cylindrical in shape
• Have softer cartilages	• Have harder cartilages
• The narrowest part is the sub-glottis	• The narrowest part is the glottis
• Lamina propria is not well developed	• Lamina propria is well developed

IMPORTANT CONGENITAL ANOMALIES OF THE PHARYNX AND LARYNX

Thyroglossal Cyst

Thyroglossal cyst is the cystic swelling of the persisting thyroglossal duct.

It could be present in the suprahyoid region or infrahyoid region.

The most common presentation is **"midline cystic swelling which moves on protruding the tongue".**

Treatment

Surgical excision is the treatment of choice.

The surgery of choice is **Sistrunk's operation.**

Tracheo-Esophageal Fistula (TOF)

These are of different types and are often associated with oesophageal atresia.

The food that the child takes in make enter the trachea.

Laryngomalacia

The most common congenital disease of larynx is ***laryngomalacia***.

In this; the child is born with extremely soft and flabby laryngeal cartilages.

This may involve all the cartilages but the mainly involved are ***epiglottis and the aryepiglottic folds.***

Main complaints

Stridor is the main presentation. The cry is normal.

The stridor is mainly *inspiratory* and increases during supine position but decreases during prone position.

Important point of stridor in infants

- *Laryngomalacia is the most common cause of stridor in newborn*
- *An infant with stridor is most probably having laryngomalacia*
- *Most common cause of stridor in infants is laryngomalacia*
- The most common congenital disease causing *expiratory stridor* is *subglottic vascular anomaly, i.e. subglottic hemangioma.*

Stridor

Stridors are of three types

1. *Inspiratory stridor*—when the obstruction is in the supraglottis.
2. *Expiratory stridor*—when the obstruction is in the subglottis.
3. *Biphasic stridor*—when the obstruction is in the glottis.

Examination

Laryngoscopric findings—direct laryngoscopy is the most important examination.

The finding is long and tubular epiglottis with curled up tip.

This is called ***Omega-shaped epiglottis***.

Omega shaped epiglottis is diagnostic of laryngomalacia.

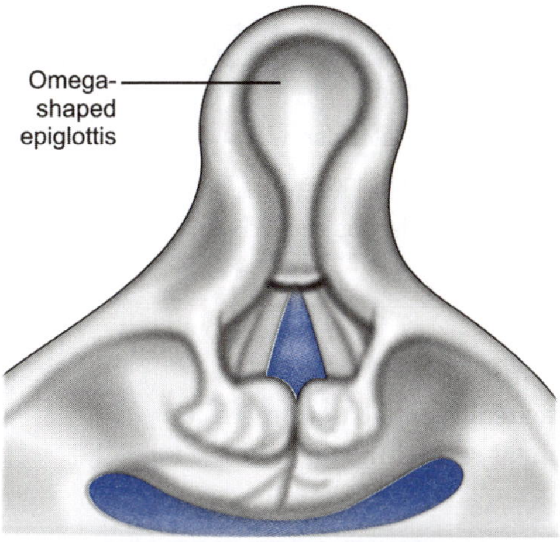

Fig. 1: Omega-shaped epiglottis

Fibroptic laryngoscopy may be done.

When patient has severe stridor, **microlaryngoscopy and bronchoscopy** should be done under general anaesthesia to rule out any other airway disease

Treatment

- Laryngomalacia is a self-healing disease but may take two years to heal.
- Hence, the parents need ***Reassurance (main treatment)***.
- Severe cases of laryngomalacia may lead to serious conditions like **Cor Pulmonale and pectus excavatum.**
- Such cases can be avoided by
- **Tracheostomy**
- **Aryepiglottoplasty/Supraglottoplasty**.

LARYNGEAL WEBS

This is due to incomplete canalization of larynx in the embryonic stage.

Anterior webs are more common but sometimes posterior webs may also be seen.

Presentation

- Inspiratory stridor
- High pitch squeaky voice
- Weak cry with recurrent attacks of croup.

Treatment

Endoscopic excision of web with CO_2 laser with/without keel placement is the best treatment.

In case of thick web; excision with laryngofissure with keel placement.

SUBGLOTTIC STENOSIS

Subglottic stenosis is formed due to incomplete canalization of the cricoids cartilage.

• Incomplete canalization of larynx	• Laryngeal web
• Incomplete canalization of cricoids/subglottic area	• Subglottic stenosis

Causes of Subglottic Stenosis

Two common causes of subglottic stenosis are:

- Congenital stenosis, and
- Intubation trauma (acquired stenosis)

The most common presentation is biphasic stridor.

Myer-Cotton grading of stenosis	
Grade I	0–5% stenosed
Grade II	50–70% stenosed
Grade III	70–99% stenosed
Grade IV	Complete obstruction

Treatment of Subglottic Stenosis

- Grade I stenosis may require no treatment
- The surgery of choice is **laryngotracheal reconstruction (LTR)**
- Another option is **partial cricotracheal resection (PCTR)**
- Tracheostomy may also be useful.

Last minute revision

- *Main structures from 1st arch are Meckel's cartilage, malleus, incus, maxilla, mandible*
- *Main structures from 2nd arch are Reichert's cartilage, stapes, facial muscles*
- *Larynx develops from IVth and VIth arch except epiglottis*
- *Epiglottis develops hypobranchial eminence of IIIrd arch*
- *Laryngomalacia is most common congenital disease of larynx*
- *Laryngomalacia is most common cause of stridor in newborns*
- *Omega-shaped epiglottis is the diagnostic finding in laryngomalacia*
- *Tracheal stenosis may require laryngo-tracheal reconstruction or partial cricotracheal resection.*

QUESTIONS

1. A 3-month-old child presents with intermittent stridor. Most likely cause is:
   a. Laryngotracheobronchitis
   b. Laryngomalacia
   c Respiratory obstruction
   d. Foreign body aspiraton
2. Rajesh, a 7-month-old child, presents with failure of gaining weight and noisy breathing which becomes worse when the child cries. Laryngoscopy shows a reddish mass in subglottis. Treatment modality may include all, except:
   a. Radiation b. Steroids
   c. Tracheostomy
   d. Carbon dioxide laser treatment
3. Most common case of stridor in neonates is:
   a. Laryngeal web b. Laryngomalacia
   c. Pneumonia d. Epiglottitis
4. Most common congenital abnormality of the larynx is:
   a. Laryngomalacia b. Laryngeal web
   c. Subglottic stenosis
   d. Subglottic haemangioma
5. Most common cause of stridor in children is:
   a. Laryngomalacia
   b. Congenital laryngeal paralysis
   c. Foreign body in larynx
   d. Congenital laryngeal tumours
6. Most common mode of treatment for laryngomalacia is:
   a. Reassurance b. Medical
   c. Surgery d. Wait and watch
7. Chromosome affected in laryngeal web is:
   a. 22q11 b. 22p11
   c. 16q12 d. 16p12
8. A four years old child presents with hoarseness for 4 months and stridor for 4 days. The most likely diagnosis is:
   a. Laryngomalacia b. Foreign body aspiration
   c. Epiglottitis
   d. Laryngeal papillomatosis
9. About laryngomalacia, all are true *except:*
   a. Is most common neonatal laryngeal anomaly
   b. Decreased symptoms during prone position
   c. Self limiting by 2–3 years
   d. Tracheostomy should be done
10. An infant is brought with stridor. He is diagnosed with laryngomalacia. The following will be found in this except:
    a. Stridor will be inspiratory
    b. Floppy AE folds
    c. Prominent arytenoids
    d. Hoarse cry
11. A child is born with 80% subglottic stridor. What grade stenosis is this?
    a. Grade I b. Grade II
    c. Grade III d. Grade IV
12. Cotton's grading is used for?
    a. Subglottic stenosis b. Laryngeal carcinoma
    c. Angiofibroma d. Vocal cord palsy
13. A 25-year-old female presented with gradually increasing respiratory distress since 4 days. She gives history of hospitalization and mechanical ventilation with orotracheal intubation for 2 weeks. Now she is diagnosed as having severe laryngotracheal stenosis. Management is:
    a. Laser excision b. Steroids
    c. Tracheal dilation
    d. Resection and end to end anastomosis
14. Topical mitomycin C is used for:
    a. Endoscopic treatment of angiofibroma
    b. Laryngotracheal stenosis
    c. Skull base osteomyelitis
    d. Tonsillectomy
15. A small child came with complaints of cough with expiratory wheeze. He gave history of tracheo-esophageal fistula formation. Most likely diagnosis is?
    a. Cough variant asthma b. Subglottic stenosis
    c. Tracheomalacia d. Vocal nodule

IMAGE BASED QUESTIONS

16. Look at this picture and answer the following question:

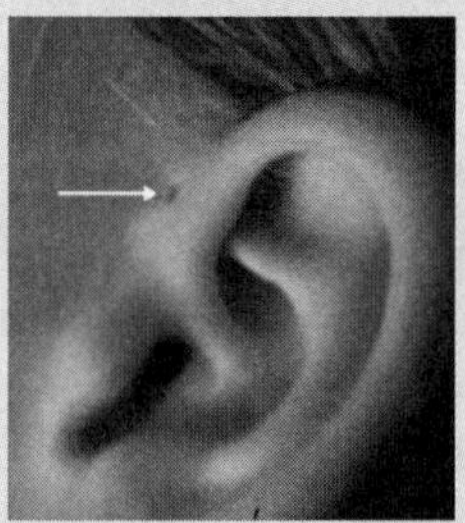

    a. It is a picture of preauricular sinus
    b. This is the most common arch anomaly
    c. It presents soon after birth
    d. All are true
17. An 8 months old child was brought to the clinic with mild stridor for the past one week. There was no history of fever, dyshagia excessive crying. The direct laryngoscopic finding is shown in the picture. Which of the following in NOT true?

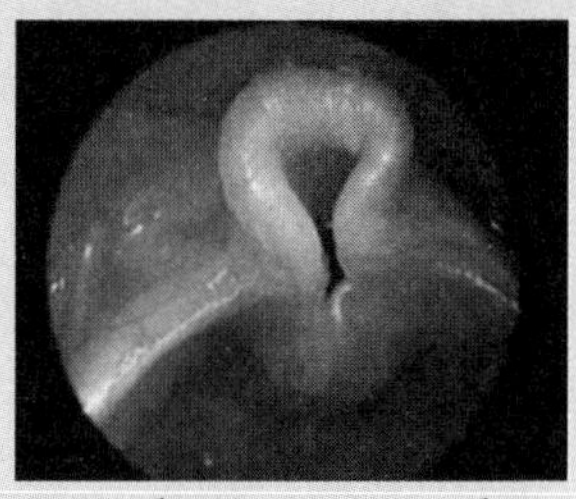

    a. The picture shows omega-shaped epiglottis
    b. In this case stridor is equal during inspirations and expiration
    c. This is the most common cause of stridor in infants
    d. No active intervention is required in this case

ANSWERS AND EXPLANATIONS

1. **b. Laryngomalacia**

Laryngomalacia is the most common congenital disease of larynx. It presents as stridor soon after birth. Hence, when a few months old child presents with intermittent stridor; it is probably laryngomalacia unless proven otherwise.

Important point of stridor in infants

- *Laryngomalacia is the most common cause of stridor in newborn*
- *An infant with stridor is most probably having laryngomalacia.*
- *Most common cause of stridor in infants is laryngomalacia*
- The most common congenital disease causing *expiratory stridor* is *subglottic vascular anomaly, i.e. subglottic hemangioma*

2. **a. Radiation**

The commonest subglottic reddish mass in infants is benign vascular tumour. It is usually a ***subglottic haemangioma***.

Subglottic haemangioma can be a congenital disease of the subglottis which presents as ***stridor between 6 months and 1 year of age.***

Treatment of subglottic haemangioma

- ***Tracheostomy*** may be required in most patients.
- Systemic steroid is given to relieve acute respiratory obstruction and regression of tumour.
- Intralesional steroids may be useful.
- CO_2 laser vaporization is done for small lesions.
- Radiotherapy may induce thyroid malignancy.

3. **b. Laryngomalacia**
4. **a. Laryngomalacia**
5. **a. Laryngomalacia**

The three questions are similar and so I have answered them together..

An infant presenting with stridor or recurrent stridor is most probably a case of laryngomalacia.

In larngomalacia, the stridor increases during:
- Supination,
- Feeding and
- Crying.

Stridor decreases when the patient is made to lie in
- Prone position.

Laryngoscopic finding is ***omega-shaped epiglottis***.

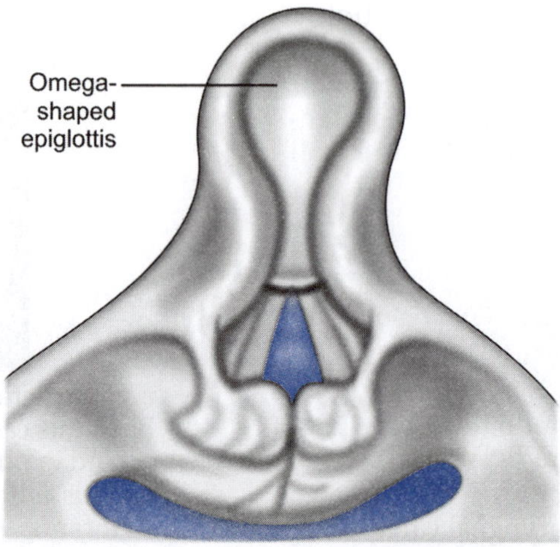

PART 3: THROAT

In this condition, the stridor is mainly during inspiration. Most common cause of expiratory stridor in new born child is subglottic vascular anomalies like hemangioma.

Causes of stridor in children
Congenital • Laryngomalacia • Stenosis • Subglottis web • Cysts • Vocal cord palsy
Acquired • Infections (epiglottitis, croup, etc.) • Foreign bodies • Subglottic haemangioma • Hereditary angioedema • Epidermolysis bullosa • Trauma (intubation, accidental, etc.)

6. **a. Reassurance**
Laryngomalacia does not require any treatment and is relieved of the problem by age of 2 yrs.
This has to be explained to the parent of the child. This is called reassurance.

7. **a. 22q11**
In laryngeal web, chromosome affected is 22q11.
Laryngeal web is a congenital anomaly of the larynx due to incomplete canalization of larynx in the embryonic stage.
The chromosomal defect responsible for it is 22q11.

Presentation

- Inspiratory stridor
- High pitch squeaky voice
- Weak cry with recurrent attacks of croup.

Treatment

- ***Endoscopic excision of web with CO_2 laser with/without keel placement is the best treatment.***

8. **d. Laryngeal papillomatosis**
From the history we understand that the child is suffering from a long duration disease of larynx (hoarseness for 4 months), which is progressive in nature (stridor for 4 days).
   - Laryngomalacia is the most common congenital disease of larynx and does NOT cause voice change or hoarseness.
   - Foreign body aspiration is an acute problem. It will NOT have 4 months old history of hoarseness.
   - Epiglottitis is an acute infective disease of epiglottis caused by *H. influenzae*. The child is around 5 years old and has fever, stridor, dysphagia with drooling.
   - Laryngeal papillomatosis is the ***most common laryngeal tumour in children.*** They are multiple in numbers and can cause symptoms like hoarseness and stridor. Since this is a benign tumour, the history can be of long duration.

9. **d. Tracheostomy should be done.**
Laryngomalacia is a self remitting condition. Hence, reassurance of the parents is the treatment.

10. **d. Hoarse cry**
The only problem in the child with laryngomalacia is inspiratory stridor. The mainly affected part is the supra-glottis.
Hoarseness is a symptom of glottis diseases and hence will NOT be present in laryngomalacia.

11. **c. Grade III**

Myer-Cotton grading of subglottic stenosis	
Grade I	0–5% stenosed
Grade II	50–70% stensed
Grade III	70–99% stenosed
Grade IV	Complete obstruction

12. **a. Subglottic stenosis**
Please refer to the table in the above answer.

13. **d. Resection and end to end anastomosis**
As mentioned in the question, the patient has severe stenosis. The management of severe stenosis is ***resection and end to end anastomosis.***

14. **b. Laryngotracheal stenosis**
The mitomycins are a family of aziridine-containing natural products isolated from Streptomyces caespitosus or Streptomyces lavendulae.
They can help reduce the formation of fibrosis and adhesions.
Application of mitomycin C onto the mucosa immediately following dilatation will decrease restenosis by decreasing the production of fibroblasts and scar tissue.
Apart from laryngotracheal stenosis, it is also used in nasal stenosis (as already discussed in Chapter 19).

15. **a. Cough variant asthma**
Cough and wheeze suggests distal respiratory problems, i.e. asthma.
Stenosis and tracheomalacia will cause stridor and respiratory distress.
Vocal cord nodules will cause hoarseness of voice.

IMAGE BASED ANSWERS

16. **a. It is a picture of preauricular sinus**
The most common arch anomaly is the 2nd arch anomaly.
Although it is a congenital defect, it present at adolescent.

17. **b. In this case stridor is equal during inspirations and expiration**
The picture is clearly showing **omega-shaped (Ω) epiglottis**. Therefore, this is a case of **laryngomalacia**.
In laryngomalacia is mainly present during inspiration and NOT during expiration.

CHAPTER 26

Mouth and Oral Cavity

Throat or pharynx is divided into three parts:

Three parts of pharynx	Diagram to show three parts
1. Nasopharynx 2. Oropharynx 3. Laryngopharynx	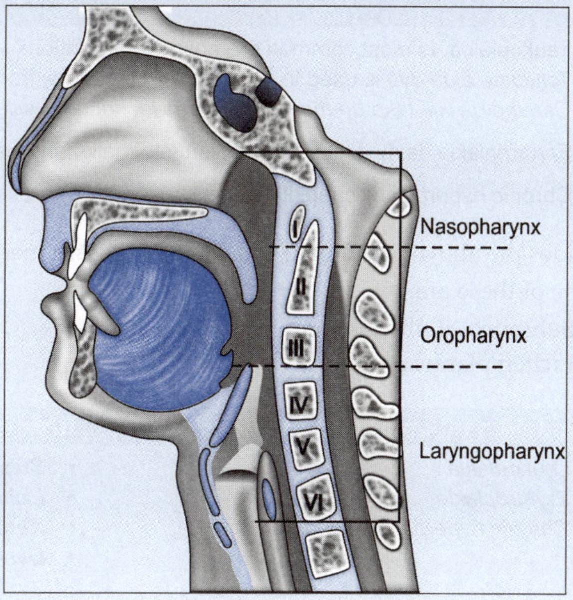

In this chapter we will discuss diseases of oral cavity.

SOME OF THE IMPORTANT TOPICS OF ORAL CAVITY ARE DISCUSSED BELOW

Fordyce's Spots

Fordyce's spots are also called **Fordyce's granules.**

Fordyce's spots are **prominent salivary glands or hypertrophied salivary gland** in the oral cavity.

The most common site is the buccal mucosa.

It appears as multiple small yellowish grains in the buccal mucosa.

Treatment

No treatment is required.

Sometimes re-assurance is needed.

Torus Mandibularis and Torus Palatinus

These are bony growths of the mandible and palate respectively.

Torus mandibularis is more common compared to torus palatinus.

They appear as small bony projection or growth in the respective bones.

No treatment is required.

Quincke's Disease

Quincke's disease is **an isolated and non-hereditary oedema of the uvula.**

It can be caused by angioneurotic oedema.

One of the important causes of non-hereditary angioneurotic oedema is deficiency of C1 estrase inhibitor enzyme.

The treatment is oral antihistamine and steroids.

This should not be confused with Quincy; which is abscess of the peritonsillar space.

PREMALIGNANT DISEASES OF ORAL CAVITY AND PHARYNX

The three important premalignant diseases of the oral cavity and rest of the throat are:

Premalignant diseases of the throat
1. Leukoplakia. Is most common premalignant condition. *Toluidine blue dye* is used to differentiate carcinoma from leukoplakia. *Carcinoma will take up the dye whereas leukoplakia will not take up the dye.*
2. Erythroplakia. Is most likely to convert into malignancy, and
3. Chronic hyperplastic candidiasis

Besides the above mentioned conditions there are many risk factors for malignancy.

Some of these are:

- Submucosal fibrosis
- Lichen planus etc.

Premalignant condition of throat	Risk factors for throat
• *Leukoplakia* • *Erythroplakia* • *Chronic hyperplastic candidiasis*	• *Submucosal fibrosis* • *Lichen planus* • *Xeroderma pigmentosa* • *Dyskeratosis congenita*

SUBMUCOSAL FIBROSIS

As the name suggests, in this condition there is fibrosis of the submucosal layers of the oral cavity.

Aetiology

It is caused by the combination of betel leaves, areca nut, lime and tobacco.

The incident increases in a patient with deficiency of vitamin A and zinc.

Presentation

It presents as gradually progressive trismus with increased sensitivity to spicy food.

Any habitual chewer of tobacco or "Pan" with gradual trismus should raise the suspicion of submucosal fibrosis.

Treatment

Till date, NO treatment has shown to improve the situation.

However, few options that we try are:

- Topical steroid injections
- Injections of proteolytic enzymes
- In severe cases surgical excision of the fibrotic tissue is done.

Dentigerous cyst:
It is a type of odontogenic cyst.
It arises from the epithelial tissue around the crown of unerupted teeth.
Most commonly arises from the 3rd molar

Nasolabial cyst (Klestadt'scyst) is the cyst of nasolacrimal duct.

Ameloblastoma:
It is benign odontogenic tumour of the lower jaw.
It presents as smooth swelling of the jaw in adults (20–50 yrs.)
Surgical excision is the treatment option.

ACUTE NECROTIZING ULCERATIVE GINGIVITIS (ANUG)

It is also called **trench mouth.**
It is called **Vincent's Angina** (when the tonsils are also involved).

Pathogens

It is caused by two pathogens:
- ***Fusiformis***
- ***Borrelia vincentii***

Presentation

It causes pain, bleeding and bad smell from the mouth (halitosis).
There is ulceration, necrosis and bleeding in the gums and inter dental papillae.

Treatment

- Debridement of necrosed tissue and
- Metronidazole

Carcinoma of the Oral Cavity

The most common site of carcinoma in Indian males is the oral cavity carcinoma.
The most common site is:
- **Gingivobuccal sulcus/**buccal mucosa/gingiva (all are same) is most common site in India.
- Lateral border of tongue is most common site in rest of the world.

Treatment

- Surgical excision of the tumour followed by radiotherapy is the most common option.
- For small tumours, the treatment option is ***partial glossectomy***
- For bigger tumours ***partial glossectomy along with supraomohyoid neck dissection*** is done.
- In case of large tumours, ***radiotherapy is added to the above mentioned treatment.***
- When radiotherapy is planned; one option for anterior 2/3 tongue is ***brachytherapy.***
- In **brachytherapy**; a radioactive wire **(192-Iridium)** is inserted into the tumour.
- This gives local radiotherapy only, thus restricting complications.

SALIVARY GLANDS

Embryology of Salivary Gland

The first gland to develop is the parotid gland.
Salivary glands arise from the epithelium of the oropharynx and are therefore mainly ***ectodermal in origin.***
These tissues proliferate and grow into the surrounding mesenchyma.
As the parotid grows into the surrounding mesenchyma, this surrounding mesenchyma develops into facial nerve and lymph nodes.

Anatomy of Salivary Gland

Salivary glands can be divided into:

1. Major glands like
   - Parotid gland
   - Submandibular gland
   - Sublingual gland
2. Minor glands
   - They are 600–1000 in number
   - Weber's gland are above the tonsils
   - Von Ebner's gland are in the posterior 1/3 of tongue

The basic secretory unit of a salivary gland is the ***acinus.***

Acinus has different types of secretory cells which rest on myoepithelium.

The various types of secretory cells are:

- Serous cells
- Mucin producing cells
- Seromucinous cells

The acini have ducts, which join to form intercalated duct.

The intercalated ducts join to form striated duct which in turn open into excretory duct.

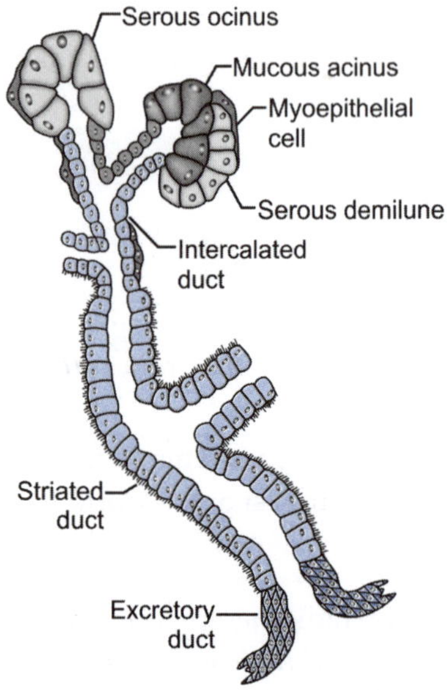

Fig. 1: Microanatomy of salivary gland cells

Major Salivary Glands and Their Ducts

Gland	Duct name	Important points
Parotid gland	Stensen's duct	It opens on the buccal mucosa, opposite the crown of second upper molar
Submandibular gland	Wharton's duct	Important nerves closely related to Wharton's duct are: • *Lingual nerve (above)* • *Hypoglossal nerve (below)*
Sublingual gland	Duct of Rivinus	When they join together then it is called ***Bartholin's duct***

Salivary calculi/Stones are most commonly seen in the ***Wharton's duct.***

Nerve Supply of Salivary Glands

- All the major salivary glands like parotid, lacrimal, submandibular and sublingual glands have sensory supply by the trigeminal nerve.
- The parasympathetic/secretomotor supply of lacrimal, submadibular and sublingual glands are from the ***facial nerve.***
- The parasympathetic/secretomotor supply of parotid gland is supplied by the ***glossopharyngeal nerve.***

FREY'S SYNDROME

It is also called *gustatory sweating.*

It is usually seen after parotid surgery in which the ***auriculotemporal nerve*** gets damaged.

As discussed above, the parasympathetic of parotid gland comes from IXth nerve.

Parasympathetic of parotid gland
Inferior salivary nucleus ↓
Glossopharyngeal nerve (IX nerve) ↓
Tympanic branch/Jacobsen's nerve ↓
Tympanic plexus ↓
Lesser petrosal nerve ↓
Otic ganglion ↓
Auriculotemporal nerve (branch of Vth nerve) ↓
Parotid gland

Treatment

- *Placing graft between parotid gland and the skin*
- *Injections of* ***botox***
- ***Tympanic neurectomy***

KIMURA DISEASE

This is slow and gradual growing painless mass in the major salivary gland.

The most common gland having this is the parotid gland.

It is seen in males above 20 years of age.

Presentation

- Enlargement of parotid gland along with cervical lymphadenopathy.
- Elevated eosinophil level and IgE level.

Treatment

- Parotidectomy is the treatment of choice
- Recurrence is common

Tumours of Salivary Glands

- Benign tumours are more common
- ***Minor salivary glands*** *have malignancy more commonly than the major glands.*

- The most common tumour of salivary gland is ***Pleomorphic adenoma.***
  It is more common in females.
  It is most commonly seen in the ***parotid gland.***
  The treatment is ***Superficial Parotidectomy.***
  During superficial parotidectomy, the following structures are encountered:
  - ***Facial nerve is most superficial structure***
  - ***Superficial temporal vein and retromandibular vein are next***
  - ***Superficial temporal artery is the last structure.***
- The most common malignant tumour is ***mucoepidermoid carcinoma.***
- ***Adenoid cystic carcinoma*** *is known to have* ***perineural spread.***

RANULA

This is discussed in Chapter no. 29.

Last minute revision

- *Fordyce's spots are hypertrophied salivary glands*
- *Premalignant diseases are:*
  - *Leukoplakia*
  - *Erythroplakia*
  - *Chronic hyperplastic candidiasis*
- *Acute necrotizing ulcerative gingivitis (ANUG) is caused by borrelia vincentii an fusiformis*
- *In India, most common site of oral cavity carcinoma is the gingivobuccal sulcus*
- *Most common salivary gland tumour is pleomorphic adenoma*
- *Most common malignant tumour of salivary gland is mucoepidermoid carcinoma*
- *Adenocystic carcinoma has perineural spread.*

QUESTIONS

1. **Fordyce's (spots) granules in oral cavity arise from:**
   a. Mucous glands b. Sebaceous glands
   c. Taste buds d. Minor salivary glands
2. **A patient has carcinoma of right tongue on its lateral border of anterior 2/3rd, with lymph node of size 4 cm in level 3 on left side of the neck, stage of disease is:**
   a. N0 b. N1
   c. N2 d. N3
3. **Not included in the oral cavity cancers:**
   a. Base of tongue b. Gingivobuccal sulcus
   c. Hard palate d. Buccal mucosa
4. **Which of these is true of aphthous ulcers?**
   a. Viral predisposition b. Recurrent ulcers
   c. Deep ulcers d. Steroids are useful
5. **All statement about Plummer-Vinson syndrome are true *except:***
   a. Commonly causes carcinoma of lower third of oesophagus
   b. Common with iron deficiency anaemia
   c. Common in females
   d. Is premalignant
6. **Which of these is not a premalignant condition of oral cavity?**
   a. Leukoplakia
   b. Erythroplakia
   c. Sub mucosal fibrosis
   d. Diffuse aphthous ulcer
7. **Most common site of squamous carcinoma in the oral cavity is:**
   a. Tongue
   b. Floor of mouth
   c. Upper and lower alveolus
   d. Buccal mucosa
8. **Carcinoma of buccal mucosa should drain to which of these lymph nodes?**
   a. Submental b. Submandibular
   c. Supraclavicular d. Mediastinal
9. **True about AJCC staging of oral cavity carcinoma is:**
   a. Involvement of pterygoid plate is T_3
   b. Involvement of pterygoid plate is T_4
   c. Involvement of lateral pterygoid muscle is T_4
   d. Involvement of medial pterygoid muscle is T_4
10. **An adult male with long history of smoking presents with a fungating papillary growth in the oral cavity. Biopsy of the lesion shows hyperkeratosis and acanthosis. No palpable lymph nodes. This could be:**
    a. Verrucous carcinoma
    b. Squamous cell carcinoma
    c. Mucosal melanoma
    d. Adenocarcinoma
11. **Woman with vitamin B_{12} deficiency presents with dysphagia and anaemia. What is the syndrome mentioned in this question?**
    a. Plummer-Vinson syndrome
    b. Eagle syndrome
    c. Job's syndrome
    d. Treacher Collins syndrome
12. **Treatment of leukoplakia is:**
    a. Local excision
    b. Excision and radiotherapy
    c. Topical chemotherapy
    d. Repositioning the ill-fitted dentures
13. **All are true statement about oral carcinoma, *except:***
    a. Most common in buccal mucosa
    b. Lymphatic metastasis uncommon
    c. Surgery is the treatment of choice
    d. Smoking is predisposing factor
14. **Which carcinoma has the best prognosis?**
    a. CA lip b. CA tongue
    c. CA palate d. CA cheek

IMAGE BASED QUESTIONS

15. **A 6 years old child presented with fever, dry cough and throat pain for 5–6 days. On examination the child had rashes all over the body with buccal mucosa having irregular patchy erythema with tiny central white 'grains in salt' appearance as shown in the picture. Which of these is true?**

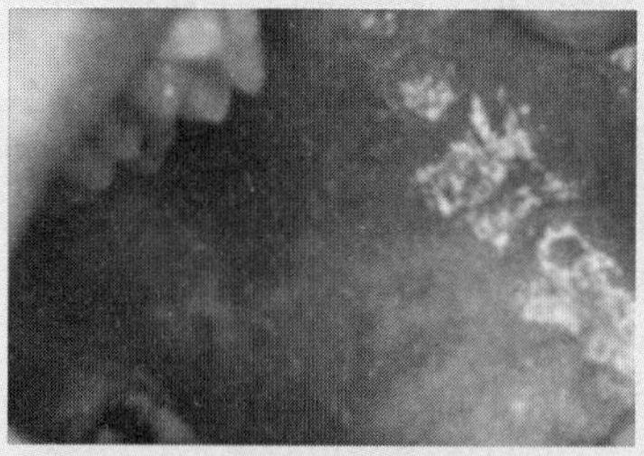

    a. The buccal mucosa findings is Foydce's granules
    b. The buccal mucosa findings is Koplik spots
    c. This is normal finding in the buccal mucosa
    d. This is erythroplakia
16. **A 35-year-old gentleman noticed some spots in the buccal mucosa, as shown in the picture. Look at the picture and pick the correct answer.**

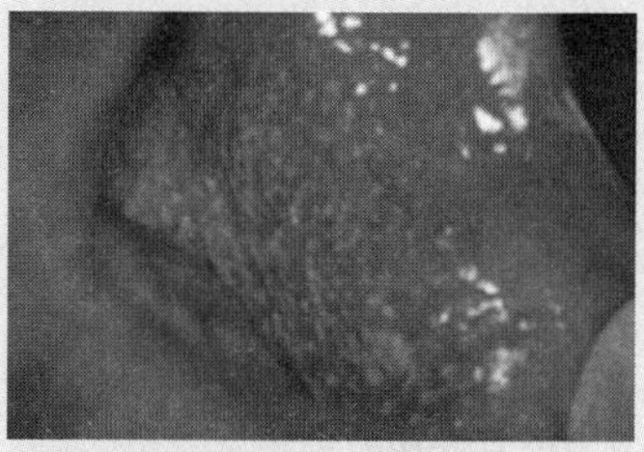

    a. This is Fordyce's granules
    b. It is hypertrophy of sebaceous glands in the cheek mucosa
    c. No treatment is required
    d. All are ture

ANSWERS AND EXPLANATIONS

1. **b. Sebaceous glands**
   Fordyce's spots are ectopic sebaceous glands. They are seen as small elevated, yellow spots on the cheek and lip in the oral cavity.
2. **c. N2**
   The choices given are neck nodes (lymph nodes) and not the disease stage.
   There are two lymph node staging
   1. UICC
   2. AJC.

   According to UICC classification, a lymph node of 4 cm on the contralateral side of disease is N2C or N2.
   According to AJC classification, it is N3C or N3:
   Hence the correct answer will depend on which classification to follow. The more accepted is UICC so the answer is N2.
3. **a. Base of tongue**
   Base of tongue is the other name of posterior 1/3 of the tongue. This part of the tongue is included in the oropharynx and NOT the oral cavity. That is the reason, this part of the tongue is supplied by glossopharyngeal nerve.
   Cancer of base of the tongue is an oropharyngeal cancer and NOT oral cavity cancer.
4. **d. Steroids are useful**
   Aphthous ulcers ***are recurrent superficial ulcers of oral cavity mucosa.***

Causes

- Cause is NOT known. However few possible causes are given.
- ***It is immunological disease. T-cell immune mediated.***
- ***Nutritional deficiency especially vitamin B_{12} deficiency.***
- ***Associated with syndromes like Behcet's disease etc.***
- ***No confirmed viral etiology known.***

Treatment

Steroid along with vitamin B_{12} is the best treatment option.

5. **a. Commonly causes carcinoma of lower third of oesophagus**
   Plummer-Vinson syndrome has the triad of:
   - Iron deficiency anaemia
   - Oesophageal webs, and
   - Post-cricoids dysphagia

   It is more common in females and is a premalignant disease.
   It may lead to ***carcinoma of the post-cricoids area in the hypopharynx in about 10–15% of patients.***
6. **d. Diffuse aphthous ulcer**

The Important Pre-Malignant Conditions of the Oral Cavity are

- ***Leukoplakia***
- ***Erythroplakia***
- ***Chronic hyperplastic candidiasis***

Important Risk Factors for Carcinoma are

- ***Submucosal fibrosis***
- ***Lichen planus***

Therefore, aphthous ulcer is neither a premalignant condition nor a risk factor for oral cavity carcinoma.

7. **d. Buccal mucosa**
   In the western countries and most of the world, the most common site of oral cavity carcinoma is ***lateral border of the tongue.***
   In India, because of the habit of tobacco chewing, the commonest site is lower gingivobuccal sulcus (alveolar-buccal sulcus).

The Three Correct Acceptable Answers are (they are nearly the same)

- ***Lower gingivobuccal sulcus (alveolar-buccal sulcus)***

- *Buccal mucosa*
- *Alveolus/gingival*

8. **b. Submandibular**
The lymphatic drainage from most of the lateral side of oral cavity including the buccal mucosa, drain into the submandibular lymph nodes.

9. **b. Involvement of pterygoid plate is T_4**
AJC staging of oral carcinoma is given below (main points of T only):

Tumour	Spread
T1	Tumour 2 cm or less in greatest diameter
T2	Tumour more than 2 cm but not more than 4 cm in greatest diameter
T3	Tumour more than 4 cm in greatest diameter
$T4_a$	Tumour invades adjacent structures • Deep muscles of tongue • Maxillary sinus • Skin of face
$T4_b$	Tumour invades • Masticator space • Pterygoid plates • Skull base • Encases internal carotid artery

From the above table it is clear that involvement of pterygoid muscles is included in AJC staging of oral cavity carcinoma.
However, the involvement of pterygoid muscles are included in the staging of oropharyngeal carcinoma (this sometimes creates confusion).

10. **a. Verrucous carcinoma**
Verrucous is a special variant of squamous cell carcinoma.
It presents as warty or papillary growth with hyperkeratosis and acanthosis and no deep invasion. Lymph nodes are not involved.
Surgical excision is the best treatment.

11. **a. Plummer-Vinson syndrome**
Three features of Plummer-Vinson syndrome are:
- *Dysphagia*
- *Anaemia, and*
- *Oesophageal web.*

Eagle syndrome	Job's syndrome	Treacher Collins syndrome
Enlarged styloid process	Hyperimmunoglobulin E	Hypoplasia of 1st arch structures like maxilla and mandible

12. **a. Local excision**
Most cases of leukoplakia are mild and therefore require NO specific treatment other than regular follow-up. However, in more severe cases of leukoplakia, treatment may be needed. The best option is local excision of the leukoplakia patch.

13. **b. Lymphatic metastasis uncommon**

14. **a. CA lip**

IMAGE BASED ANSWERS

15. **b. The buccal mucosa findings is Koplik spots**
The history suggests that the child has some acute infective disease with rashes on the body and koplik spots on the buccal mucosa.
Foydce's granules do not have fever or rashes over the body. They have NO erythema on the buccal mucosa.
Erythroplacia is a premalignant condition seen in adults. It presents as a patch on the buccal mucosa and not as 'granis on salt' appearance.

16. **d. All are ture**
This is a picture of fordyce granules which is prominence of sebaceous glands. No treatment is required in this case.

CHAPTER

27 Oropharynx, Tonsils and Hypopharynx

Oropharynx is the part of the pharynx that lies between the nasopharynx and laryngopharynx.

It is continuous with the oral cavity via the oropharyngeal isthmus.

Oropharyngeal isthmus is the border between oral cavity and the oropharynx.

This isthmus is formed by the following:

- Junction between the soft palate and the hard palate
- Both anterior tonsillar pillars, and
- The circumvalate papillae

Like rest of the pharynx, the oropharynx also has four layers.

The four layers of the pharynx are:	
1. **Mucosal layer**	**This is the inner most layer.** **This layer has lymphoid tissue of the pharynx.** **This lymphoid tissue of the pharyngeal mucosa is called "mucosa associated lymphoid tissue (MALT)"** **These lymphoid tissues are present in groups called 'tonsils'**
2. Pharyngobasilar fascia	This is second layer. This layer forms **capsule of the tonsil.**
3. Muscular layer	This is the third layer. The main muscles are the three constrictors. This layer also forms the Passavant's ridge.
4. Buccopharyngeal fascia	This is the outer most layer of pharynx. Persistence of this layer may be one of the causes of **choanal atresia.**

The most important contents of oropharynx are the palatine tonsils.

These are part of the **Waldeyer's ring**.

The other important structure in the oropharynx is the **base of tongue (posterior 1/3 tongue).**

WALDEYER'S RING

The subepithelial/submucosal layer of pharynx has a circle of lymphoid tissue.

These lymphoid tissues are aggregated/collected in groups at many places.

These aggregations/collections of lymphoid tissues are called tonsils.

All the tonsils of the pharyngeal mucosa form a ring of tonsils.

This ring of tonsils is called the ***Waldeyer's ring***.

Tonsils of the Waldeyer's ring	
Palatine tonsils or faucial tonsils	These are the main tonsils.
*Adenoids or **Lushka's tonsils*** *Nasopharyngeal tonsils*	
*Tubal tonsils or **Gerlach's tonsils***	These are near the Eustachian tube
Pharyngeal tonsils	
Lingual tonsils	They are at the base of tongue

ADENOIDS

Adenoids are also called **Lushka's tonsils.**

Adenoid is a type of tonsils and is part of Waldeyer's ring.

They are located at the junction posterior wall of nasopharynx and the roof of nasopharynx.

Growth Pattern of Adenoids

- Adenoid begins to enlarge *at 2-3 years of age and attends the maximum size by 5-6 years.*
- *Then it remains the same size for another 3-4 years.*
- *After this, they begin to regress in size.*

Therefore, adenoidectomy is usually **not** done before three years of age.

As we can guess, it is common for a child to have enlarged adenoid.

PRESENTATION OF ADENOID HYPERTROPHY

- Breathing difficulty.
- As a result of this, the child becomes **mouth breather**
- If this continuous for a long time, it leads to **adenoid facies.** The feature of adenoid facies are
  - Elongated face with dull expressions
  - Open mouth
  - Crowded upper teeth
  - High arched palate
  - Pinched nose
- Enlarged adenoid may block the Eustachian tube and cause **glue ear/serous otitis media**
- Adenoid hypertrophy is the commonest cause of glue ear in children.
- In adult with unilateral glue ear, we must rule out ***nasopharyngeal carcinoma.***
- In some patients it can cause obstructive sleep apnea syndrome **(OSAS)**

NOTE: The best age for adenoidectomy is 5–8 years.

Note: If adenoid like mass is seen in a child less than 3 years of old, then *meningocele/meningo-encephalocele* should be ruled out.

*Meningocele may have positive **Furstenberg sign.***
Furstenberg sign- There is pulsation in the meningocele when the child/patient starts crying

DIFFERENTIAL DIAGNOSIS OF NASOPHARYNGEAL MASS

- ***Adenoid hypertrophy***
- ***Meningo-encephalocele***
- ***Thornwaldt's disease-*** it is also called *nasopharyngeal bursitis.*
- It is infection of the *notochord remnant of primitive pharynx.*
- *The treatment is **marsupialisation.***
- Nasopharyngeal angiofibroma

PALATINE TONSILS

Palatine tonsils are the main tonsils in the Waldeyer's ring.

It is located on the tonsillar bed between the anterior tonsillar pillar and the posterior tonsillar pillar.

- *Tonsillar bed is formed by **superior constrictor muscle***
- *Anterior tonsillar pillar is formed by **palatoglossal muscle***
- *Posterior tonsillar pillar is formed by **palatopharyngeal muscle.***

It is lined by non-keratinising squamous epithelium and has a number of crypts.

The largest crypt of tonsil is called ***the crypta magna.***

NOTE: The crypta magna represents the VENTRAL PART OF 2ND BRANCHIAL POUCH.

Blood Supply of Tonsils

It is supplied by five arteries. These are:

- *Tonsillar branch of facial artery- the main artery of tonsils*
- *Ascending pharyngeal artery*
- *Ascending palatine artery*
- *Descending palatine artery, and*
- *Dorsal lingual artery.*

  It drains into the tonsillar plexus of veins and thus into pharyngeal plexus of veins.

  This venous system has many names:
- Tonsillar plexus of veins
- External palatine vein

Nerve Supply

- Tonsil is supplied by glossopharyngeal nerve.
- A small part is supplied by trigeminal (lesser palatine nerve)

DIFFERENCE BETWEEN TONSILS AND ADENOID

Tonsils	Adenoids
Are two in number	Single
Lined by non-keratinising squamous epithelium	Lined by ciliated columnar epithelium
Has crypts	Does not have crypts
Has capsule	No capsule

Tonsillitis

Tonsillitis is inflammation of the tonsils. This is usually seen with other conditions like

- Pharyngitis- it causes pharyngotonsillitis.
- Adenoiditis- this causes adenotonsillitis
- Obsessive compulsive disorders with tics- this causes ***Pediatric Autoimmune Neuropsychiatric Disorder associated with Streptococcal infection (PANDAS).*** This is caused by the antibodies of the streptococcus that causes tonsillitis. In this, the child has obsessive compulsive disorder and tics following GABHS tonsillitis.

Types of tonsillitis	Features
Acute catarrhal tonsillitis	This type is a part viral tonsillo-pharyngitis. This is the most common type of tonsillitis.
Follicular tonsillitis	*This can be either* • *Acute or* • *Chronic type.* *There is pus collection in the crypts.* *Therefore pus-points are seen at the mouth of crypts.*
Parenchymatous tonsillitis	*In this the tonsillar tissue is involved*
Membranous tonsillitis or Streptococcal tonsillitis	*This can be* • *Acute or* • *Chronic* ***The pus-points join to form a membrane on the tonsil*** *This is the* ***most common cause of membrane on the throat***
Fibroid tonsillitis	*This is seen only in the chronic form.* *The size of tonsil is reduced due to fibrosis* *Pus comes on pressing the tonsils.* *This is called* ***Irwin Moore's sign****.*

Causes of membrane in the throat

- *Membranous tonsillitis- This is the most common cause of membrane in the throat*
- *Diphtheria*
- *Vincent's angina*
- *Agranulocytosis*
- *Infectious mononucleosis*
  - *Candidiasis-***is controversial. Not accepted by every author.**
  - *Aphthous ulcer-***is controversial. Not accepted by every author.**

Aphthous ulcer may be associated with Behcet's Syndrome

Behcet's Syndrome is also called ***Oculo-oro-genital syndrome.*** It has three features:

- *Aphthous ulcer*
- *Genital ulcers, and*
- *Uveitis*

Indications for tonsillectomy

- *Recurrent tonsillitis-* ***This is the most common indication.***
- *Rheumatic tonsillitis*
- *Haemorrhagic tonsillitis*
- *Large tonsils causing obstruction*
- *Suspicion of malignancy of tonsil-* ***unilateral enlarged tonsils especially in adults should raise the suspicion***
- ***Quincy/Peritonsillar abscess***
- *Eagle's disease. This is enlarged styloid process. It impinges into tonsillar tissue and causes compression of the IXth cranial nerve. This results in throat pain. This pain is called* ***stylalgia.***
- *Long term management of* ***IgA nephropathy***
- *Severe infectious mononucleosis of the upper respiratory tract*
- *As a initial stage of other surgeries like*
  - *Glossopharyngeal neurectomy*
  - *Removal of styloid process/****Eagle's disease causing styalgia.***
  - *Uvulopalatopharyngoplasty (UPPP)-* ***A surgery done for*** *obstructive sleep apnea syndrome (OSAS)*

Comparison of Styalgia and Anterior Ethmoidal Neuralgia

Styalgia	Anterior ethmoidal neuralgia
Caused by Eagle's disease or enlarged styloid process	**Caused by DNS or septal spur**
Styloid process impinges into tonsil	**Septum impinges into middle turbinate**
Anterior ethmoidal nerve is compressed	**Glossopharyngeal nerve is compressed**
Referred pain in the forehead	**Referred pain in the oropharynx and ear**

Important Contraindications for Tonsillectomy

- Acute infection of tonsil and pharynx
- Bleeding disorders
- Epidemic of polio
- Submucosal cleft palate, etc.

Important Points about the Surgery - Tonsillectomy

Position of patient during tonsillectomy is ***"Rose position/morning sniff position"***

Part of pharynx to be operated	Surgical position
1. Nasopharynx and Oropharynx **This position is called** "Rose position"	• Extension of atlanto-occipital joint and • Extension of cervical spine/neck. • This is used for: – Tonsillectomy and – Adenoidectomy

Part of pharynx to be operated	Surgical position
2. Larynx and hypopharynx **This position is called** "Boyce-Jackson position"	• Extension of atlanto-occipital joint but • Flexion of cervical spine/neck. • This is used for: – Laryngoscopy – Bronchoscopy – Oesophagoscopy – Microlaryngeal surgery (MLS)

VARIOUS METHODS/TECHNIQUES FOR TONSILLECTOMY

Conventionally, tonsillectomy is done by dissection followed by crushing and cutting method.

Eve's tonsillar snare is used for this.

With time many new technologies have been used for this surgery.

You must know few important ones. They are given below.

Name of the technique	Important points about these techniques
• Cold knife tonsillectomy	This is the conventional surgery. It involves blunt dissection followed by crushing and cutting The main instruments are: • Boyle's Davis mouth gag and • Eve's tonsillar snare • Haemorrhage is the main complication
• Diathermy/electrocautery tonsillectomy	Is painful and healing is slow
• Hormonal knife tonsillectomy (ultrasound)	
• Laser tonsillectomy	KTP laser and CO_2 laser are used to evaporate the tonsils
• Microdebrider tonsillectomy	It is intracapsular tonsillectomy. The capsule of the tonsil is not removed. • Regrowth/recurrence may happen.
• Radiofrequency tonsillectomy. • These are newer technologies. – Somnoplasty tonsillectomy – Co-ablation tonsillectomy – Argon plasma tonsillectomy	This is also intracapsular tonsillectomy. Advantages are: • Less pain • Faster recovery • Bleeding may be less

COMPLICATIONS

The most common complication of tonsillectomy is ***Bleeding or haemorrhage***.

We are discussing only the important complication.

Bleeding

This is the most common complication of tonsillectomy

Bleeding can be three types:

- Primary bleeding
- Reactionary bleeding, and
- Secondary bleeding

Primary bleeding– is bleeding during the surgery

The most common source bleeding during the surgery is:

- ***Tonsillar plexus of veins or pharyngeal plexus of veins***
- Arterial bleeding is from the *tonsillary branch of facial artery*.

Reactionary bleeding- is bleeding within the first 24 hours. The cause of this is

- ***Slippage of ligature, or***
- ***Dislodgment of clots***

Secondary bleeding- is bleeding after 24 hours.

.The cause of this is *infection*

Most commonly, secondary bleeding takes place between 5th and 8th day.

Treatment of secondary bleeding is:

- ***Immediate ligation under general anaesthesia/re-operate.***

SUBLUXATION OF ATLANTO-AXIAL JOINT

Atraumatic subluxation of atlantoaxial joint is also called **"Grisel's syndrome".**

This happens due to inflammation of cervical ligament post tonsillectomy and adenoidectomy.

CREUTZFELDT-JAKOB DISEASE

The new variant of Creutzfeldt-Jakob prion (vCJD) usually concentrates in lymphoid tissue like tonsils.

During the surgery of tonsillectomy, they get attached to the surgical instruments and may get transmitted to the next patient.

Quincy

Quincy is also called **peritonsillar abscess.**

Note: it is **not** paratonsillar abscess

In this disease, the pus collects between:

- ***Capsule of tonsil, and***
- ***Bed of tonsil/Superior constrictor muscle***

Quincy is usually caused by mixed organisms

Presentation

- It is a very painful condition. Patient is unable to speak properly and has ***"hot potato voice/plummy voice"***
- *Unable to swallow even their own saliva.*
  Sometimes, there is *drooling of saliva.*
- ***Trismus*** may be seen.
  This is due to *contraction of* ***medial pterygoid muscle.***

Finding

When the following findings are together, it is diagnostic of quincy:

- *Tonsil is pushed* ***antero-medially***
- Uvula is pushed onto the ***opposite side***

Treatment

Immediate ***incision and drainage with antibiotics; followed by interval tonsillectomy.***

However, in case of children or patient having trismus or both; the following is done

1. ***Start antibiotics***
2. ***After 24-48 hours , incision and drainage is done***
3. ***After 4-6 weeks, tonsillectomy is done.***

This tonsillectomy, since it is done after a long gap, is called ***interval tonsillectomy.***

Vincent's angina

Vincent's angina is also called

- ***Trench mouth***
- ***Acute necrotizing gingivo-tonsillitis***
- ***Acute necrotizing ulcerative gingivitis (ANUG),*** when only gingival is involved.

It is a painful condition with membrane on the tonsils and gingival.

Note: Ludwig's angina is "cellulitis of submandibular space". This is discussed in Chapter 29.

Organisms

- ***Borrelia vincentii-*** *a type of spirochaete, and*
- ***Fusiform bacillus***

Treatment

- *Debridement of the necrosed tissue*
- *Metronidazole is very effective*
- **Penicillin when the patient is pregnant.**

Obstructive Sleep Apnea Syndrome (OSAS)

Is described as ***"more than five episodes of apnea-hypopnea in one hour of sleep"***

Apnea is described as *"cessation of breathing for more than ten seconds"*

It is the most common type of sleep disorder.

Presentation

The common presentations are:
- Snoring
- Excessive day time sleeping
- Morning headache
- Weight gain
- Mood disorders etc.

Investigations

The most important investigation is ***polysomnography/sleep study***

Overnight Oxymetry

Muller's maneuver may also be used for diagnosis.

Muller's maneuver is also called **reverse valsalvae.**

X-ray and CT Scan may be required

Treatment

- ***Weight loss.*** *Because obesity is one of the main cause of OSAS*
- ***Oral devices.*** *They usually advance the mandible thereby increasing the space posterior to the tongue.*
- ***C-PAP machine*** *(Continuous positive airway pressure)*
- ***Bi-PAP machine*** *(Bi level positive airway pressure)*
- ***Mandibular repositioning splints (MRS)***
- ***Surgeries*** *may be required if the above mentioned options fail.*

The types of surgery done depends on the cause of obstruction.

Types of surgery for OSAS	Feature of surgery
• ***Uvulopalatopharyngoplasty (UPPP)***	• *Tonsillectomy done* • *Size of soft palate and uvula is reduced* • *Done when the cause of obstruction is palate and tonsils*
• *Laser assisted uvulopalatoplasty (LAUP)*	• *Same as above but laser is used.* • *The results are better*
• *Radiofrequency tissue volume reduction (somnoplasty)*	• *The technology is similar to the one discussed for tonsillectomy* • *Done when large tongue base is the cause*
• *Trans-oral robotic surgery (TORS) for base tongue resection*	• *It is a robotic surgery* • *Done when large tongue base is the cause of obstruction*
• *Mandibular myotomy*	• *Muscle of mandible is resected* • *Attachment between hyoid and mandible is snapped*

Important Points about Tumours of Oropharynx

There are three important sites for tumours in the oropharynx:

1. Tonsils and pillars of tonsil is the most common site.

   If this is not given in the choices, then lateral wall of oropharynx is also accepted because tonsils are on the lateral wall.

Base of the tongue/posterior 1/3 of tongue is the second common site

Soft palate which also has the salivary glands.

The most common malignant tumour of oropharynx is:

- ***Squamous cell carcinoma. It is most common on the tonsils.***
- ***Non-Hodgkin's lymphoma*** *is also a common tumour.*

Aetiology

The four important aetiological factors are:

1. Smoking
2. Alcohol
3. **Human papilloma virus (HPV) type 2, 11 and 16.**
4. **Vitamin A deficiency**

Presentation

Oropharyngeal carcinomas are more common in males and pain in the throat is the common presentation.

This pain may be referred to the ear (Earache), because the middle ear and oropharynx have nerve supply from the same nerve i.e. Glossopharyngeal nerve (IXth).

Diagnosis

A simple clinical examination may reveal the tumour in most cases.

However, there are two points that should be kept in mind in case of oropharyngeal tumours:

1. Often the tumous are **sub-mucosal** and hence may be missed in clinical examination.
2. Oropharyngeal carcinomas the ***most common tumours with synchronous tumour or second carcinoma (along with oropharynx some other site also has a tumour).***

The most common site of second tumour is **hypopharynx or oesophagus.**

Therefore, in these patients we should do:

- **Triple endoscopy and**
- **Positron emission tomography (PET)** using 2-(F18) fluoro-2-deoxy-D-glucose.

TRIPLE ENDOSCOPY

As the same suggests three different endoscopies are done in this
1. Nasopharyngoscopy
2. Laryngoscopy and bronchscopy
3. Hypopharyngoscopy and oesophagoscopy **Indication of triple endoscopy are:** • Suspicion of second primary as in oropharyngeal carcinoma • Unknown primary in case of positive neck node.

Treatment

For early stage carcinomas, **transoral CO_2 laser excision is best option.**

If this is not possible, radiotherapy is indicated.

For higher stage tumours, surgery and radiotherapy with treatment of the neck nodes is done.

The second option for these tumours is concomitant radiotherapy and chemotherapy.

HYPOPHARYNX

Hypopharynx is a part of laryngopharynx and is located behind the larynx.

Hypopharynx has three parts. They are:

- Pyriform fossa
- Post cricoids area, and
- Posterior pharyngeal wall.

Like the rest of the pharynx, the hypopharynx also has four layers. The muscular layer is made of inferior constrictor muscle.

The main function of hypopharynx is swallowing of food.

Killian's Dehiscence

Killian's dehiscence is a weak area between the two fibres of inferior constrictor muscle.

1. Thyropharyngeus muscle and
2. Cricopharyngeus muscle.

"Killian's" is a very important name in ENT

• Killian's speculum	Used for anterior rhinoscopy and nasal surgeries
• Killian's incision	Incision used during submucosal resection (SMR)
• Killian's polyp	Is another name for maxillary polyp
• Killian's dehiscence	Is a site for Zenker's diverticulum

ZENKER'S DIVERTICULUM

Zenker's diverticulum is the herniation of pharyngeal mucosa through the Killian's dehiscence to form a pharyngeal pouch.

It is usually seen in old and weak people.

Presentation

- *Dysphagia*
- *Regurgitation of food*
- *Halitosis or bad smell from mouth*

Diagnosis

Barium swallow is usually diagnostic investigation

Treatment

- *Endoscopic stippling is the best option for small pouch*
- *Dohlman's operation is an option*
- *Laser excision can also be done.*

Last minute revision

- *Capsule of tonsil is formed by pharyngobasilar fascia*
- *Largest cryp of tonsil is called crypta magna*
- *Main artery of tonsil is facial artery*
- *Most common bacteria causing tonsillitis is beta hemolyticus streptococcus*
- *The latest method of tonsillectomy is coablation tonsillectomy which is a type of radiofrequency surgery*
- *The commonest complication of tonsillectomy is bleeding. Most common vessel that bleeds is paratonsillar vein*
- *Grisel's syndrome is sublaxation of atlanto-axial joint. It is a complication of tonsillectomy*
- *In quincy the pus collects between the capsule and superior constrictor muscle*
- *Immediate drainage followed by interval tonsillectomy is the treatment*
- *In obstructive sleep apnea (OSAS), the apnea-hypopnea index (AHI) should be more than 5*
- *Polysomnography is the gold standard investigation*
- *Weight reduction is the first line of management of OSAS*
- *Oropharyngeal carcinoma may be caused by human papilloma virus (HPV) type 2, 11, 16*
- *Killian's dehiscence is between thyropharyngeus muscle and cricopharyngeus muscles*
- *Zenker's diverticulum takes place through this dehiscence*

QUESTIONS

1. **A 6-year-old child with recurrent URTI with mouth breathing and failure to grow with high arched palate and impaired hearing. The treatment is:**
   a. Tonsillectomy
   b. Grommet insertion
   c. Myringotomy with grommet insertion
   d. Adenoidectomy with grommet insertion
2. **Causative organism of tonsillitis is:**
   a. Streptococcus b. Staphylococcus
   c. Pseudomonas d. Homophiles
3. **A 5-year-old patient is scheduled for tonsillectomy. On the day of surgery he had running nose, temperature 37.5°C and dry cough. Which of the following should be the most appropriate decision for surgery?**
   a. Surgery should be cancelled
   b. Can proceed for surgery if chest is clear and there is no history of asthma
   c. Should get X-ray chest before proceeding for surgery
   d. Cancel surgery for 3 weeks and patient to be on antibiotic
4. **Dehiscence of Killian seen in:**
   a. Plummer Vinson syndrome
   b. Oesophageal diverticulum
   c. Pharyngeal pouch
   d. Achlasia
5. **True statement about faucial diphtheria is:**
   a. Pearly white membrane
   b. Bleeds when membrane is removed
   c. Membrane can be removed easily
   d. High grade fever with bradycardia
6. **'Trench mouth' is:**
   a. Submucosal fibrosis
   b. Tumour at uveal angle
   c. Ulcerative lesion of the tonsil
   d. Retension cyst of the tonsil
7. **Human papilloma virus (HPV) is not associated with which of the following?**
   a. CA base of tongue b. CA tonsil
   c. Nasopharyngeal CA
   d. Laryngeal papillomatosis
8. **Disease "PANDAS" is associated with which of these?**
   a. Pharyngotonsillitis
   b. Obstructive sleep apnea syndrome
   c. Schwannoma
   d. Ranula
9. **Carcinoma of pyriform fossa usually presents with:**
   a. Hoarseness b. Lump in the neck
   c. Cough d. Dysphagia
10. **Capsule of the tonsil is formed by:**
    a. Pharyngobasilar fascia
    b. Buccopharyngeal fascia
    c. Prevertebral fascia
    d. Bucconasal membrane
11. **Which of the following is called the 'Gateway of tears'?**
    a. Killian's dehiscence b. Rathke's pouch
    c. Waldeyer ring d. Sinus of Morgagni
12. **All are true of Zenker's diverticulum *except:***
    a. It is an acquired condition
    b. Is a false diverticulum
    c. Barium swallow is the investigation of choice
    d. It has outpouching from the anterior wall
13. **Which of the following structures is seen in the oropharynx?**
    a. Pharyngotympanic tube
    b. Fossa of Rosenmuller
    c. Palatine tonsils
    d. Pyriform fossa
14. **Lower limit of hypopharynx is:**
    a. Lower border of cricoids cartilage
    b. Lower border of thyroid cartilage
    c. Upper border of cricoids cartilage
    d. Upper border of thyroid cartilage
15. **Regarding adenoid hypertrophy the following is untrue:**
    a. There is failure to thrive
    b. Mouth breathing is seen
    c. High arched palate may be seen
    d. Immediate surgery should be done even for mild hypertrophy.
16. **In a child with adenoid hypertrophy and its symptoms, all are treatment options *except:***
    a. Nasal decongestants b. Antibiotics
    c. β_2 agonists d. Adenoidectomy
17. **Indications for adenoidectomy in children include all *except:***
    a. Recurrent URTI
    b. Recurrent middle ear infections with hearing loss
    c. Chronic serous otitis media
    d. Multiple adenoids
18. **In a patient with adenoid hypertrophy, the voice abnormality seen is:**
    a. Rhinolalia clausa b. Rhinolalia aperta
    c. Hot potato voice d. All
19. **Adenoidectomy is contraindicated in:**
    a. Cleft palate
    b. Cleft lip
    c. Adenoid hypertrophy
    d. Tonsil hypertrophy
20. **Referred pain from tonsils to ear is due to:**
    a. Vagus nerve
    b. Glossopharyngeal nerve
    c. Auriculotemporal nerve
    d. Greater auricular nerve
21. **All of the following causes grey white membrane on the tonsils *except:***
    a. Infectious mononucleosis
    b. Ludwig's angina
    c. Diphtheria
    d. Streptococcal tonsillitis

22. **Palatine tonsil receives its arterial supply from all of the following *except:***
    a. Tonsillar branch of facial artery
    b. Sphenopalatine artery
    c. Ascending pharyngeal artery
    d. Dorsal lingual
23. **All are indications for tonsillectomy *except:***
    a. Foreign body in tonsil
    b. Chronic tonsillitis
    c. Quincy
    d. Suspicion of malignancy
24. **Contraindications for tonsillectomy are all *except:***
    a. Submucosal fibrosis b. Bleeding disorders
    c. Epidemic of polio d. Acute tonsillitis
25. **The position adopted for tonsillectomy is also adopted for which of these procedures?**
    a. Direct laryngoscopy
    b. Indirect laryngoscopy
    c. Bronchoscopy
    d. Tracheostomy
26. **Ramu a 15 years male presents with haemorrhage 5 hours after tonsillectomy. Best treatment is:**
    a. External gauze packing
    b. Antibiotics with mouth wash
    c. Irrigation with cold saline
    d. Re-explore immediately
27. **Torrential bleeding during tonsillectomy is due to:**
    a. Tonsillar artery
    b. Paratonsillar plexus veins
    c. Lingual artery
    d. Medial meningeal artery
28. **Which of these is NOT seen in palatine tonsils?**
    a. Develops from 2nd pharyngeal pouch
    b. Branch of facial artery is the main supply
    c. Covered by fibrous capsule
    d. Leads to ear pain due to vagus nerve
29. **Laser uvulopalatoplasty is done for:**
    a. Snoring
    b. Pharyngotonsillitis
    c. Cleft palate
    d. Stammering
30. **An elderly male presents with history of dysphagia, regurgitation, foul breath, hoarseness and cough, right side lung crepts are present. Most likely diagnosis is:**
    a. Schatzki ring
    b. Zenker's diverticulum
    c. Corkscrew oesophagus
    d. Plummer Vincent Syndrome
31. **Dohlman's surgery is done for:**
    a. Vocal palsy
    b. Zenker's diverticulum
    c. Saccule of larynx
    d. None
32. **All of the following are true about obstructive sleep apnea syndrome *except:***
    a. Females have more common than males
    b. Commonly associated with hypertension
    c. Day time sleepiness is seen
    d. > 5 episodes of apnea per hour
33. **A 36 years old obese man was suffering from hypertension and snoring. Patient was a known smoker. In sleepest, there were 5 apnea/hypopneas per hour. He was given antihypertensives and advised to quit smoking. Next line of management:**
    a. Uvulopalatopharyngoplasty (UPPP)
    b. Weight reduction and diet plan
    c. Nasal CPAP
    d. Mandibular repositioning
34. **Second primary tumour of head and neck is most commonly seen as malignancy of:**
    a. Oral cavity b. Oropharynx
    c. Hypopharynx d. PNS

IMAGE BASED QUESTIONS

35. **The picture shows tonsils of Waldeyer's ring. Which is not true?**

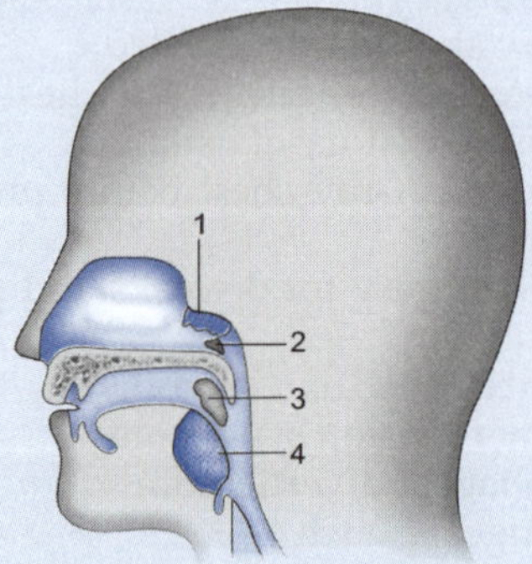

    a. Tonsil no 1 is Luschka's tonsil
    b. Tonsil no 2 is Gerlach's tonsil
    c. Tonsil no 3 is Palatine tonsil
    d. No 4 is not a tonsil
36. **In the below pictures, which of the following is being done:**

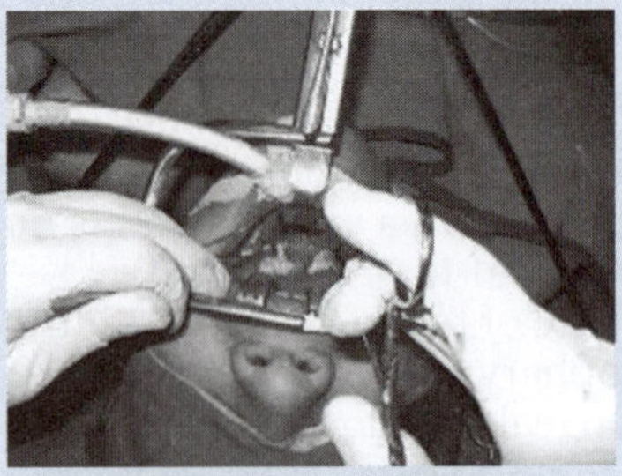

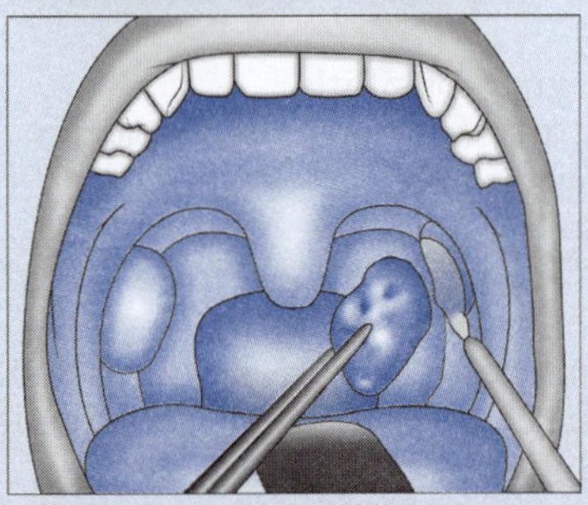

    a. Adenoidectomy
    b. Tonsillectomy
    c. Drainage of pus in quincy
    d. None of the above

PART 3: THROAT

37. Identify this instrument and answer the following question:

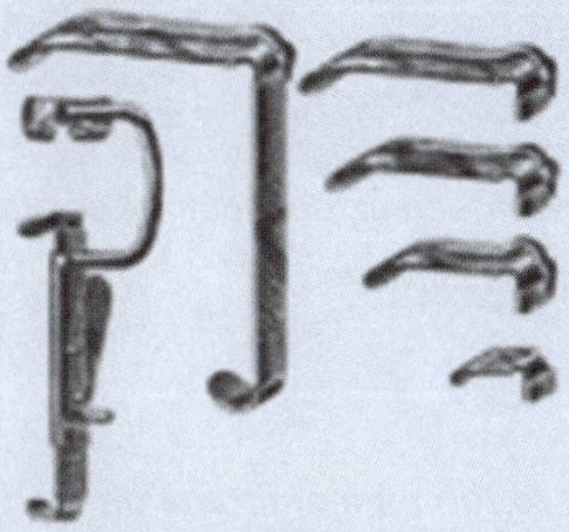

a. This is a picture of Boyles Davis mouth gag
b. It is used during adenoidectomy
c. It is used during tonsillectomy
d. All are true

38. This is a pictorial presentation of an ENT procedure being done. Which is true about this picture?

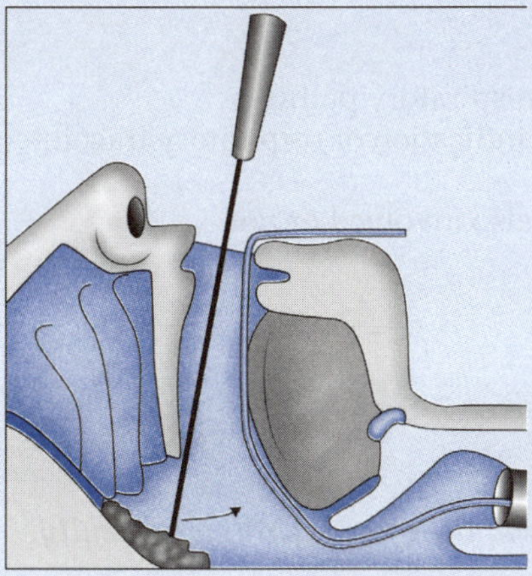

a. The procedure being done is adenoidectomy
b. Tonsillectomy is usually done along with this procedure if required
c. The instrument shown is called St. Clair Thomson Adenoid Curette
d. All are true

39. The diagnosis is:

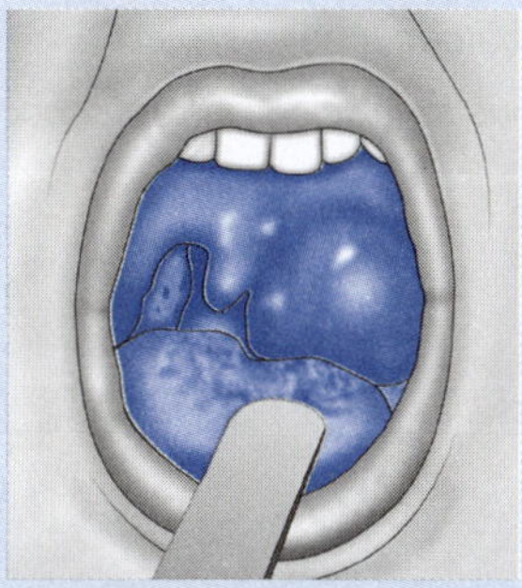

a. Acute tonsillitis
b. Quincy/peritonsillar abscess
c. Parapharyngeal abscess
d. Oral cavity carcinoma

40. Pick the right answer based on the picture given below:

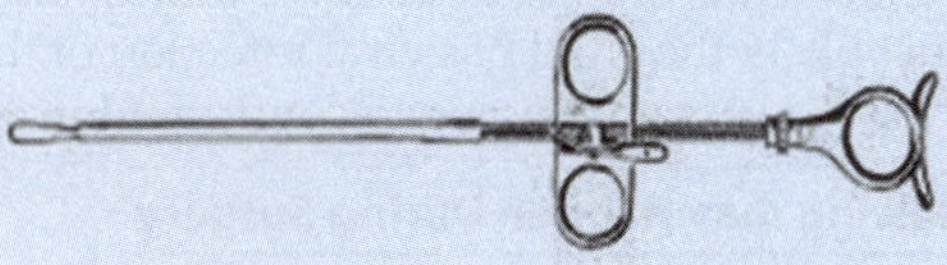

a. It is called Eve's tonsillar snare
b. It can be used for tonsillectomy as well as adenoidectomy
c. This is one of the latest technologies for tonsillectomy
d. It can be used for tonsillectomy in children only, NOT in adults

ANSWERS AND EXPLANATIONS

1. **d. Adenoidectomy with grommet insertion**
A child with mouth breathing and high arched palate has adenoid facies. If this child is having impaired hearing then he must be having glue ear.
Therefore the diagnosis clearly is ***adenoid hypertrophy with glue ear (SOM)***
In a child with serous otitis media (SOM), adenoid hypertrophy should be ruled out
In an adult with serous otitis media (SOM), nasopharyngeal carcinoma should be ruled out.
In such a case adenoidectomy with grommet insertion has to be done.

OTHER FEATURES OF ADENOID FACIES ARE

1. Elongated face with dull expression
2. Open mouth
3. Crowding of upper teeth and
4. Pinched nose.

2. **a. Streptococcus**
Tonsillitis is the inflammation of palatine tonsils.
Tonsillitis can be of the following types:

Acute catarrhal tonsillitis	This type is a part viral tonsillo-pharyngitis This is the most common type of tonsillitis.
Follicular tonsillitis	*This can be either* • *Acute or* • *Chronic type.* *There is pus collection in the crypts.* *Therefore pus-points are seen at the mouth of crypts*
Parenchymatous tonsillitis	*In this the tonsillar tissue is involved*
Membranous tonsillitis or Streptococcal tonsillitis	*This can be* • *Acute or* • *Chronic* ***This pus-points join to form a membrane on the tonsil*** This is the ***most common cause of membrane on the throat***
Fibroid tonsillitis	*This is seen only in the chronic form* *The size of tonsil is reduced due to fibrosis* *Pus comes on pressing the tonsils.* *This is called* ***Irwin Moore's sign***

Bacterial tonsilllitis is most commonly caused by Streptococcus.
This can sometimes lead to ***rheumatic diseases.***

3. **d. Cancel surgery for 3 weeks and patient to be on antibiotic**
Tonsillectomy is a surgery of oropharynx. Oropharynx is in the respiratory pathway.
A child with running nose, fever (mild) and dry cough has clear indication of respiratory tract infection.
Most likely the child has viral infection of the respiratory tract.
Chest X-ray is only going to confirm if lower respiratory tract is also involved or not.

The Following may Happen During Surgery

- ***Larynx may go into laryngospasm during intubation***
- ***The surgical wound may allow the deep spread of the pathogen.***
- ***This may cause systemic infection***
- ***Bleeding will be massive during surgery***
- ***It may lead to excessive oedema of the airway post-surgery and therefore breathing difficulty.***
- ***It may lead to secondary bacterial infection.***
- ***Some of the above mentioned conditions can be life threatening.***

In a child with respiratory infection, surgery in the pathway i.e. tonsillectomy should be postponed till the infection is fully controlled.

4. **c. Pharyngeal pouch**
Killian's dehiscence is a week point of pharynx which falls between the fibres of:
- Thyropharyngeus muscle and
- Cricopharyngeus muscle.
- This weak point is also called *gateway of tears*.

In rare cases the mucosa of pharynx may herniate through this weak point to form a pouch called pharyngeal pouch.
This pouch is called ***Zenker's diverticulum.***
More commonly tears are seen in this area during procedures like esophagoscopy.
Hence, the name *"Gateway of tears"*.

5. **b. Bleeds when membrane is removed**
Faucal diphtheria is one of the most important causes of membrane in the throat. However, the most common cause of membrane in the throat is streptococcal tonsillitis.
In cases of diphtheria, the membrane is described as dirty grey white and is difficult to remove and it bleeds on removal.

Other Causes of Membrane in the Throat are

Streptococcal tonsillitis/membranous tonsillitis (most common cause)
Diphtheria

PART 3: THROAT

Vincent's angina
Infectious mononucleosis
Leukemias etc

6. **c. Ulcerative lesion of the tonsil**
Trench mouth is another name of **Vincent's** angina which is also called acute necrotizing ulcerative gingivitis (ANUG).
It is caused by:
- Borrelia vincenti and
- Fusiform bacillus.

The drug of choice in this case is metronidazole and penicillin.
This condition is one of the causes of membrane in the throat.

7. **c. Nasopharyngeal CA**
Nasopharyngeal carcinoma is caused by Epstein-Barr virus (EBV).
Oropharyngeal carcinomas like tumours of base of tongue and tonsil are known to be caused by HPV stains 16 and 18.
Laryngeal papilloma is benign disease of larynx and is believed to be caused by HPV stains 6 and 11.

Viruses that causes head and neck cancers	
Nasopharyngeal carcinoma	*Epstein barr virus (EBV)*
Oropharyngeal carcinoma	*Human papilloma virus (HPV) 16 and 18*
Recurrent respiratory papillomatosis (RRP)	*Human papilloma virus (HPV) 6 and 11*
Laryngeal carcinoma	*No virus implicated*

8. **a. Pharyngotonsillitis**
"PANDAS" stand for ***Pediatric Autoimmune Neuropsychiatric Disorder associated with Streptococcal infection.***
It is usually due to antibodies of streptococcus of the pharyngotonsillitis.
These antibodies cross into the brains and cause damage especially in the basal ganglion.
The child has obsessive compulsive disorder and tics.

9. **d. Dysphagia**
Pyriform fossa is a part of hypopharynx. Hypopharynx has three parts. They are:
- ***Post cricoids***
- ***Posterior pharyngeal wall***
- ***Pyriform fossa.***

Carcinoma of hypopharynx is most common in the pyriform fossa.
- Carcinoma of all three areas of hypopharynx present most commonly as **dysphagia**.
- The second common complain is hoarseness of voice.
- Post cricoid carcinomas are associated with Plummer Vincent syndrome and so are more common in females.

10. **a. Pharyngobasilar fascia**
Pharyngeal wall is formed of four layers:
- Mucosal layer
- Pharyngobasilar fascia
- Muscular layers, and
- Buccopharyngeal fascia

Tonsil is lymphoid tissue and is a part of MALT (***mucosa associated lymphoid tissue***).
As the name suggests, tonsil is lymphoid tissue and mixed in mucosal layer. The mucosal layer in the tonsil forms two membranes over the tonsil. They are:
1. Plica semilunaris and
2. Plica triangularis

- Deep to the tonsil is the second layer of pharyngeal wall i.e. ***pharyngobasilar fascia. This forms the capsule of tonsil.***
- The third layer is the muscular layer and then the buccopharyngeal fascia.

11. **a. Killian's dehiscence**
    Killian's dehiscence is a triangular space between the two fibres of ***inferior constrictor muscle:***
    - ***Thyropharyngeus (vertical fibres) and***
    - ***Cricopharyngeus (horizontal fibres)***

    This is a weak area and can lead to following problems:
    - Formation of Zenker's diverticulum
    - Accidental trauma or tear during oesophagoscopy.
12. **d. It has outpouching from the anterior wall**
    Zenker's diverticulum is a false diverticulum from the posterior wall of laryngopharynx. It is seen through **Killian's dehiscence** between two muscles:
    - ***Above cricopharyngeus and***
    - ***Thyropharyngeus***
13. **c. Palatine tonsils**
    Palatine tonsil is one of the three tonsillar groups present in the oropharynx. Rest of the two groups are in the nasopharynx.
    Pharyngotympanic tube (Eustachian tube) and Fossa of Rosenmuller are present in the nasopharynx and the pyriform fossa is one of the three parts of hypopharynx.
14. **a. Lower border of cricoids cartilage**
    Hypopharynx has three parts. They are:
    - Pyriform fossa
    - Post cricoids area, and
    - Posterior pharyngeal wall.

    It extends from the hyoid to the lower border of cricoids cartilage.
15. **d. Immediate surgery should be done even for mild hypertrophy**
    It is common to have mild hypertrophy of adenoids in children. Most of these patients do NOT have any problems and therefore NO surgery is required.
    Surgeries are done only if adenoids causes severe symptoms like failure to thrive, sleeping with open mouth, glue ear etc.
16. **c. β_2 agonists**
    β_2 agonists are usually used for bronchoconstriction. Rest of the options given is commonly used for adenoid hypertrophy.
17. **d. Multiple adenoids**
    We have only one Adenoids which is in the midline of nasopharynx. Multiple adenoids are not possible.
    Rest of the options given are common indications for adenoidectomy.
18. **a. Rhinolalia clausa**

Causes of Rhinolalia Clausa/Hyponasality are

- Any condition causing nasal blockade like polyps, tumors etc.
- Any condition causing nasopharyngeal obstruction like adenoid hypertrophy

Causes of Hypernasality are

- *Cleft palate*
- *Oroantral fistula*
- *Soft palate palsy*
- *Post adenoidectomy*
- *After UPPP*
- *Velopharyngeal insufficiency*

Hot Potato Voice is Seen in Inflammatory Condition of Oropharynx Like

- Quincy

19. **a. Cleft palate**
Cleft palate and related conditions (*bifid uvula, submucosal cleft palate etc.)* are some of the most important contraindications of adenoidectomy.
Other important contraindications are:
- Acute infection
- Velopharyngeal insufficiency etc.

20. **b. Glossopharyngeal nerve**
The entire oropharynx (along with tonsils) is mainly supplied by the glossopharyngeal nerve.
Therefore, any referred pain from oropharynx/tonsils can happen only via this nerve.
Middle ear is also supplied by ***tympanic branch (Jacobsen's nerve)*** of glossopharyngeal nerve.
This common nerve **(glossopharyngeal nerve)** supply causes referred pain from tonsils to the ear.

21. **b. Ludwig's angina**
We should NOT confuse Ludwig's angina with Vincent's angina.
Vincent's angina is infection of oral cavity and oropharynx caused by ***Borrelia vincenti and fusoformis*** and can cause grey white membrane on tonsils.
Ludwig's angina, on the other hand, is ***cellulitis of the submandibular space*** caused by mixed pathogens.

Causes of membrane in the throat

- *Membranous tonsillitis- This is the most common cause of membrane in the throat*
- *Diphtheria*
- *Vincent's angina*
- *Agranulocytosis*
- *Infectious mononucleosis*
  - Candidiasis- is controversial. Not accepted by every author.
  - Apthous ulcer- is controversial. Not accepted by every author.

22. **b. Sphenopalatine artery**
Remember the artery supply of two important areas of ENT.

Artery supply of septum/nose	Artery supply of tonsils
1. Sphenopalatine artery	1. Tonsillar branch of facial artery
2. Greater palatine artery	2. Ascending pharyngeal artery
3. Superior labial artery	3. Ascending palatine artery
4. Anterior ethmoidal artery	4. Descending palatine artery
5. Posterior ethmoidal artery	5. Dorsal lingual artery

23. **a. Foreign body in tonsil**
Foreign body in tonsil can easily be removed and so tonsillectomy is usually not required.

24. **a. Submucosal fibrosis**
In Submucosal fibrosis, tonsillectomy is very difficult to do but it is NOT contraindicated.

25. **d. Tracheostomy**
Position of the patient during tonsillectomy is called **Rose Position.**
This position is used for:
- ***Procedures of oropharynx like tonsillectomy***
- ***Procedures of nasopharynx like adenoidectomy***
- ***Procedures on the neck like tracheostomy***

Note: Rest of the procedures mentioned (laryngoscopy, brochoscopy) are procedures of laryngopharynx, and therefore this position will NOT be suitable.

26. **d. Re-explore immediately**
This is a case of reactionary haemorrhage.
Treatment of reactionary haemorrhage and secondary haemorrhage post tonsillectomy is ***immediate re-exploration and ligation of the bleeding vessel.***

27. **a. Tonsillar artery**
We know that during tonsillectomy, bleeding is the most common complication.
During this complication, bleeding is most commonly from paratonsillar plexus of veins.
However, if there is torrential bleeding, then it is most common from **tonsillar branch of facial artery** especially when this is an **aberrant tonsillar artery.**

28. **d. Leads to ear pain due to vagus nerve**
Any pain from **oropharynx/tonsils** is referred to ear through the glossopharyngeal nerve.
Note: Pain from **larynx** to the ear is via vagus nerve.

29. **a. Snoring**
Laser uvulopalatoplasty is done for ***obstructive sleep apnea syndrome (OSAS) and snoring.***

30. **b. Zenker's diverticulum**
The above mentioned presentation is almost classical presentation of Zenker's diverticulum.
Foul breath and lung crepts are NOT seen in rest of the conditions mentioned.
Schatzki ring and corkscrew oesophagus presents with dysphagia and heart burns.
Plummer Vincent syndrome has anaemia with dysphagia. It can sometimes be premalignant.

31. **b. Zenker's diverticulum.**

32. **a. Females have more common than males**

33. **b. Weight reduction and diet plan**
Obstructive sleep apnea syndrome (OSAS) is diagnosed when the ***apnea/hypopnea index (AHI) is more than 5 per hour.***
This diagnostic criteria is based on ***polysomnography (sleep study).***

Severity of OSAS Based on Polysomnography

Apnea/hypopnea index	Severity
Between 5 and 15	Mild OSAS
Between 15 and 30	Moderate OSAS
>30	Severe OSAS

Causes

- Almost twice more common in males
- Obesity is the most important cause
- Other are contributing factors like hypertension, alcohol etc.

Important Investigations

- Overnight oxymetry
- Polysomnography (gold standard investigation)
- Cephalometry/EEG etc.

Treatment

- Stop smoking/alcohol
- Weight reduction
- Continuous positive airway pressure devices (CPAP)
- Mandibular repositioning splints
- Uvulopalatopharyngoplasty (UPPP)
- Trans oral robotic surgery (TORS) etc.

34. **b. Oropharynx**
Oropharyngeal carcinomas are the most common carcinomas in the head and neck region having second primaries.

The most common site having second in the head and neck region is the oesophagus. If oesophagus is not given in the choices, then ***hypopharynx*** is an acceptable answer for most common site of second primary.

Note:

- *Oropharyngeal carcinomas are most common carcinomas having second primaries*
- *The most common site of second primary is Oesophagus/hypopharynx.*

IMAGE BASED ANSWERS

35. **d. No 4 is not a tonsil**
    - Tonsil no 1 is adenoid, also called Luschka's tonsil
    - Tonsil no 2 is tubal tonsil of Gerlach

    Tonsil no 4 is lingual tonsil.

36. **b. Tonsillectomy**
    In the first picture, the patient is seen in **Rose position**. This position is used in adenoidectomy and tonsillectomy and NOT during drainage of quincy.
    In the second picture, tonsil is clearly being cut and removed.

37. **d. All are true**
    This is Boyles Davis mouth gag with different size blades for different age groups.
    It is used during adenoidectomy as well as tonsillectomy.

38. **d. All are true**
    This is a pictorial diagram of adenoidectomy being doe with the curette called St. Clair Thomson Adenoid Curette.
    The actual of St. Clair Thomson Adenoid Curette is:

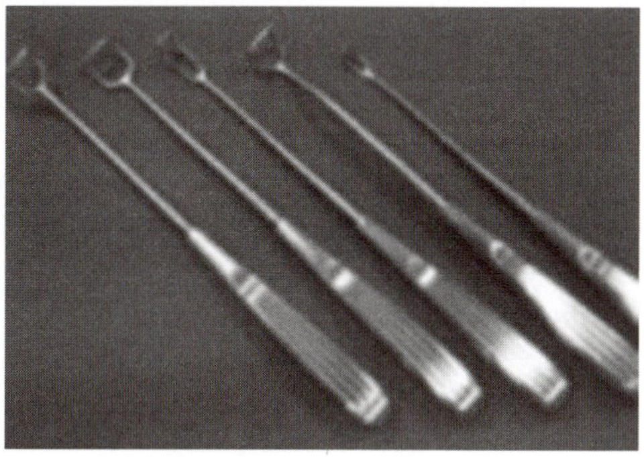

When needed, adenoidectomy and tonsillectomy are done together.

39. **b. Quincy/peritonsillar abscess**
    The picture shows left tonsil pushed anteromedially and the uvula is pushed onto the right side. This is classical findings of quincy.

40. **a. It is called Eve's tonsillar snare**
    This is the ***Eve's tonsillar snare*** which is one of the oldest methods of doing tonsillectomy in adults as well as children.

CHAPTER

28 Nasopharynx

Nasopharynx is a vault/space behind the nasal cavity and above the oropharynx.

Its dimentions are:

- Height – 3-4 cm
- Width – 4 cm, and
- Depth – 2 cm.

The anterior boundary is **choana.**

It may lead to **choanal atresia** if bucconasal membrane is persisting after birth.

The floor has **Passavant's ridge.**

> *Passavant's ridge is formed by horizontal fibres of palatopharyngeus muscle and superior constrictor muscle.*
> *Vertical fibres of palatopharyngeus muscle forms posterior pillar of tonsil.*
> Defect of Passavant's ridge may lead to Velopharyngeal insufficiency.

The roof and posterior is skull base and the most important structure here is adenoid. Adenoid is a type of tonsil that we have already discussed.

Lateral walls of nasopharynx have the following important structures:

- Eustachian tube opening. It is ***1.25 cm below and behind the inferior turbinate***
- **Torus tubaris.** This is bulge on the nasopharyngeal end of Eustachian tube.
  Torus tubaris is formed by the
  - ***Cartilage of the Eustachian tube and***
  - ***Tensor vali palatini muscle***

  Other muscles which may contribute to the torus tubarius are:
  - Levator palatini muscle and
  - Salpingopharyngeus muscle
- Near the torus tubarius is the **tubal tonsil of Gerlach.** It is part of Waldeyer's ring.
- Behind this is **fossa of Rosenmuller.**

Fossa of Rosenmuller is the **most common site of nasopharyngeal carcinoma.**

STRUCTURES AROUND NASOPHARYNX

There are lots of important areas around nasopharynx that might be affected by diseases of nasopharynx.

- Foramen lacerum is near the roof, connecting it with cranial cavity.
- Retropharyngeal space containing the ***sentinel lymph nodes*** of nasopharynx.
- The lateral most lymph node is called **Node of Rouviere.**
- Parapharyngeal spaces with ***last four cranial nerves*** are located lateral to nasopharynx.
- ***Sinus of Morgagni*** is present posterosuperiorly.

Sinus of morgagni is a space between the base of skull and superior constrictor muscle

The structures passing through it are:

- **Eustachian tube**
- **Ascending palatine artery**
- **Levator palate muscle**

When nasopharyngeal carcinoma spreads into this sinus, it will involve these structures causing sinus of Morgagni syndrome also called **Trotter's triad.**

IMPORTANT DISEASES OF NASOPHARYNX

Many of the diseases of nasopharynx (like ***Adenoids***) have already been discussed in the previous chapters. We are now going to discuss the remaining few.

Rathke's Pouch Cyst and Tumour

Rathke's pouch is a point in the nasopharynx from where the ectodermal part (adenohypophysis) of the pituitary gland develops.

This may give rise to two pathologies:

- ***Rathke's pouch cyst***
- ***Craniopharyngioma.*** It is a benign tumour arising from tissue of pituitary gland which may be present in the nasopharynx.

Thornwald's Cyst

The midline of nasopharynx has a bursa called nasopharyngeal bursa also called **Thornwald's bursa.**

This bursa represents the site of the cranial end of primitive notochord.

Sometimes it may give rise to a cyst called ***Thornwald's cyst.***

Treatment is marsupialization.

Nasopharyngeal Angiofibroma

It is also called **Juvenile Angiofibroma**

Juvenile angiofibroma is a benign and vascular tumour which spreads aggressively.

Histopathology

Juvenile angiofibroma has proliferating and irregular blood vessels intertwined in fibrous tissue.

Most common vessel supplying blood to the tumour is **Sphenopalatine artery.**

It is branch of **maxillary artery.**

The middle layer of these vessels, which is smooth muscle, is absent.

Aetiology

Aetiology is very clear. These two factors are important for you to remember:

1. These tumours have ***androgen receptors.***
2. *They are more common in patients with* ***familial adenomatous polyposis.***

Site of origin

The most common site of origin is posterosuperior wall of **Sphenopalatine Foramen**.

Presentation

- It is usually seen in **males in juvenile or adolescent**.
- The most common presentation is ***severe or recurrent nasal bleeding in juvenile males.***

Note: This is a differential diagnosis of *bleeding nasal mass.*

Spread of Angiofibroma	
• **Nasal spread**	It may spread into the nasal cavity and present as ***bleeding nasal mass***.
• **Pterygopalatine fossa extension**	Angiofibroma can extent laterally into pterygopalatine fossa. From here it can spread further lateral into infratemporal fossa. This may increase the gap between maxilla and mandible. This is called **hondusa sign**
• **Orbital extension**	From pterygopalatine fossa it can spread into ***orbit via infra orbital fissure***. In this case it may cause *proptosis*. This condition is called ***frog like face***.

Spread of Angiofibroma

• **Intracranial extension**	• It may extend into the cranial cavity from the nasopharynx. In this case it will land up in the *anterior cranial fossa.* • This may show **Crescent sign/Dodd's sign** (discussed below) • It may extend into the cranial cavity from the pterygopalatine fossa. In this case it will land up in the *middle cranial fossa*
• **Maxillary extension**	From pterygopalatine fossa it may push posterior wall of maxilla in the anterior direction. It is called ***anterior bowing of post maxillary wall.*** This can be seen on a scan. This finding of scan is called **Antral Sign** which is also called **Holman Miller Sign.**

STAGING OF NASOPHARYNGEAL ANGIOFIBROMA

There are many types of staging for angiofibroma.

The most important is **fisch staging of nasopharyngeal angiofibroma.**

If you recall, **Fisch staging** is also done for **glomus tumour in ear.**

Investigation

The investigation modality depends on the aim.

- X-ray shows **Hondousa Sign,** in which there is widening of gap between the maxilla and the mandible.
- This suggests involvement of Infratemporal fossa.
- **Dodd's sign:** This is an X-ray finding, in which there is a crescent-shaped space between the antrochoanal polyp and posterior pharyngeal wall.
- This is also called the **Crescent sign.**
- This is used to differentiate between ***nasal polyp and angiofibroma***.
- **CECT-** This modality used to be most commonly used.
- It delineates the bony erosion very well. It may show **Holman Miller sign.**
- **MRI-** This is better investigation for intracranial extension of tumour and soft tissue spread.
- In MRI, angiofibroma appears like a *"bag of worms"*.
- **Angiography** – This is preferred to see the vascularity of the tumour and when *embolization* is considered.
- Therefore, ***the best investigation modality is CT scan.***

Advantages of CT Scan

Tumour arises from a bony foramen called ***"pterygopalatine foramen"***. The scan can show the bony foramen

Various bony sign like ***antral sign, hondousa sign, crescent sign*** are better seen in CT scan.

Erosion of greater wing of sphenoid and through that the cranial spread is seen better in a CT scan.

Biopsy and FNAC are contraindicated.

Histopathology Findings

- ***It appears as unencapsulated stroma of fibroblast and collagen with thin walled blood vessels in it. The muscular layers of blood vessels are absent.***

Treatment

The main treatment modality is ***surgical excision.***

The following may be added to surgery:

- ***Radiotherapy***- especially in case of intracranial spread. It reduces the vascularity of the tumour as well shrinks the size.
- ***Chemotherapy***—may be used to shrink the size of tumour.
- ***Embolisation***—this is increasingly used as a pre-operative procedure to cut down the blood supply of the tumour.
- **Sphenopalatine artery is embolised.**
- ***Hormonal therapy***—this is a controversial topic, and hence, not used commonly.

Surgical approaches

1. Tumour confined to nasopharynx:	• *Per oral approach* • *Transpalatal approach* • *Endoscopic intranasal approach (FESS)*	Only when the tumour is very small and confined to nasopharynx Only after embolization.

2. Tumour has spread into the pterygopalatine fossa:	• ***Facial degloving approach***
	• *Lateral rhinotomy approach*
	  – *Moure's incision*
	  – *Weber Fergusson incision*
	• *Infratemporal approach*
		No external scar seen
		In these, the following method can be used:
		• Intranasal transantral approach
		• Maxillary swing approach
		• Sardana's approach
		When tumour spreads to infratemporal fossa

NASOPHARYNGEAL CARCINOMA

Most common site of nasopharyngeal carcinoma is ***fossa of Rosenmuller.***

Aetiology

- It is believed to be caused by ***Ebstein Barr virus*** **(EBV)**
- It is seen in patients who are ***genetically predisposed.***
  The loci involved are:
  - HLA-A
  - HLA-B
  - HLA-DR. They are on short arm of chromosome 6.
- It is caused by ***nitrosamine,*** present in smoked fish that the Chinese eat.

Histology

According to WHO classification, they are of two types:

Grade I	Keratinizing squamous cell carcinoma
Grade II	Nonkeratinizing squamous carcinoma and Undifferentiated squamous cell carcinoma

The most common type of nasopharyngeal carcinoma is ***undifferentiated carcinoma***.

Presentation

- It is most commonly seen in *Chinese population or South East Asia.*
- The most common presentation is ***cervical lymphadenopathy.***
  The lymph node that presents are the ***group II nodes also called jugulodigastric nodes.***
  Although the jugulodigastric lymphadenopathy is the first presentation, the ***sentinel lymph node for nasopharyngeal carcinoma is the retropharyngeal lymph node (node of Rouviere)***
  When jugulodigastric lymph nodes are palpable, it is called **Wood's sign**
  Wood's sign is seen in conditions like:
  - Tonsillitis
  - Nasopharyngeal carcinoma
- Other important presentations are
  - Nasal obstruction
  - Nasal bleeding
  - ***Unilateral glue ear in adult*** leading to *conductive hearing loss.*
  - ***Horner's syndrome*** due to involvement of cervical sympathetic chain
  - **Trotter's triad.** It is also called ***Sinus of Morgagni Syndrome.***

Trotter's triad has three features:	
1. Ipsilateral soft palate palsy	Due to involvement of levator palate muscle
2. Conductive hearing loss	Due to involvement of eustachian tube
3. Ipsilateral headache or facial pain.	Due to involvement of mandibular nerve
The facial pain in this case is due to mandibular nerve and hence is called *mandibular neuralgia*	

- Endocrinal changes like
  1. *Cushing's syndrome*
  2. *Eaton-Lambert syndrome, etc.*
- Cranial nerve palsies. All the nerves from 3rd to 12th can be involved.

Important points about cranial nerve involvement in nasopharyngeal carcinoma
• These nerves are involved when the tumour spreads into parapharyngeal space. • Please recollect that the same nerves are also involved in glomus jugulare tumour. • In glomus jugulare these nerves are involved in jugular fossa
• Most commonly involved nerves nasopharyngeal carcinoma are Vth and VIth nerves
• Involvement of the last four nerves may cause some syndrome. Some of these important syndromes are given in the next table:

Important syndromes when cranial nerves are involved. These syndromes are seen in nasopharyngeal carcinoma and glomus tumour

Syndromes	Nerves involved
Vernet syndrome (jugular fossa syndrome)	IX, X, XI
Collet-Sicard syndrome (intercondylar space syndrome)	IX, X, XI, XII
Villaret's syndrome (retropharyngeal space syndrome)	IX, X, XI, XII (last four) and sympathetic chain (Horner's syndrome)

Investigation

CT scan and biopsy are the most important investigations

Anti-EBV serology. The relevant antibodies are:

- ***IgA against viral capsid antigen (VCA)- it is more sensitive***
- ***IgA against early antigen (EA)—it is more specific.***

TNM Classification and Staging of Nasopharyngeal Carcinoma

Primary Tumour (T)

	Tumor confined to the nasopharynx
T2 T2a T2b	Tumor extends to soft tissues of oropharynx and/or nasal fossa • Without parapharyngeal extension • With parapharyngeal extension
T3	Tumor invades bony structures and/or paranasal sinuses
T4	Tumor with intracranial extension and/or involvement of • Cranial nerves • Infratemporal fossa • Hypopharynx • Orbit • Masticator space

Lymph Nodes (N) Classification

Note: The lymph nodes classification of nasopharyngeal carcinoma is different from rest of the head and neck cancers like laryngeal ca, oral ca etc. This is because lymphatic involvement in nasopharyngeal ca is more commonly involved as nasopharynx has good lymphatic supply.

Nx	Regional lymph nodes cannot be assessed
N0	No regional lymph node metastasis
N1	Unilateral metastasis in lymph node(s), 6 cm or less in greatest dimension, above the supraclavicular fossa
N2	Bilateral metastasis in lymph node(s), 6 cm or less in greatest dimension, above the supraclavicular fossa
N3	Metastasis in a lymph node(s) >6 cm and/or to supraclavicular fossa
N3a	Greater than 6 cm in dimension
N3b	Extension to the supraclavicular fossa

Treatment

- The most important treatment is ***radiotherapy.***

  Nasopharyngeal carcinoma is one of the ***most radiosensitive*** carcinomas of the head and neck region.

However, glottic carcinoma have better prognosis with radiotherapy. This is because glottis does **not** have the lymphatic supply.

- Surgery is done either for radiosensitive tumours or for recurrence.
- ***Photodynamic therapy (PDT)*** is an alternative.

  In photodynamic therapy, injection of ***photofrin*** is given to the patient.

  Photofrin is selectively taken up by the malignant cells.

  Photofrin is also light sensitive.

  This photosensitive agent releases active oxygen when irradiated with non-thermal laser light of some wavelength.

  The free oxygen radical causes cell death.

Last minute revision

- *Passavant's ridge is formed by horizontal fibres of palatopharyngeus muscles*
- *Torus tubarius is formed by cartilage of Eustachian tube and tensor veli palatini muscle*
- *Craniopharyngioma a tumour of pituitary gland may arise from rathke's pouch*
- *Juvenile angiofibroma arises from sphenopalatine foramen*
- *It is supplied by sphenopalatine artery, which is a branch of internal maxillary artery*
- *It presents as severe epistaxis in a juvenile male*
- *Important signs in angiofibroma are Holman Miller sign, Hondusa sign, frog face etc.*
- *Investigation of choice for angiofibroma is CECT*
- *Nasopharyngeal carcinoma arises form fossa of Rosenmuller*
- *The most common type is undifferentiated carcinoma*
- *It is caused by EBV and is seen in China*
- *Cervical lymphadenopathy is the most common presentation*
- *Trotter's triad has soft palate palsy, facial pain and hearing loss*
- *Adult with unilateral glue ear, we should rule out nasopharyngeal carcinoma by doing nasopharyngoscopy*
- *Radiotherapy is the treatment of choice in this*

QUESTIONS

1. Unilateral secretory otitis media in an adult is associated with:
a. Mastoiditis
b. CSOM
c. Carcinoma nasopharynx
d. Foreign body

2. Nasopharyngeal angiofibroma presents as:
a. Recurrent attacks of epistaxis
b. Deep cervical lymphadenopathy
c. Odynophagia
d. Difficulty in respiration

3. Treatment of carcinoma of nasopharynx is:
a. Radiotherapy
b. Chemotherapy
c. Surgery and radiotherapy
d. Radiotherapy and chemotherapy

4. Chandu a 15 years aged boy presents with unilateral nasal blockade, mass in the cheek and epistaxis: likely diagnosis is:
a. Nasopharyngeal ca
b. Angiofibroma
c. Inverted papilloma
d. None of the above

5. Most radiosensitive tumour of the following is:
a. Supraglottic ca
b. Ca glottis
c. Ca nasopharynx
d. Subglottic ca

6. Radiotherapy is the treatment of choice for which of these:
a. Nasopharyngeal CA T3N1
b. Supraglottis CA T3N0
c. Glottis CA T3N1
d. Subglottis CA T3N0

7. Most appropriate investigation for angiofibroma:
a. Angiography
b. CT scan
c. MRI scan
d. Plain X-ray

8. 12/M presented with bleeding and epistaxis. Hb-6.5 gm%, with normocytic hypochromic RBCs. Which is the most probable diagnosis?
a. Antrochoanal polyp
b. Juvenile angiofibroma
c. ethmoidal polyp
d. Inferior turbinate hypertrophy

9. Plasmacytoma of the nasopharynx is best treated by:
a. Radiotherapy
b. Chemotherapy
c. Surgery
d. Surgery plus radiotherapy

10. The main vessel involved in bleeding from juvenile nasopharyngeal angiofibroma:
a. Facial artery
b. Ascending pharyngeal artery
c. Internal maxillary artery
d. Anterior ethmoidal artery

11. In nasopharyngeal angiofibroma, all are true, *except:*
a. Common in females
b. Most common presentation is epistaxis
c. Arises from sphenopalatine foramen
d. It may cause frog face

12. A 10-year-old boy presents with nasal obstruction and intermittent profuse epistaxis. He has a firm pinkish mass in the nasopharynx. All of the following investigations are done in this case, *except:*
a. X-ray of skull base
b. CECT
c. Carotid angiography
d. Biopsy

13. Angiofibroma bleeds excessively because:
a. It lacks a capsule
b. Vessels lack a contractile component
c. It has multiple sites of origin
d. all

14. An 18-year-old boy presented with repeated epistaxis and there is a mass extending into the nose and nasopharynx. It was decided to operate on him. All of the following are true of the management, *except:*
a. Pre-operative radiotherapy is advised
b. Lateral rhinotomy approach may be used
c. Transmaxillary approach may be used
d. Transpalatine approach may be used

15. Which is the best treatment in angiofibroma in stage 2B?
a. Radiotherapy b. Chemotherapy
c. Surgery d. None

16. Antral sign is seen in:
a. Juvenile angiofibroma
b. Otosclerosis
c. Nasopharyngeal carcinoma
d. CSOM

17. A 10-year-old boy presents with unilateral nasal obstruction, cheek swelling and epistaxis. Most likely diagnosis:
a. Angiofibroma
b. AC polyp
c. Foreign body of nose
d. Inverted papilloma

18. Most common presentation of nasopharyngeal carcinoma is:
a. Neck mass
b. Epistaxis
c. Nasal stuffiness
d. Hoarseness of voice

19. True of Trotter's sign are A/E:
a. Conductive hearing loss
b. Involves Vth cranial nerve
c. Seen in angiofibroma
d. Palatal palsy

20. Branch of trigeminal nerve involved in nasopharyngeal CA
a. Mandibular b. Maxillary
c. Ophthalmic d. ALL

21. Category of non-keratinized squamous cancer of nasopharynx according to WHO is:
a. Grade I b. Grade II
c. Grade III d. Grade IV

22. Nasopharyngeal carcinoma is caused by:
a. EBV b. HPV
c. Herpes d. Adeno virus

23. Horner' syndrome is caused by:
a. Nasopharyngeal carcinoma metastasis
b. Ethmoidal polyp
c. Maxillary sinusitis
d. Angiofibroma

24. Type of speech seen in nasopharyngeal CA:
a. Rhinolalia aperta b. Rhinolalia clausa
c. Hot potato voice d. Hoarse voice

25. Thornwaldt's cyst is:
a. Nasopharyngeal cyst b. Laryngeal cyst
c. Oropharyngeal cyst d. Hypopharyngeal cyst

ANSWERS AND EXPLANATIONS

1. **c. Carcinoma nasopharynx**

Secretory otitis media (SOM) is a disease of middle ear which is usually caused due to blockade of eustachian tube.

Causes of eustachian tube blockade could be many. Important causes of eustachian tube blockade are:

1. **Adenoid hypertrophy**. This is more common in children.
2. **Nasopharyngeal carcinoma**. This is more common in adults.

SOM is more common in children and is bilateral.

However, it may also be seen in adults but is usually bilateral (like in children).

If secretory otitis media (SOM) is seen in adults and is unilateral then it should raise the suspension of nasopharyngeal carcinoma.

This is because the most common site of nasopharyngeal carcinoma is ***fossa of Rosenmuller, which is just behind the Eustachian tube.***

Hence, CA of this area may block the tube leading to unilateral secretory otitis media in adults.

Therefore, in all adults with unilateral secretory otitis media, nasopharyngeal carcinoma should be ruled out either by:

- CT Scan or
- Nasopharyngoscopy.

2. **a. Recurrent attacks of epistaxis**

Nasopharyngeal angiofibroma which is a **vascular tumour** is seen in juvenile males,

The vessels of the tumour usually ***do not have the muscular layers and hence the contractile properties of the vessels of the tumour are lost.***

Therefore, the tumour has tendency to bleed either heavily or recurrently.

Note: A 13 to 17-year-old male with nasal bleed should be investigated for nasopharyngeal angiofibroma by either CT Scan or venography.

- Nasopharyngeal carcinoma presents as cervical lymphadenopathy.
- Odynophagia is caused by diseases of ***oropharynx and hypopharynx and NOT nasopharynx***
- Difficulty in breathing may be late presentation of angiofibroma.

3. **a. Radiotherapy**

Carcinoma of nasopharynx is most commonly seen in the fossa of Rosenmuller which is very closely to related the parapharyngeal space, mandibular nerve and internal carotid artery.

The treatment of choice is radiotherapy of the tumour and the draining lymph nodes.

Chemotherapy may be added for stage III and stage IV CA.

Surgeries are also being tried specially for resistant tumours.

4. **b. Angiofibroma**

Angiofibroma is more common in juvenile male patient. Therefore, in a 15 years old male patient with epistaxis, angiofibroma should be ruled out. Cheek swelling in such a patient is seen when angiofibroma extends into the infratemporal fossa.

The other two choices i.e. nasopharyngeal CA and inverted papilloma are seen in adults.

5. **c. Ca nasopharynx**
Nasopharyngeal carcinoma are usually of the following type.
WHO classification of nasopharyngeal carcinoma
   1. Keratinizing squamous cell carcinoma.
      - Well differentiated
      - Moderately differentiated
      - Poorly differentiated
   2. Non-keratinizing carcinoma
   3. Undifferentiated carcinoma of nasopharyngeal type (lymphoepithelioma)

The most common is the lymphoepithelioma. This is the most radiosensitive of the above mentioned carcinoma. However glottic CA responds best to radiotherapy not because it is more radiosensitive than nasopharyngeal CA but because glottis has no lymphatic supply and so nodal metastasis is not seen.

6. **a. Nasopharynx CA T3N1**
Nasopharyngeal carcinoma is most commonly arises from fossa of Rosenmuller.
The most common type of nasopharyngeal carcinoma is ***undifferentiated squamous cell carcinoma.***
This is the ***most radiosensitive carcinoma in the head and neck region.*** Hence, radiotherapy is the treatment of choice in most nasopharyngeal carcinoma including stage T3N1.
In most of laryngeal carcinoma surgery is the preferred option.
Radiotherapy is the second option in most of early laryngeal carcinoma.

7. **b. CT scan**
Diagnosis of angiofibroma is based on two things:
   1. Clinical examination, and
   2. Radiological findings

The investigation modality depends on the aim. Various options are:
- X-ray shows **Hondousa Sign,** in which there is widening of gap between the maxilla and the mandible. This suggests involvement of Infratemporal fossa.
- **Dodd's sign:** This is an X-ray finding, in which there is a crescent shaped space between the antrochoanal polyp and posterior pharyngeal wall.
  This is also called the **Crescent sign.**
- **CECT**—This modality used to be most commonly used.
  It delineates the bony erosion very well. It may show **Holman Miller sign.**
  The above mentioned X-ray signs can also be seen in a CT scan.
- **MRI**—This is better investigation for intracranial extension of tumour and soft tissue spread
- In MRI, angiofibroma appears like a ***"bag of worms"***.
- **Angiography**—This is preferred to see the vascularity of the tumour and when ***preoperative embolization*** is considered.
- Therefore, the best investigation modality is ***CT scan.***

ADVANTAGES OF CT SCAN

- Tumour arises from a bony foramen called ***"pterygopalatine foramen"***. The scan can show the bony foramen.
- Various bony sign like ***antral sign, hondusa sign, crescent sign*** are better seen in CT scan.
- Erosion of greater wing of sphenoid and through that the cranial spread is seen better in a CT scan.

8. **b. Juvenile angiofibroma**
It is clear from the question that a juvenile child has iron deficiency anaemia.
This can also result from excessive bleeding. The only condition from the above list that can cause bleeding is ***juvenile angiofibroma.***

9. **a. Radiotherapy**
Plasmacytoma is a malignant plasma cell tumour that grows:
- Within soft tissue, or
- Within axial skeleton.

In nasopharynx hey are not very common. If present, it is extramadullary plasmacytoma.

The treatment of choice for this is ***radiotherapy.***

Note: For undifferentiated carcinoma of the nasopharynx (this is most common carcinoma of nasopharynx), ***the treatment of choice is radiotherapy.***

10. **c. Internal maxillary artery**

Juvenile nasopharyngeal angiofibroma is a vascular tumour with fibrous tissue in it.

The blood vessels supplying this tumour are:

	Community	Arteries
	• **Most common artery**	Sphenopalatine artery. This is a branch of ***intermal maxillary artery***
	• **Second common artery**	Ascending pharyngeal artery
	• **Third common artery**	Branches from internal carotid artery

11. **a. Common in females**

It is seen in juvenile males and NOT females.

Rest of the features are true of angiofibroma.

12. **d. Biopsy**

INVESTIGATIONS FOR ANGIOFIBROMA

The investigation modality depends on the aim.

- X-ray shows **Hondousa Sign,** in which there is widening of gap between the maxilla and the mandible.
- This suggests involvement of Infratemporal fossa.
- **Dodd's sign:** This is an X-ray finding, in which there is a crescent shaped space between the antrochoanal polyp and posterior pharyngeal wall.
- This is also called the **Crescent sign.**
- This is used to differentiate between ***nasal polyp and angiofibroma.***
- **CECT**—This modality used to be most commonly used.
- It delineates the bony erosion very well. It may show **Holman miller sign.**
- **MRI**—This is better investigation for intracranial extension of tumour and soft tissue spread.
- In MRI, angiofibroma appears like a ***"bag of worms"***.
- **Carotid Angiography –** This is preferred to see the vascularity of the tumour and when *embolization* is considered.

Therefore, ***the best investigation modality is CT scan.***

ADVANTAGES OF CT SCAN

Tumour arises from a bony foramen called ***"pterygopalatine foramen"***. The scan can show the bony foramen various bony sign like ***antral sign, hondusa sign, crescent sign*** are better seen in CT scan.

Erosion of greater wing of sphenoid and through that the cranial spread is seen better in a CT scan.

- **Biopsy- should be avoided.** *The blood vessels of this tumour lack the middle muscular/fibrous layer and so may result in severe bleeding,*

13. **b. Vessels lack a contractile component**

The blood vessels of this tumour lack the middle muscular/fibrous layer contractile layer) and so may result in severe bleeding,

Angiofibroma do lack a capsule unlike tonsils which has a fibrous capsule. But this in NOT the reason for bleeding in angiofibroma.

14. **a. Pre-operative radiotherapy is advised**

TREATMENT OF ANGIOFIBROMA

The main treatment modality is ***surgical excision.***

The following may be added to surgery:

- ***Radiotherapy-*** **ONLY** in case of intracranial spread. It reduces the vascularity of the tumour as well shrinks the size.

- *Chemotherapy*—may be used to shrink the size of tumour.
- *Embolisation*—this is increasingly used as a pre-operative procedure to cut down the blood supply of the tumour.
- **Sphenopalatine artery is embolised.**
- *Hormonal therapy*—this is a controversial topic, and hence, not used commonly.

Surgical approaches

1. Tumour confined to nasopharynx:	• *Per oral approach* • ***Transpalatal*** *approach* • *Endoscopic intranasal approach (FESS)*	Only when the tumour is very small and confined to nasopharynx Only after embolization.
2. Tumour has spread into the pterygopalatine fossa:	• *Facial degloving approach* • ***Lateral rhinotomy*** *approach* – Moure's incision – Weber ferguson incision • Infratemporal approach	No external scar seen In these, the following method can be used: • *Intranasal* ***transmaxillary*** *approach* • *Maxillary swing approach* • *Sardana's approach* When tumour spreads to infratemporal fossa

15. **c. Surgery**
Refer to the above explanation.

16. **a. Juvenile angiofibroma**
Antral sign also called Holman miller sign is seen when angiofibroma spreads into the pterygopalatine fossa. In this sign, there is ***anterior bowing of posterior maxillary wall.***

17. **a. Angiofibroma**
This is a classical presentation of angiofibroma. Cheek swelling suggests that the tumour has spread to infratemporal fossa. Such a spread will, most likely, show **antral sign and hondusa sign** also.
    - AC polyp (antrochoanal polyp) does not bleed as nasal polyps have very poor blood supply.
    - Inverted papilloma/Ringertz tumour is seen in **adult males** and not in children.
    - Foreign body is usually seen in very small child and will not cause cheek swelling.

18. **a. Neck mass**
Jugulodigastric/Group II lymph node enlargement is the commonest presentation in nearly ¾ of these patients.
    - First lymph node involved in nasopharyngeal carcinoma is ***retropharyngeal node/node of Rouviere***
    - First lymph node that presents in nasopharyngeal carcinoma is ***jugulodigastric lymph node/neck mass.***

19. **c. Seen in angiofibroma**
Trotter's triad. It is also called ***Sinus of Morgagni Syndrome.***

Trotter's triad has three features:

1. Ipsilateral soft palate palsy	Due to involvement of levator palate muscle
2. Conductive hearing loss	Due to involvement of Eustachian tube
3. Ipsilateral head ache or facial pain.	Due to involvement of mandibular nerve

- **The facial pain in this case is due to mandibular nerve and hence is called** *mandibular neuralgia*

20. **a. Mandibular**
Please refer to the explanation in the previous answer.

21. **b. Grade II**
According to WHO classification, they are of two types:

Grade I	Keratinizing squamous cell carcinoma
Grade II	Nonkeratinizing squamous carcinoma and Undifferentiated squamous cell carcinoma

22. **a. EBV**

ENT tumours	Viruses causing them
1. Nasopharyngeal CA	EBV
2. Oropharyngeal CA	HPV 16, 18
3. Laryngeal papilloma	HPV 6, 11

23. **a. Nasopharyngeal carcinoma metastasis**
Horner's syndrome is caused when sympathetic chain is involved by nasopharyngeal carcinoma invading the parapharyngeal space.

24. **b. Rhinolalia clausa**

Causes of Rhinolalia Clausa/Hyponasality

- Any condition causing nasal blockade like polyps, tumors, etc.
- Any condition causing nasopharyngeal obstruction like adenoid hypertrophy, nasopharyngeal CA etc.

Causes of Hypernasality

- *Cleft palate*
- *Oroantral fistula*
- *Soft palate palsy*
- *Post adenoidectomy*
- *After UPPP*
- *Velopharyngeal insufficiency*

Hot Potato Voice is Seen in Inflammatory Condition of Oropharynx Like

- Quincy

Causes of Hoarse Voice

- Conditions of vocal cord like vocal nodule, vocal polyp, Rienke's oedema, etc.

25. **a. Nasopharyngeal cyst**
The midline of nasopharynx has a bursa called nasopharyngeal bursa also called **Thornwald's bursa.**
This bursa represents the site of the cranial end of primitive notochord.
Sometimes it may give rise to a cyst called ***Thornwald's cyst.***

CHAPTER

29 Neck Spaces and Abscesses

Head and neck region has many types of cervical fascia. Sometimes these cervical fascia have spaces between them. These spaces are called neck spaces.

The important neck spaces are:

1. Retropharyngeal space
2. Prevertebral space
3. Danger space of neck
4. Parapharyngeal space
5. Submandibular space
6. Peritonsillar space

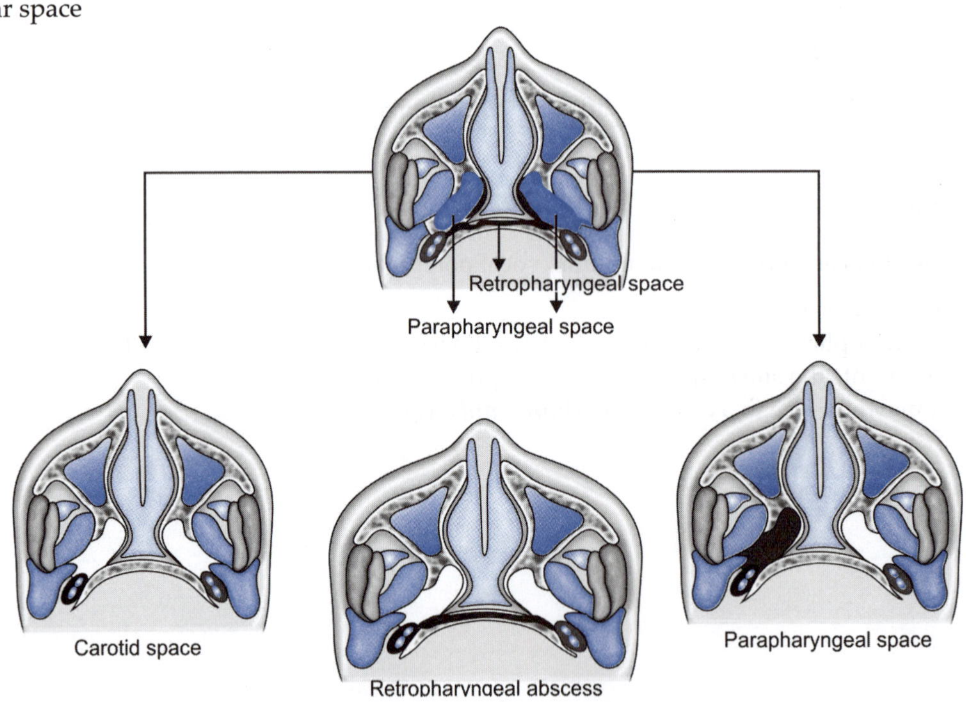

Fig. 1: Various spaces of neck

RETROPHARYNGEAL SPACE AND ABSCESS

Retropharyngeal space is also called ***space of Gillette.***

These are two in number, one on each side of midline

Boundaries

- Posterior boundary is formed by *prevertebral fascia* or *alar fascia*
- Anterior boundary is formed by *buccopharygeal fascia,* and
- Laterally are the *carotid sheaths*

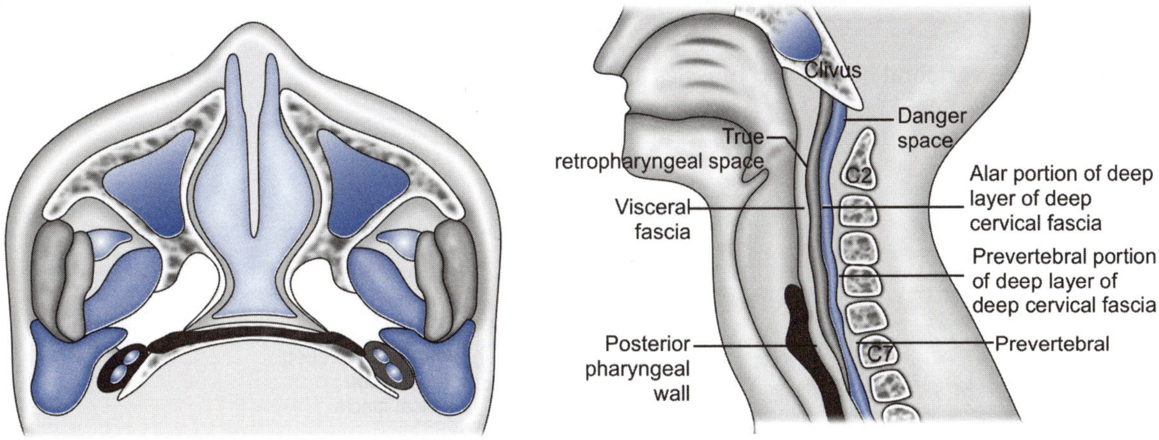

Fig. 2: Retropharyngeal space

Content of Space

It has retropharyngeal lymph nodes.

The most superior of these nodes are called the ***Nodes of Rouviere.***

Nasopharynx drains into these nodes.

Therefore, in nasopharyngeal carcinoma, ***retropharyngeal nodes are the sentinel nodes.***

Various Nodes of Head and Neck Area

Nodes of Rouviere	Retropharyngeal space
Krause's nodes	Jugular fossa
Nodes of Delphian	Prelaryngeal nodes

Causes of Abscess

- *Acute abscess in children is caused by* ***lymphadenitis.***
- *Acute abscess in adults is caused by* ***foreign body trauma.***
- *Chronic infection in both children and adult is caused by* ***tuberculosis.***

Presentation

Fever with *dysphasia and odynophagia with restricted neck mobility*

These symptoms are more severe in sitting position and less severe in supine position.

There is bulge on the lateral side of posterior pharyngeal wall with loss of normal curvature of spine.

This bulge is present in the ***paramedian position because there are two parapharyngeal spaces which are divided in the midline.***

Investigation

X-ray shows ***widening of prevertebral soft tissue shadow.***

Note: *Various books give values of the widening, which varies from book to book. There is no consistency in the value, hence, should not be memorized.*

MRI *is the best investigation.*

Treatment

- If tubercular, antitubercular therapy is given.
- Otherwise, incision and drainage may be required.

PREVERTEBRAL SPACE AND ABSCESS

It is bounded:

- Posteriorly by the vertebral bodies and muscles and
- Anteriorly by prevertebral fascia.

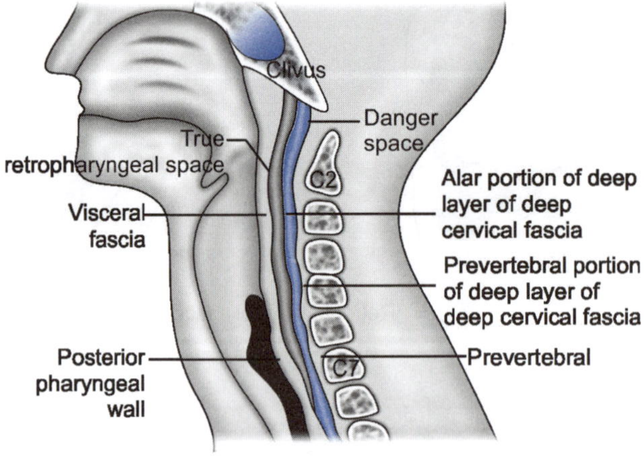

Fig. 3: Prevertebral space

Abscess is usually caused *secondary to caries of the spine.*

Presentation is similar to the retropharyngeal abscess.

Treatment is antitubercular therapy.

DANGER SPACE OF THE NECK

- Danger space of the neck lies between the prevertebral space and the retropharyngeal space.
- The posterior boundary formed by ***prevertebral fascia.***
- Anterior boundary is formed by ***alar fascia.***
- ***The infection of this space spreads into the mediastinum and so is called danger space.***
- *Abscess of this space is also called* **Grodinsky's abscess.**
- *Rest of the features of this space are similar to retropharyngeal space.*

SUBMANDIBULAR SPACE

Submandibular space has two parts which are separated by ***mylohyoid muscle.***

These parts are:

- ***Sublingual space, and***
- ***Submaxillary space.***

Content of Submandibular Space

- Submandibular gland and its duct (***Wharton's duct)***
- Sublingual gland and its duct ***(Duct of Rivinus/Bartholin's duct)***
- Lingual nerve and hypoglossal nerve

Relation between structures of submandibular space

Wharton's duct, lingual nerve and hypoglossal nerve run parallel to each other.

- Lingual nerve is at the top
- Wharton's duct is in the middle
- Hypoglossal nerve is the at bottom

PART 3: THROAT

Two important diseases that arise in this space are:
1. Ludwig's angina and
2. Ranula

LUDWIG'S ANGINA

Ludwig's angina is ***cellulite of submandibular space.***
Grodinsky proposed four criteria to distinguish Ludwig's angina from other forms of deep neck abscesses.

Grodinsky's Criteria for Ludwig's Angina are

- The infection must occur bilaterally in more than one space
- Product gangrenous serosanguineous infiltration with or NO pus
- Involve connective tissues fascia and muscle but NOT glandular structures, and
- Spread by continuity and not by lymphatics

Causes

- It is usually caused secondary to ***dental infection.***
- It is caused by ***mixed infection.***
- The main pathogen is ***alpha hemolyticus Streptococcus.***

Treatment

CT scan should be done
The treatment is medicinal, the antibiotic is of the penicillin group.
The dental infections should also be treated.
In some cases, incision and drainage may be required.

RANULA

Ranula is the retention cyst of the sublingual gland.
It is present in the sublingual space.
Sometimes, it crosses the mylohyoid muscle and spreads deep into the neck.
Such a ranula is called ***plunging ranula.***

Presentation

It presents as a cystic swelling on one side of the floor of the mouth.
This swelling has a very thin capsule which may appear ***blue in color.***

Treatment

- ***Excision of the cyst wherever possible***
- ***Marsupialization of the cyst when excision is not possible.***

PARAPHARYNGEAL SPACE AND ABSCESS

Parapharyngeal space is of the shape of an *inverted pyramid.*

Boundaries

- Posterior boundary is formed by ***prevertebral fascia***
- Medial boundary is formed by ***buccopharyngeal fascia***
- Lateral boundary is formed
  - ***Posteriorly by pterygoid muscles, and***
  - ***Anteriorly by mandible and parotid gland***

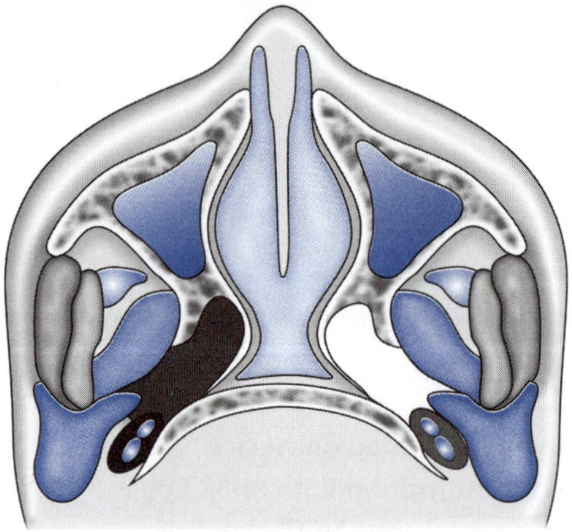

Fig. 4: Parapharyngeal space

Content

- ***Styloid process*** divides this space into two parts:
  - Pre-styloid compartment, and
  - Post-styloid compartment.
- Last four cranial nerves i.e. IX, X, XI, XII
  Therefore, spread of nasopharyngeal carcinoma into this space may involve these nerves and cause syndromes like Vernet syndrome, Collet-Sicard syndrome, vellaret syndrome, etc.
- ***Carotid artery***
- ***Jugular vein***
- ***Cervical sympathetic chain***
- ***Prestyloid space has mandibular nerve***
- Out of these, the following are within the ***carotid sheath (which is also a content of this space)***
  - ***Carotid artery***
  - ***Jugular vein***
  - ***Vagus nerve (X)***

ABSCESS

Abscess is usually secondary to abscess of other spaces, with which it is connected, mainly the *submandibular space abscess and peritonsillar space.*

Presentation

- *Dysphagia and odynophagia*
- *Trismus.* Trismus is due to spasm of ***medial pterygoid muscle.***
- *Fullness behind the angle of mandible*
- *Tonsil is pushed medially*

Note: *In case of peritonsillar abscess, the tonsil is pushed anteromedially, whereas in parapharyngeal space abscess, it is pushed medially.*

Investigation

CT scan is the most important investigation.

Treatment

Is mainly incision and drainage through external route.

Antibiotics have to be added.

PERITONSILLAR SPACE

Peritonsillar space is discussed with oropharynx and tonsils.

Last minute revision

- *Retropharyngeal space is also called Space of Gillette*
- *It contains nodes of Rouviere which are sentinel nodes in nasopharyngeal carcinoma*
- *Abscess of parapharyngeal space causes bulge in the paramedian area*
- *Danger space lies between prevertebral fascia and alar fascia*
- *The abscess of this space may extend into the mediastinum*
- *Ludwig's angina is a cellulitis of submandibular space*
- *Ranula is a retention cyst of sublingual gland in the sublingual space*
- *Marsupialization is the treatment*
- *Parapharyngeal space is also called pharyngomaxillary space*
- *It contains last four cranial nerves, great vessels, sympathetic chain and styloid process*
- *Abscess of this space causes bulge on medial wall of pharynx and trismus due to medial pterygoid muscle*

QUESTIONS

1. **Quinsy is:**
   a. Peritonsillar abscess b. Common in adults
   c. Retropharyngeal abscess
   d. Peritonsilitis
2. **Which of the following locations shows collection of pus in 'quinsy'?**
   a. Peritonsillar space
   b. Parapharyngeal space
   c. Retropharyngeal space
   d. Within the tonsil
3. **Quinsy is synonymous with:**
   a. Parapharyngeal abscess
   b. Retropharyngeal abscess
   c. Peritonsillar abscess d. Paratonsillar abscess
4. **A 7-year-old child has peritonisillar abscess present with trismus. The best treatment is:**
   a. Immediate abscess drain orally
   b. Drainage externally
   c. Systemic antibiotics up to 48 hours, then drainage
   d. Tracheostomy
5. **True statement regarding Ludwig's angina is:**
   a. Aphthous ulcers in the pharynx region
   b. Caused by Gram -ve bacilli
   c. Cellulitis of the floor of the mouth and submandibular space
   d. Incision and drainage of the abscess is done
6. **Peritonsillar abscess can extend posteriorly into:**
   a. Anterior triangle of neck
   b. Parapharyngeal space
   c. Posterior triangle on neck
   d. Submaxillary space
7. **Lateral retropharyngeal lymph node of Rouviere is involved in carcinoma of:**
   a. Glottis b. Oropharynx
   c. Esophagus d. Nasopharynx
8. **A medially bulging swelling in lateral pharyngeal wall is suggestive of:**
   a. Peritonsillar abscess
   b. Pharyngomaxillary abscess
   c. Retropharyngeal abscess
   d. Mastoid abscess
9. **Middle-aged diabetic presents with tooth extraction, ipsilateral swelling over the upper one-third of sternocleidomastoid and displacement of ipsilateral tonsils towards the opposite side. Diagnosis is:**
   a. Parapharyngeal abscess
   b. Retropharyngeal abscess
   c. Ludwig's angina d. None
10. **A 30-year-male underwent tooth extraction for dental caries. Now he has fever and trismus. Tonsil is pushed medially and has a swelling in the upper part of sternocleidomastoid. Diagnosis is:**
    a. Parapharyngeal abscess
    b. Retropharyngeal abscess
    c. Ludwig's angina d. None
11. **Regarding ranula, all are true *except:***
    a. Retention cyst
    b. Arises from submandibular gland
    c. Is translucent
    d. Plunging may be a feature
12. **The ideal time for operation of quincy after an acute attack of tonsillitis is:**
    a. 2 weeks b. 4 weeks
    c. 6 weeks d. 12 weeks
13. **Which of the following is not true about acute retropharyngeal abscess?**
    a. Dysphagia
    b. Swelling in posterior wall of pharynx
    c. Torticollis
    d. Caries of spine is the usual cause
14. **All are true about retropharyngeal abscess *except:***
    a. Confined to one side of midline
    b. Can be palpated per orally
    c. Lies behind the prevertebral fascia
    d. Presents with dysphagia and breathing difficulty
15. **"Ludwig's angina" is characterized by all except:**
    a. Cellulitis in the floor of mouth
    b. Caused by anerobic organisms
    c. Aphthous ulcer in the pharynx
    d. Infection spreads to hyoglossus muscle
16. **Cranial nerve not at risk during surgery of submandibular salivary gland is:**
    a. Glossopharyngeal nerve
    b. Marginal mandibular nerve
    c. Hypoglossal nerve d. Lingual nerve
17. **Ranula is:**
    a. Hypertrophied lymphoid tissue
    b. Arises from floor of mouth
    c. Hard and hemorrhagic
    d. An abscess
18. **Ranula is:**
    a. Leukoplakia b. Retention cyst
    c. Premalignant
    d. Arises from submandibular gland

IMAGE BASED QUESTION

19. **Answer the following question based on the picture given below:**

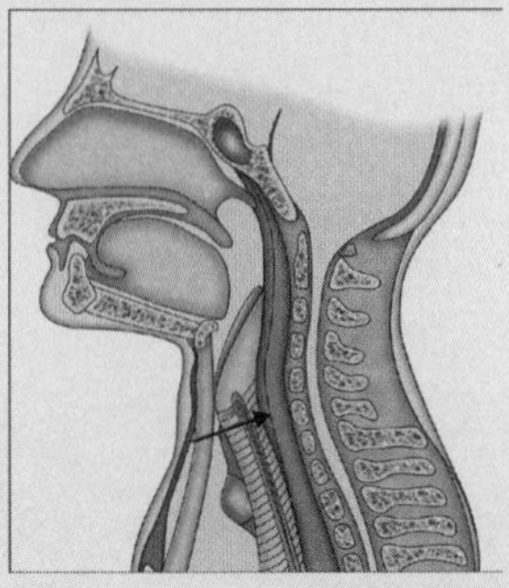

    a. The arrow marked space is danger space of the neck.
    b. The abscess of this space is called Grodinsky's abscess
    c. The abscess of this space may spread into the mediastinum
    d. All are true

ANSWERS AND EXPLANATIONS

1. **a. Peritonsillar abscess**
2. **a. Peritonsillar space**
3. **c. Peritonsillar abscess**
4. **c. Systemic antibiotics up to 48 hours, then drainage**
   Peritonsillar abscess, also called quincy, is a very painful condition and so is also described as "hot potato" condition. Hence, immediate I and D should be done to relieve this painful condition.
   However, there are ***two situations of quincy where antibiotics should be gven for 24-48 hrs and then I and D*** *done*.

   These are:
   1. Quincy with trismus (as asked in the question)
   2. Quincy in small children.
   3. Small child with trismus.

   In the above-mentioned case, the patient is a child as well as has trismus. Hence, antibiotics up to 48 hours, then drainage
5. **c. Cellulitis of the floor of the mouth and submandibular space**
   Ludwig's angina is the cellulitis (not an abscess) of the floor of mouth and the submandibular space, which is usually secondary to the teeth infection.
   Grodinsky proposed four criteria to distinguish Ludwig's angina from other forms of deep neck abscesses.
   Grodinsky's criteria for Ludwig's angina are:
   - The infection must occur bilaterally in more than one space
   - Product gangrenous serosanguineous infiltration with or NO pus
   - Involve connective tissue fascia and muscle but NOT glandular structures, and
   - Spread by continuity and not by lymphatics

   This condition usually has mixed infections and presents with:
   - Odynophagia,
   - Trismus,
   - Raised floor of mouth and
   - The **feel is woody**.

   Medicines are required for the treatment and since it is not an abscess, incision and drainage may sometimes be required.
6. **b. Parapharyngeal space**
   Peritonsillar absess is an abscess where the pus collects between:
   - The tonsillar capsule and
   - The superior constrictor muscle.

   The pus from here can spread into the parapharyngeal space causing parapharyngeal abscess.
   It is believed that every peritonsillar abscess is a potential parapharyngeal abscess waiting to happen.
   Peritonsillar abscess, also called quincy, presents as hot potato voice and immediate incision and drainage is the treatment.
   Parapharyngeal space can be prestyloid or post-styloid, depending on whether the pus collects in front of styloid process or behind the styloid process.
7. **d. Nasopharynx**
   Lateral retropharyngeal lymph nodes of Rouviere are drained by the nasopharynx.
   Nasopharyngeal carcinoma involves nodes of Rouviere and from there it spreads to upper jugulodigastric lymph nodes (also called upper deep cervical nodes).
   NOTE: The most common presentation of carcinoma of nasopharynx is upper deep cervical lymphadenopathy. This means that the nodes of Rouviere are often involved before the patient presents to his doctor.

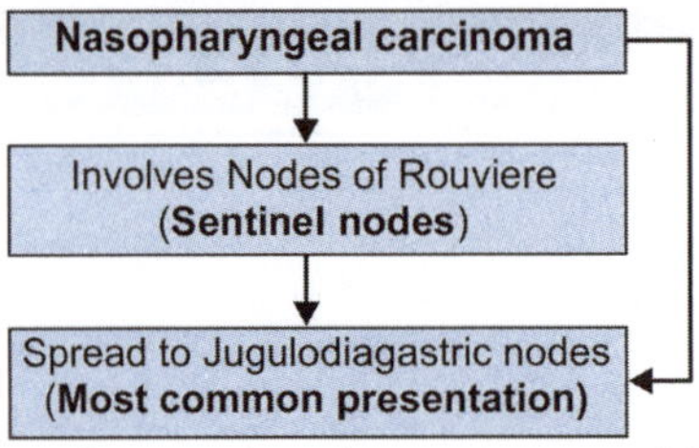

1. Nasopharyngeal carcinoma may spread to jugulodigastric nodes either directly or
2. It first spreads to Nodes of Rouviere and from there to jugulodigastric nodes.

- ***Jugulodigastric lymphadenopathy is the most common presentation of nasopharyngeal carcinoma.***
- ***Lateral retropharyngeal lymph node of Rouviere is the sentinel (first node involved) of nasopharyngeal carcinoma.***

8. **b. Pharyngomaxillary abscess**

Pharyngomaxillary abscess is abscess of pharyngomaxillary space. This space is also called ***parapharyngeal space.***

Parapharyngeal space is of the shape of an *inverted pyramid.*

Boundaries of Parapharyngeal Space

- Posterior boundary is formed by ***prevertebral fascia***
- Medial boundary is formed by ***buccopharyngeal fascia and superior constrictor muscle***
- Lateral boundary is formed
  - ***Posteriorly by pterygoid muscles, and***
  - ***Anteriorly by mandible and parotid gland***
- Inferiorly is the apex of this space which ends at ***hyoid bone.***

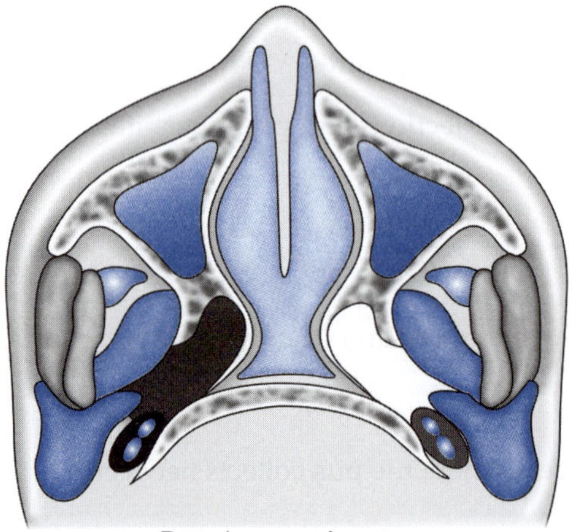

Parapharyngeal space

Since this space is lateral to the pharynx, abscess of this space may cause bulge in the lateral pharyngeal wall.

PRESENTATION OF PHARYNGOMAXILLARY ABSCESS

- *Dysphagia and odynophagia*
- *Trismus:* Trismus is due to spasm of ***medial pterygoid muscle.***
- *Fullness behind the angle of mandible*
- *Tonsil and lateral pharyngeal wall are pushed medially*

SITE OF BULGE IN OTHER ABSCESSES OF NECK

- In peritonsillar abscess (Quincy), the tonsil is pushed ***anteromedially.***
- In retropharyngeal abscess, the bulge is seen in the ***paramedial position*** of the posterior pharyngeal wall.

- In prevertebral abscess and abscess of danger space, the posterior pharyngeal wall has a ***bulge in the midline.***
- In cellulitis of submandibular space (Ludwig's angina), bulge is seen in the ***floor of the mouth.***
- In mastoiditis, bulge in seen in the post-auricular region.

9. **a. Parapharyngeal abscess**
10. **a. Parapharyngeal abscess**
11. **b. Arises from submandibular gland**
    Ranula is retention of sublingual gland and presents as a translucent swelling in the floor of the mouth with blue capsule around it.
    It may plunge deep to mylohyoid muscle and then is called plunging ranula.
12. **c. 6 weeks**
    The ideal time is between 4 weeks and 6 weeks. This is called ***interval tonsillectomy.***
    If one has to select between 4 weeks and 6 weeks, then 6 weeks is the better answer.
13. **d. Caries of spine is the usual cause**

CAUSES OF ABSCESS

- *Acute abscess in children is caused by* ***lymphadenitis***
- *Acute abscess in adults is caused by* ***foreign body trauma***
- *Chronic infection in both children and adults is caused by* ***tuberculosis/caries of cervical spine.***

From the above, mentioned fact, we can see that ***caries will cause chronic abscess and not acute abscess.***

14. **c. Lies behind the prevertebral fascia**
    Retropharyngeal space is also called *space of Gillette*
    These are two in number, one on each side of midline.

BOUNDARIES

- Posterior boundary is formed by *prevertebral fascia or alar fascia*
- Anterior boundary is formed by *buccopharygeal fascia, and*
- Laterally are the *carotid sheaths*

As we can see, it lies anterior to the prevertebral fascia.

15. **c. Aphthous ulcer in the pharynx**
    Ludwig's angina is cellulitis of the submandibular space.
    It is caused by anerobic organisms.

Grodinsky's Criteria for Ludwig's Angina are

- The infection must occur bilaterally in more than one space
- Product gangrenous serosanguinous infiltration with or NO pus
- Involve connective tissues fascia and muscle (like hyoglossus) but NOT glandular structures, and
- Spread by continuity (along muscles and fascia) and not by lymphatics

Note: Apthous ulcer is NOT seen in Ludwig's angina.
Apthous ulcer is a feature of;
- ***Behcet's disease***
- ***Autoimmune diseases of GIT.***

16. **a. Glossopharyngeal nerve**
    The three nerves that are at risk during submandibular gland excision are:
    - Marginal mandibular nerve
    - Lingual nerve, and
    - Hypoglossal nerve
      - Marginal mandibular nerve is a branch of facial nerve and passes just below the mandible. This may be damaged while giving incision for the surgery.

This nerve can be saved by applying a low incision. The incision applied is approximately two-finger width below the ramus of mandible.

- Lingual nerve and hypoglossal nerve run parallel and close to the duct of submandibular gland (***Wharton's duct***). There is chance of damage of these two nerves while this duct is being cut.

17. **b. Arises from floor of mouth**
Ranula is retention of sublingual gland and presents as a translucent swelling in the floor of the mouth with blue capsule around it.

18. **b. Retention cyst**
Refer to the explanation in the previous question.

IMAGE BASED ANSWER

19. **d. All are true**
The arrow marked space is called **danger space** of the neck. It is so called because the abscess of this space, also called ***Grodinsky's abscess***, can spread into the mediastinum.

PART 4

Larynx

CHAPTERS

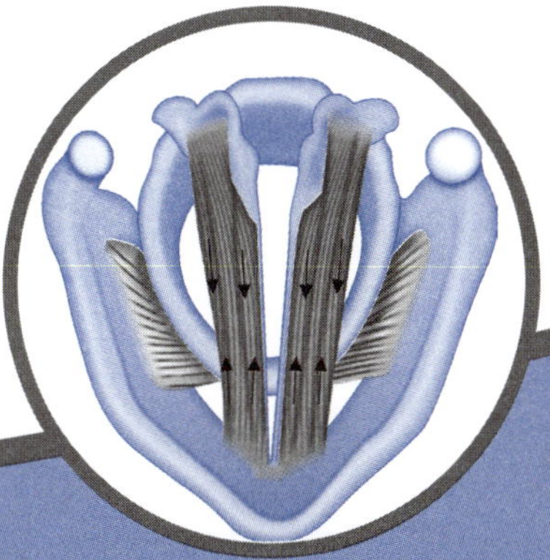

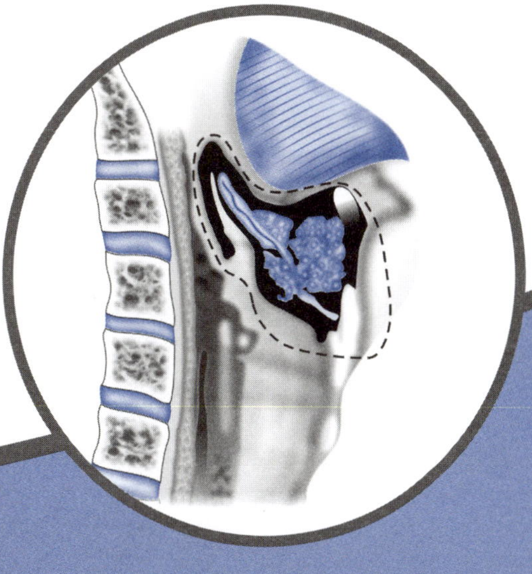

CHAPTER

30 Anatomy of Larynx

Larynx is also called voice box.

Adult larynx is described as a tube like or cylindrical organ. It is made of number of cartilages, membranes, ligaments and muscles.

The outer structure is made mainly by cartilages and membranes.

CARTILAGES OF LARYNX

Larynx has six types of cartilages, out of which three are paired and three unpaired.

Unpaired	Paired
Epiglottis	Arytenoids
Thyroid	Corniculate cartilage of Santorini
Cricoid	Cuneiform cartilage of Wrisberg
Note: A new paired cartilage called triticea is also added as 7th cartilage.	

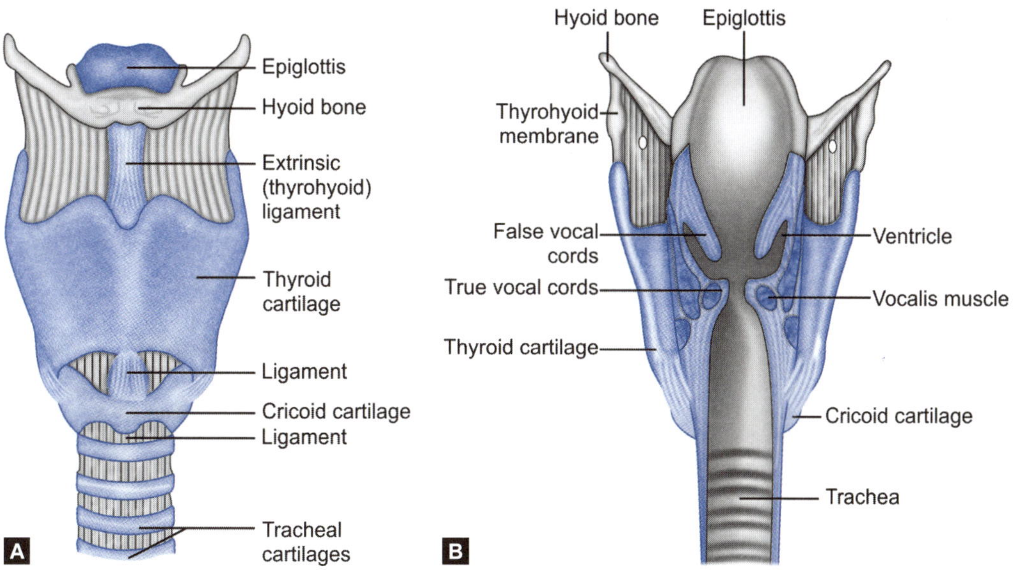

Figs. 1A and B: Cartilages of larynx

Shapes of Laryngeal Cartilages

- The **cricoid cartilage** forms a **signet-shaped ring.**
- Epiglottis is leaf like

- Thyroid is 'C'-shaped
- Arytenoids are pyramidal-shaped.

Membranes of Larynx

Laryngeal membranes are divided into
1. Extrinsic membranes
2. Intrinsic membranes

Extrinsic membranes	Intrinsic membranes
• Thyrohyoid membrane • Cricotracheal membrane	• Quadrangular membrane • Cricovocal membrane also called *conus elasticus* • Cricothyroid membrane is a part of cricovocal membrane.

Muscles of Larynx

Intrinsic muscles	Extrinsic muscle
• *Attach laryngeal cartilages to each other* • *They are supplied by recurrent laryngeal nerve except Cricothyroid* – Posterior cricoarytenoid – Lateral cricoarytenoid – Interarytenoid – Thyroarytenoid – Cricothyroid	• *Attach larynx to surrounding structures* – Stylopharyngeus – Salpingopharyngeus – Palatopharyngeus – Thyrohyoid – Mylohyoid – Digastric – Stylohyoid – Geniohyoid – Sternohyoid – Sternothyroid – Omohyoid

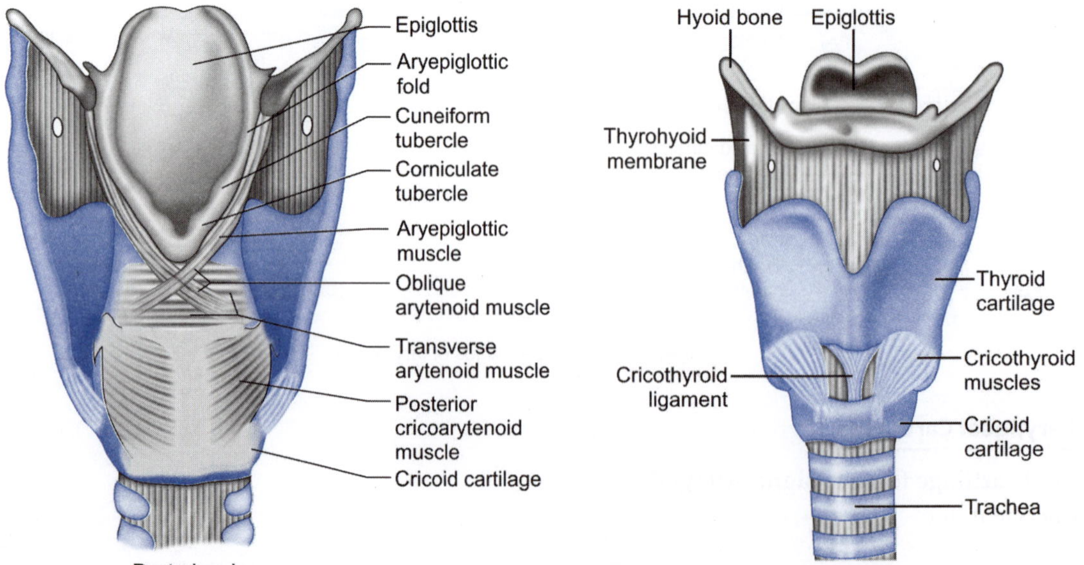

A Posterior view B

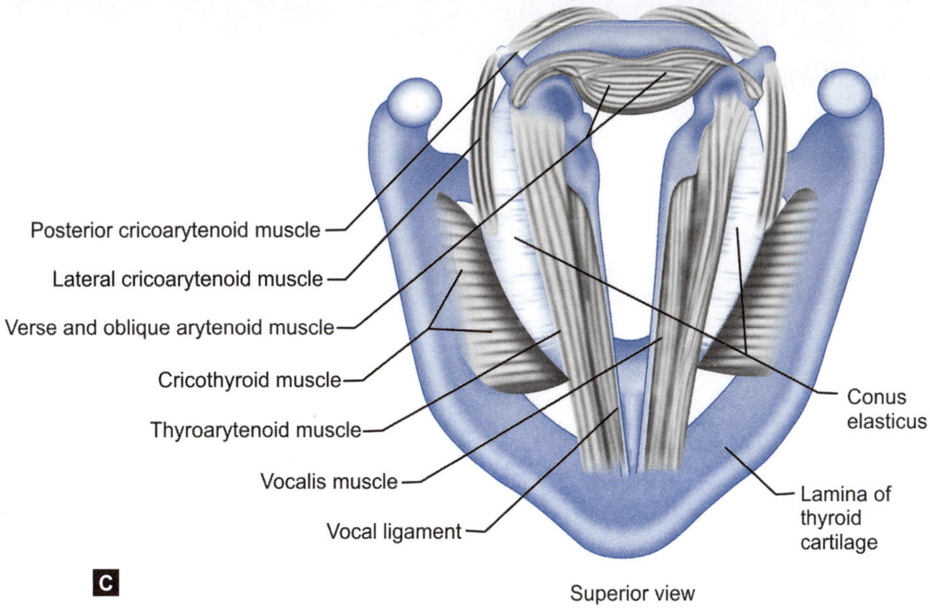

Figs. 2A to C: Muscles of vocal cord

FUNCTIONS OF MUSCLES

Elevators of larynx	Depressors of larynx
Primary elevators • Stylopharyngeus • Salpingopharyngeus • Palatopharyngeus • Thyrohyoid	• Sternohyoid • Sternothyroid • Omohyoid
Secondary elevators • Mylohyoid • Digastric • Stylohyoid • Geniohyoid	

Note: 1. Any membrane, ligament or muscle that are attached to two laryngeal cartilages are ***intrinsic structure***; whereas, those connecting a laryngeal cartilage to any other adjoining structure like trachea, sternum, hyoid, mandible, styloid process etc are ***extrinsic structure.***

2. ***Extrinsic muscles*** that connect laryngeal cartilage to structures above it like *hyoid, mandible, styloid process* will **elevate the larynx,** whereas, those that connect it to structure below it like sternum will **depress the larynx.**

Also note that *omohyoid is depressor of larynx.*

ADDUCTORS OF LARYNX

- Lateral cricoarytenoid
- Interarytenoid
- Thyroarytenoid (lateral fibres), and
- Cricothyroid

ABDUCTORS

- Posterior cricoarytenoid

TENSORS

- Thyroarytenoid (medial fibres also called **vocalis)**
- Cricothyroid

Function of Individual Muscle of Larynx

Muscles	Functions
Posterior cricoarytenoid	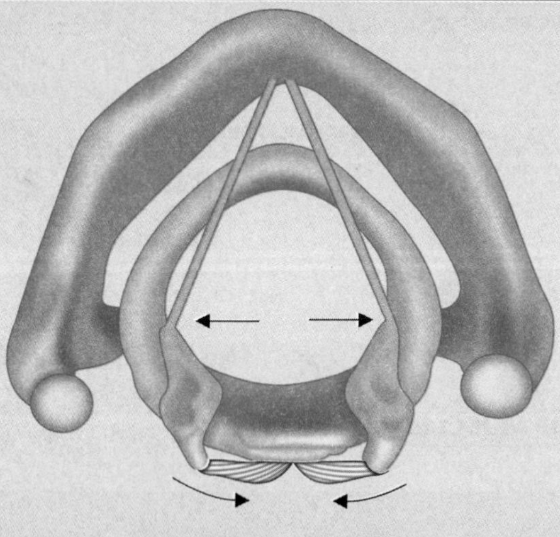 Posterior cricoarytenoid is the only abductor of vocal cord
Lateral cricoarytenoid	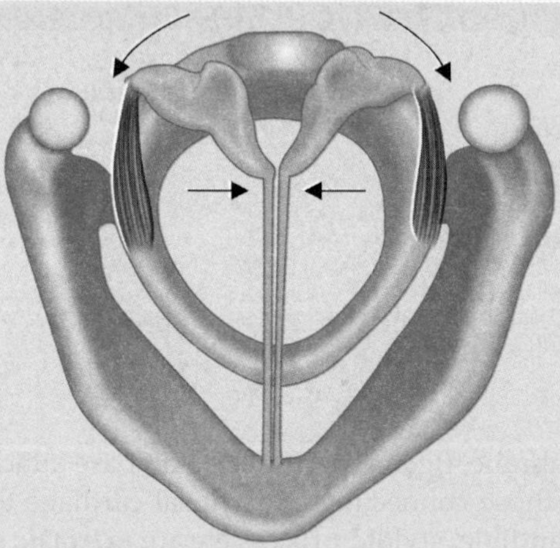 Lateral cricoarytenoid causes: • Adduction and • Lengthening
Interarytenoid	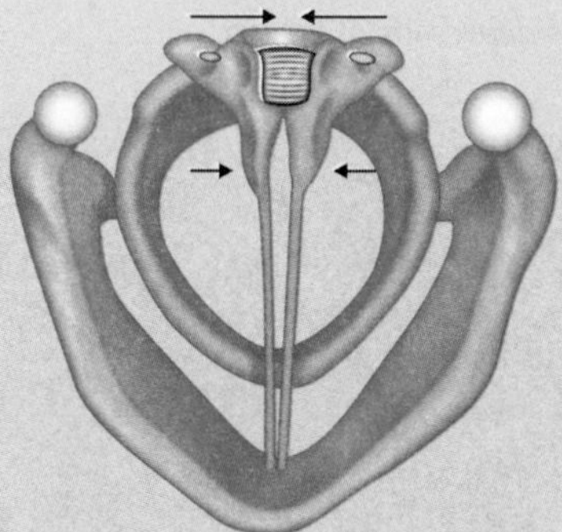 Interarytenoid is adductor of vocal cord

Contd...

Contd...

Muscles	Functions
Thyroarytenoid	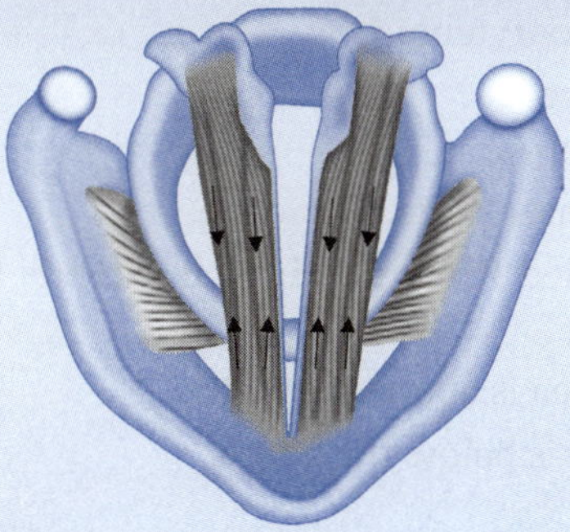 Thyroarytenoid has two parts: • Medial part called ***vocalis muscle.*** It causes – Tension and thickening of vocal cord • Lateral part which causes – Adduction and thickening
Cricothyroid	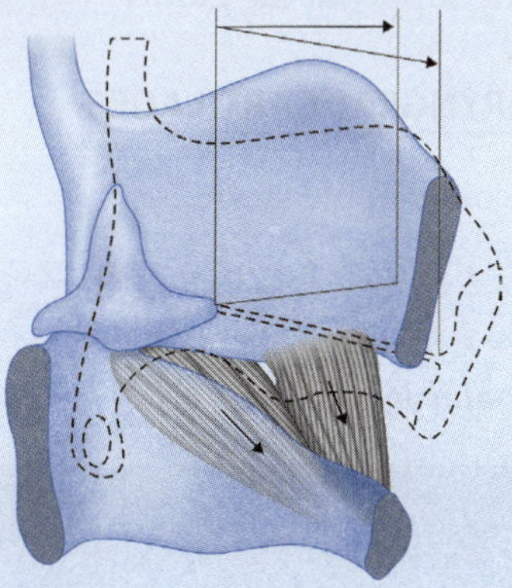 Cricothyroid causes • Tension • Mild adduction and • Lengthening

Note: 1. **Cricothyroid and thyroarytenoid** have two functions of adduction and tension
2. The only abductors of vocal folds is posterior cricoarytenoid

PARTS OF LARYNX

1. ***Laryngeal inlet***
   - This is bounded by:
     - Anteriorly by the epiglottis
     - On sides by aryepiglottic folds, and
     - Posteriorly by the mucosa between the arytenoids
2. ***Vestibular folds***
   This is also called ***false vocal cords.***
   - It contains:
     - Vestibular ligaments, which is formed by lower free end of quadrilateral membrane.
     - Mucous glands.
3. ***Ventricle***
   This is also called ***Saccule or sinus of larynx***
   It lies between the vestibular folds and the vocal folds
   It can form ***laryngocele***

4. *Vocal folds*

   This is also called ***true cords.***

   - It contains
     - Vocal ligaments, which is formed by the upper free end of cricovocal membrane
     - Fibres of thyroarytenoid
     - **Reinke's space**
   - Squamous epithelium

Larynx is divided into three parts. These are:

1. **Glottis:** It is also called **Rima glottidis.** It extends from the upper end of vocal folds to 1 cm below the vocal folds.
2. **Supraglottis:** This area is above the glottis
3. **Subglottis:** This area is below the glottis.

IMPORTANT FEATURES OF THE GLOTTIS

- This is the only area of larynx lined by *squamous epithelium*
- This is the narrowest part of adult larynx
- There are **no** lymphatic supply at the glottis

JOINTS BETWEEN LARYNGEAL CARTILAGES

There are two important joints in the larynx.

1. Cricoarytenoid joint
2. Cricothyroid joints

Both these joints are ***synovial joints.***

Nerve supply of larynx

Larynx is supplied by two nerves, both of which are branches of vagus

1. *Superior laryngeal nerve.*
   - This gives rise to two branches
     - *Internal laryngeal nerve, and*
     - *External laryngeal nerve*
2. *Recurrent laryngeal nerve*

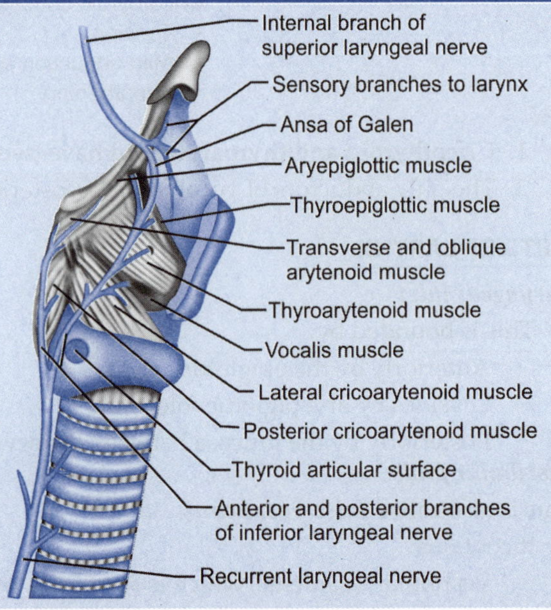

- ***External laryngeal nerve*** supplies only one muscle i.e. **Cricothyroid muscle.** Hence, this nerve is mainly responsible for tension of vocal cord.
- ***Recurrent laryngeal nerve*** supplies rest of the laryngeal muscles. Therefore, this nerve is responsible for *adduction and abduction* of vocal cords.

- It is also the sensory supply of the subglottic area
- ***Internal laryngeal nerve*** is the sensory supply of the supraglottic area
- ***Galen's anastomosis*** is present in the glottis and is formed by the joining of internal laryngeal nerve and the recurrent laryngeal nerve.
  This supplies the glottis.

MEASUREMENTS OF LARYNX

Length of vocal cords in females is **16-17 mm**
Length of vocal cords in male is **24-25 mm**
A-P length of larynx in females is **28-29 mm**
A-P length of larynx in males is **36-37 mm**

SPACES IN LARYNX

There are two spaces in larynx.

1. **Preepiglottic space:** It is also called *Space of Boyer.*
2. **Paraglottic space:** It is also called *Space of Tucker.*

Space of Boyer/preepiglottic space	Boundaries
Anteriorly	Thyrohyoid ligament and Hyoid bone
Posteriorly	Epiglottis
Superiorly	Hyoepiglottic ligament

Tucker's space/paraglottic space	Boundaries
Medially	Conus elasticus and Quadrilateral membrane
Laterally	Thyroid cartilage
Posteriorly	Mucosa of pyriform fossa

FUNCTIONS OF LARYNX

The main function of larynx is ***protection of airway***.
Functions of larynx are:

- Protection of airway/prevent aspiration
- Voice production
- Respiration
- Fixation of chest.

Last minute revision

- *Larynx has three paired cartilages and three unpaired cartilages*
- *Cricoids is signet ring-shaped cartilage. It is the only ring-shaped cartilage of larynx*
- *The only abductor of vocal cords is posterior cricoarytenoid muscle*
- *The only muscle supplied by superior laryngeal nerve is cricothyroid muscle*
- *Reinke's space is deep to squamous epithelium in the glottis*
- *Most important function of larynx is protection of airway*

QUESTIONS

1. **Which of the following laryngeal cartilage is a complete ring?**
   a. Thyroid b. Cricoid
   c. Cuneiform d. Arytenoid
2. **Only abductor of the vocal cord is:**
   a. Lateral cricoarytenoid
   b. Posterior cricoarytenoid
   c. Cricothyroid d. Thyroarytenoid
3. **Which of the following muscles is supplied by external laryngeal nerve which is a branch of superior laryngeal nerve?**
   a. Posterior cricoarytenoid
   b. Cricothyroid
   c. Lateral cricoarytenoid
   d. Thyroarytenoid
4. **True cord is lined by which type of epithelium:**
   a. Stratified squamous
   b. Cuboidal epithelium
   c. Stratified columnar
   d. Stratified columnar ciliated
5. **Trachea divides at the level of:**
   a. Upper border of Tl
   b. Lower border of T4
   c. Lower border of T7
   d. Lower border of T10
6. **Epiglottis arises from which of these:**
   a. 2nd arch b. 3rd arch
   c. 4th arch d. 6th arch
7. **True about Reinke's space is:**
   a. Located in true vocal cord
   b. Bounded by upper and lower arcuate lines
   c. Vocal polyp is associated with it
   d. All
8. **Which of the following open the inlet of larynx?**
   a. Thyroepiglotticus b. Vocalis
   c. Cricothyroid d. Thyroarytenoid
9. **A neonate while suckling milk can respire without difficulty due to:**
   a. Small soft palate b. Small tongue
   c. High larynx d. Small pharynx
10. **Elastic cartilage is present in:**
    a. Thyroid b. Epiglottis
    c. Cricoid d. Arytenoid
11. **Laryngeal crepitus is absent in all of the following conditions, *except:***
    a. Postcricoids malignancy
    b. Hypopharyngeal abscess
    c. Parapharyngeal abscess
    d. Prevertebral abscess
12. **Which of the following is the only intrinsic muscle of larynx that lie outside the laryngeal framework?**
    a. Cricothyroid
    b. Superior constrictor
    c. Cricopharyngeus
    d. Lateral cricothyroid
13. **Epilarynx include A/E:**
    a. Suprahyoid epiglottis
    b. Infrahyoid epiglottis
    c. Arytenoid
    d. Aryepiglottic folds
14. **Closure of the glottis is by all *except:***
    a. Posterior cricoarytenoids
    b. Lateral cricoarytenoids
    c. Cricothyroid
    d. Thyroarytenoids
15. **Which of the following are functions of larynx?**
    a. Respiration b. Protection of airway
    c. Fixation of chest d. All
16. **All are elevators of larynx *except:***
    a. Thyrohyoid b. Digastric
    c. Stylohyoid d. Sternohyoid
17. **Which of the following is depressor of larynx?**
    a. Mylohyoid b. Digastric
    c. Stylopharyngeus d. Sternohyoid
18. **Space of Tucker is seen in:**
    a. Larynx b. Oesophagus
    c. Femoral canal d. Hypopharynx
19. **Safety muscles of larynx are:**
    a. Posterior cricoarytenoid
    b. Thyroarytenoid
    c. Cricothyroid d. Interarytenoid
20. **True about infantile larynx as compared adult larynx:**
    a. Epiglottis is large and omega shaped.
    b. Cricoid is the narrowest part.
    c. It extends at C_4, C_5, C_6 vertebra
    d. Breathing and swallowing at the same time

IMAGE BASED QUESTION

21. **In this animated picture of the larynx, identify the arrow marked bone or cartilage:**

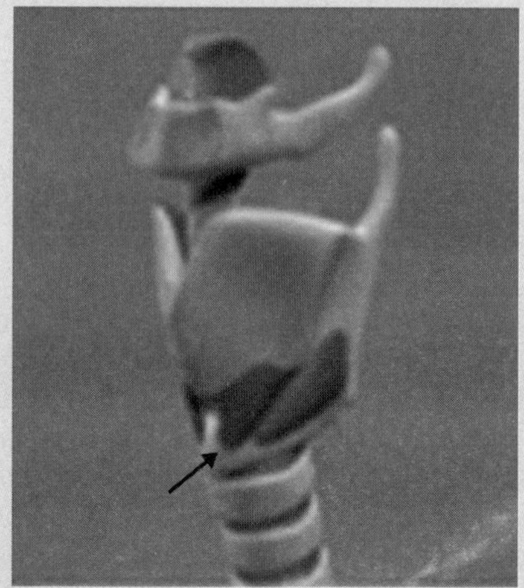

    a. Hyoid bone
    b. Thyroid cartilage
    c. Cricoid cartilage
    d. Arytenoid

ANSWERS AND EXPLANATIONS

1. **b. Cricoid**

Larynx is made of six cartilages of which three are paired and three are unpaired.

Unpaired	Paired
Epiglottis	Arytenoids
Thyroid	Corniculate cartilage of Santorini
Cricoid	Cuneiform cartilage of Wrisberg

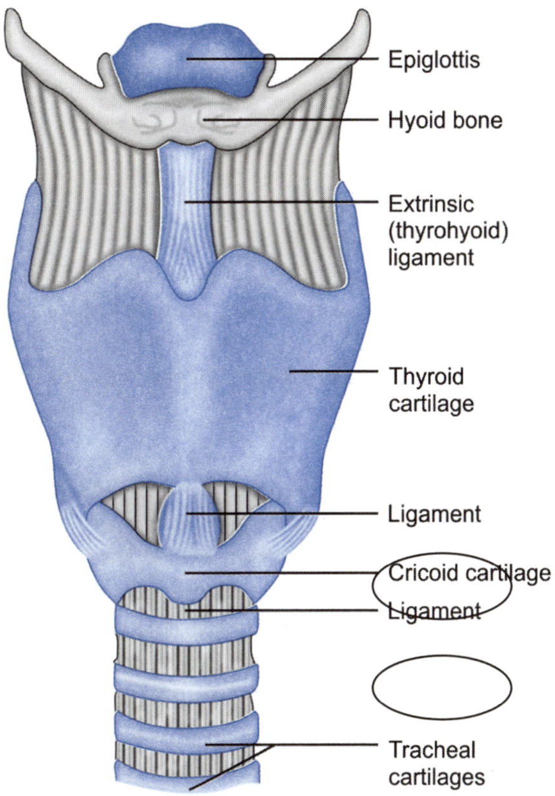

SHAPES OF LARYNGEAL CARTILAGES

- The **cricoid cartilage** forms a **signet-shaped ring.**
- Epiglottis is leaf like
- Thyroid is 'C' shaped
- Arytenoids are pyramidal shaped.

2. **b. Posterior cricoarytenoid**

Of the many muscles supplying vocal cord the only abductor is posterior cricoarytenoid, rest of the muscles are adductors. Among these adductors, two muscles i.e. interarytenoid and lateral cricoarytenoid are only adductors whereas rest of the two i.e thyroarytenoid and cricothyroid are adductors as well as tensors of vocal cord.

FUNCTION OF INDIVIDUAL MUSCLE OF LARYNX

Muscles	Functions
Posterior cricoarytenoid	Posterior cricoarytenoid is the only abductor of vocal cord
Lateral cricoarytenoid	Lateral cricoarytenoid causes: • Adduction and • Lengthening
Interarytenoid	Interarytenoid is adductor of vocal cord
Thyroarytenoid	Thyroarytenoid has two parts: • Medial part called ***vocalis muscle.*** It causes: – Tension and thickening of vocal cord • Lateral part which causes: – Adduction and thickening
Cricothyroid	Cricothyroid causes: • Tension • Mild adduction and • Lengthening

3. **b. Cricothyroid**

   All the muscles of larynx are supplied by recurrent laryngeal nerve except the cricothyroid, which is supplied by external laryngeal nerve (a branch of superior laryngeal nerve).

   The function of cricothyroid is mainly tension of the vocal cord. In addition it is also believed to be a week adductor of vocal cord.

   Hence in the case of recurrent laryngeal nerve palsy, all the muscles of the larynx are paralysed except the cricothyroid muscle.

4. **a. Stratified squamous**

   The vocal fold or true cord is made up of mucosa and muscles. The mucosa is further made up of epithelium and lamina propria. The epithelium is of stratified squamous type.

   If cross section of vocal cord is seen, it consists of four layers. They are:

   1. The deepest layer or skeleton of vocal cord is formed by the vocalis muscle which are the fibres of thyroarytenoid muscles.
   2. Around the muscles is the vocal ligaments formed by intermediate and deep layers of lamina propria.
   3. Superficial to this is the Reinke's space which is formed by superficial layer of lamina propria and is filled with loose fibrous substance and finally.
   4. The epithelial covering of stratified squamous epithelium.

   As mentioned above, the epithelium of vocal cord is stratified squamous. During voice production, waves are formed in this epithelium.

   This wave pattern of the squamous epithelium of vocal cord can be examined on ***video strobolaryngoscopy.***

5. **b. Lower border of T4**

   The dividing point of trachea called carina is between T4 and T5.

   If this not in the choice then the acceptable answer is either lower border of T4 or upper border of T5.

6. **b. 3rd arch**

   This is a very tricky question and students often get it wrong.

   It is well known that larynx develops from the fusion of 4th and 6th arch.

   - Supraglottis develops from 4th arch, and
   - Subglottis develops from 6th arch.

   From this we should infer that epiglottis which is a part of supraglottic area should develop from 4th arch. ***This is NOT true.***

   The entire supraglottis develops from 4th arch ***EXCEPT epiglottis, which develops from branchial eminence which in turn develops from 3rd arch.***

   Therefore, epiglottis develops from 3rd arch and NOT 4th arch.

PART 4: LARYNX

7. **d. All**

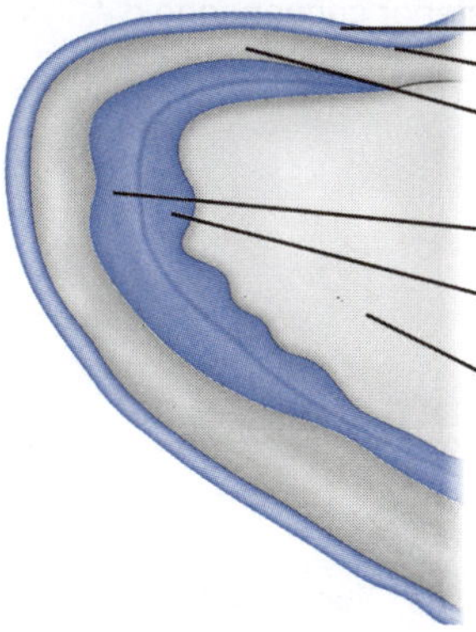

This is a cross section of vocal cord which shows Reinke's space.

- Vocal polyp arises in this space and is therefore associated with it.
- We know that larynx is mainly lined by mucosa.
- But glottis is lined by squamous epithelium
- Therefore there is transition from mucosa to squamous epithelium above the glottis. This is called upper arcuate line.
- There is transition from squamous epithelium to mucosa, below the glottis. This is called lower arcuate line.
- Glottis and therefore Reinke's space lie between the two arcuate lines.

8. **a. Thyroepiglotticus**

Inlet of larynx is the entry point of larynx. The boundaries of laryngeal inlet are:

	Boundries of inlet of larynx
• **Anteriorly**	Epiglottis
• **Sides/laterally**	Aryepiglottic fold having thyroepiglottic muscles
• **Posteriorly**	Mucosa between the arytenoids

Thyroepiglottic in the aryepiglottic folds open the inlet of larynx.

9. **c. High larynx**

Infantile larynx as compared to adults is located much higher. It is located at the level of C_2 and $C_{3.}$
Hence, air from nasopharynx can enter directly into the larynx bypassing the oropharynx.
In adults the air has to pass through the oropharynx into the larynx.
Because of this special anatomy in infants, this infant can breathe while swallowing.

10. **b. Epiglottis**

All the cartilages of larynx are made of hyaline cartilage except epiglottis, which is made of elastic cartilage.
Note: The anterior process of arytenoids to which the vocal fold are attached, are also made of elastic cartilage.

11. **c. Parapharyngeal abscess**

Laryngeal crepitus is crepitus is a normal finding caused due to friction between laryngeal cartilages against the vertebra.
This crepitus is absent swellings of any form between the larynx and vertebra. Parapharyngeal abscess is NOT in this area.

12. **a. Cricothyroid**

Rest of the mentioned muscles are extrinsic muscles of the larynx.

13. **b. Infrahyoid epiglottis**

14. **a. Posterior cricoarytenoids**

Posterior cricoarytenoid help in opening of the glottis (it is an abductor) rather than closing it.

Adductors of larynx (opens glottis)	Abductors (closes glottis)
• Lateral cricoarytenoid • Interarytenoid • Thyroarytenoid (lateral fibres), and • Cricothyroid	• Posterior cricoarytenoid

15. **d. All**

16. **d. Sternohyoid**

FUNCTIONS OF MUSCLES

Elevators of larynx	Depressors of larynx
Primary elevators • Stylopharyngeus • Salpingopharyngeus • Palatopharyngeus • Thyrohyoid	• Sternohyoid • Sternothyroid • Omohyoid
Secondary elevators • Mylohyoid • Digastric • Stylohyoid • Geniohyoid	

17. **d. Sternohyoid**

Please refer to the table given in the previous answer.

18. **a. Larynx**

SPACES IN LARYNX

There are two spaces in larynx.

1. Preepiglottic space. It is also called *Space of Boyer.*
2. Paraglottic space. It is also called *Space of Tucker.*

Space of Boyer/preepiglottic space	Boundaries
Anteriorly	Thyrohyoid ligament and Hyoid bone
Posteriorly	Epiglottis
Superiorly	Hyoepiglottic ligament

Tucker's space/paraglottic space	Boundaries
Medially	Conus elasticus and Quadrilateral membrane
Laterally	Thyroid cartilage
Posteriorly	Mucosa of pyriform fossa

19. **a. Posterior cricoarytenoid**

Posterior cricoarytenoid is the only abductor of vocal cord allowing inspiration and expiration (breathing). Bilateral palsy of this muscle may completely block the glottis and cause severe asphyxia.

20. **c. It extends at C_4, C_5, C_6 vertebra**

Difference between infantile larynx and adult larynx

Infant larynx	Adult larynx
• It is higher up at C_{2-3} vertebrae • As a result; epiglottis is close to soft palate and the two appose against each other during suckling. Therefore, an infant can swallow as well as breathe simultaneously.	• It is lower down between C_3 to C_{6-7} vertebrae
• It is cone/funnel shaped	• It is cylindrical in shape
• Have softer cartilages	• Have harder cartilages
• The narrowest part is the sub-glottis	• The narrowest part is the glottis
• Lamina propria is not well developed	• Lamina propria is well developed

IMAGE BASED ANSWER

21. **c. Cricoid cartilage**
This is the cricoids cartilage, the lower most cartilage of larynx and also the only ring-shaped cartilage.

CHAPTER 31

Common Investigations of the Larynx

Larynx is located in the anterior part of laryngopharynx.

The most common test/investigations done here are:

1. Laryngoscopy

   Laryngoscopy can be of various types:
   - Indirect laryngoscopy
   - Direct laryngoscopy
   - Fiberoptic laryngoscopy
2. Laryngostroboscopy/videolaryngostroboscopy
3. Bronchoscopy, etc.

INDIRECT LARYNGOSCOPY

Indirect laryngoscopy is done using a mirror called indirect laryngoscopy mirror.

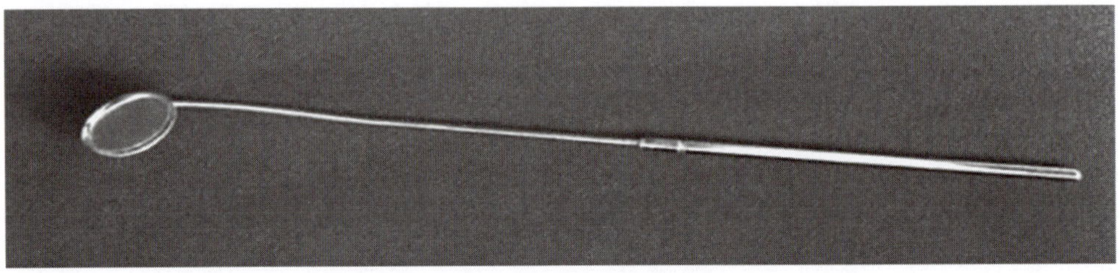

Fig. 1: Indirect laryngoscopic mirror

This mirror looks very similar to the posterior rhinoscopy mirror. Given below are the pictures of both these mirrors. You are expected to identify them by looking at pictures of these.

Indirect laryngoscopy mirror

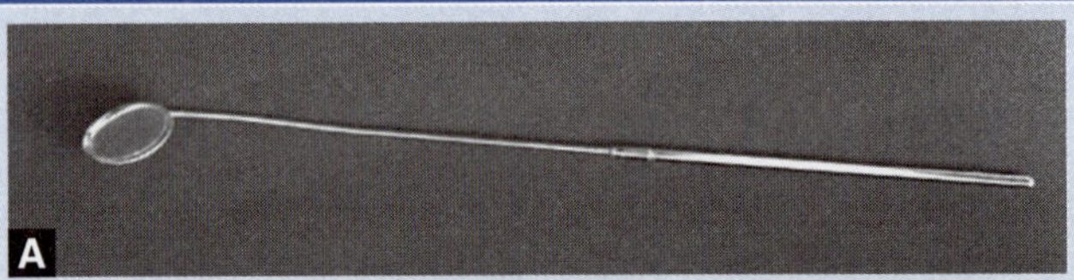

Posterior rhinoscopy mirror

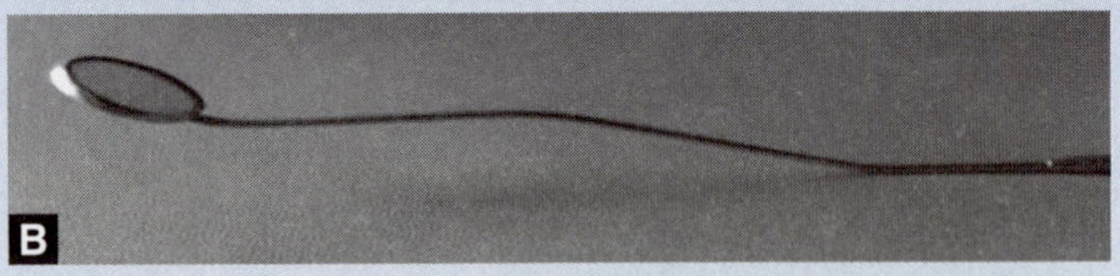

Figs 2A and B: Notice the differences between the two mirrors

Shown below is the procedure of indirect laryngoscopy.

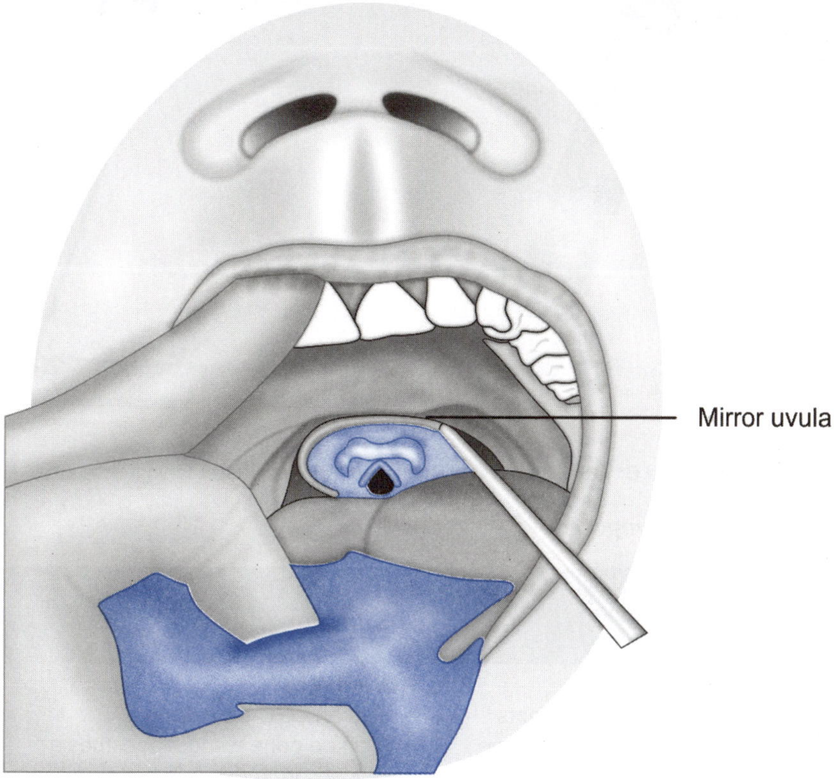

Fig. 4: Indirect laryngoscopic procedure being done'

The important structures seen during indirect laryngoscopy are:

- Base of tongue
- Vallecula
- Epiglottis
- False cords
- True cords
- Movement of the vocal folds, etc.

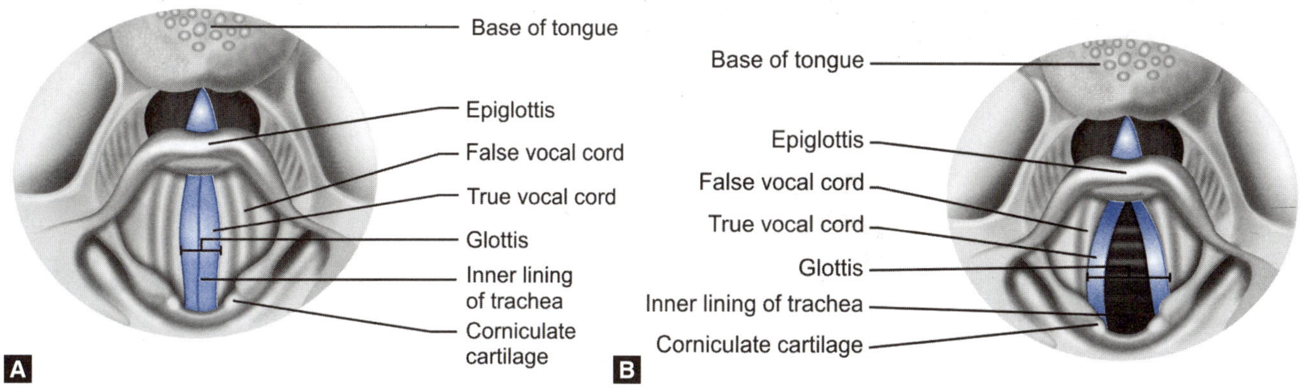

Figs 5A and B: Vocal cord structures during laryngoscopy

DIRECT LARYNGOSCOPY

During direct laryngoscopy, the patient is placed in ***Boyce-Jackson position.*** Direct laryngoscopy is done using direct laryngoscopes.

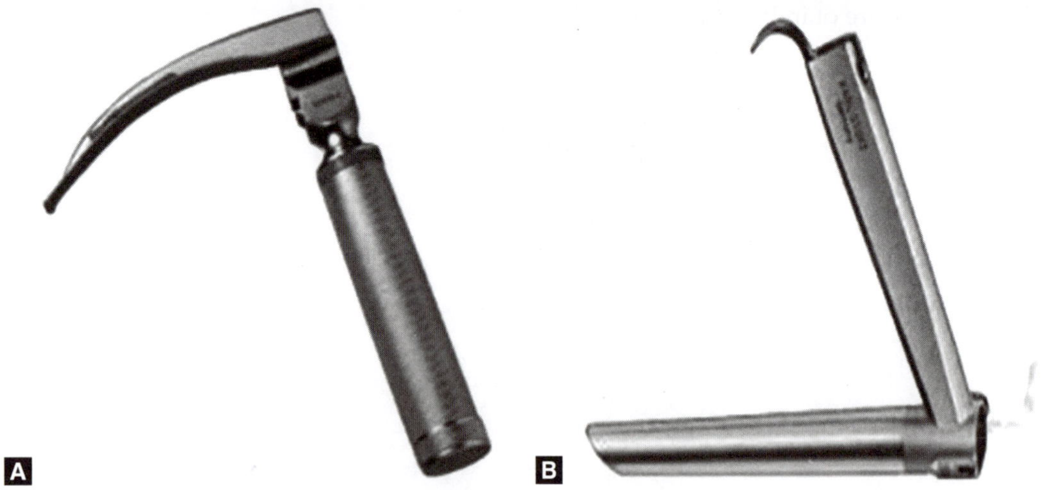

Figs. 6A and B: (A) Macintosh laryngoscope; (B) Kleinsasser laryngoscope

Advantages of direct and indirect laryngoscopy:

Direct laryngoscopy	Indirect laryngoscopy
Advantages: • Can be done in children and uncooperative patients • Procedures like biopsy and laryngogram can be done • Entire larynx can be seen including the hidden areas of larynx	**Advantages:** • It is an OPD procedure • Can be done without anesthesia • *Vocal cord mobility* is better assessed during indirect laryngoscopy

KLEINSASSER'S SELF RETAINING LARYNGOSCOPE

This laryngoscope is fixed on the chest of the patient and the doctor does not need to hold it.

In this way, both the hands of the doctor are free to perform procedures.

The self retaining laryngoscope is usually used for procedures like microlaryngeal surgery (MLS).

This laryngoscope has two parts:

Self-retaining laryngoscope		
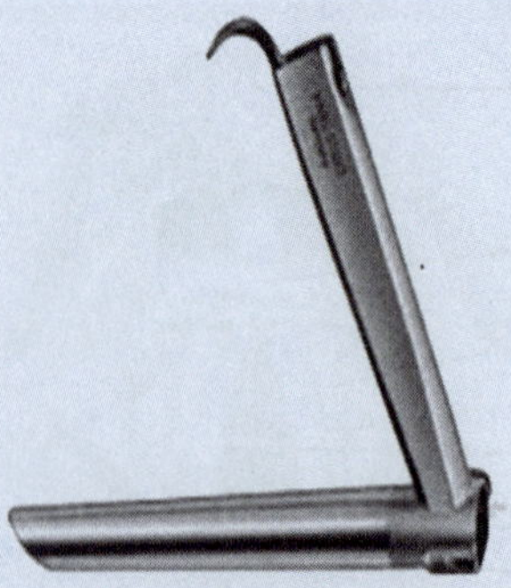 **Fig. 7:** Kleinsasser laryngoscope	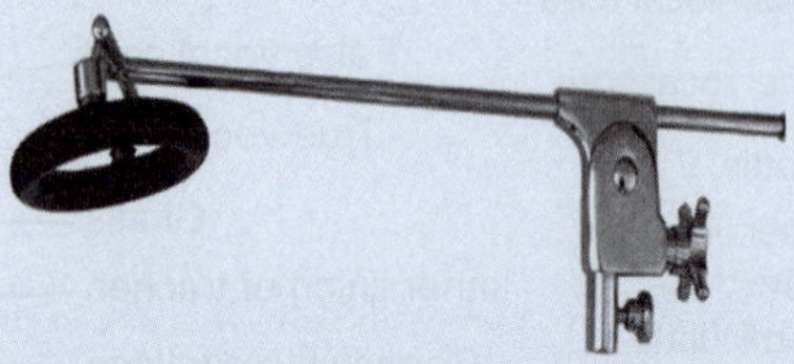 **Fig. 8:** Self-retaining stand	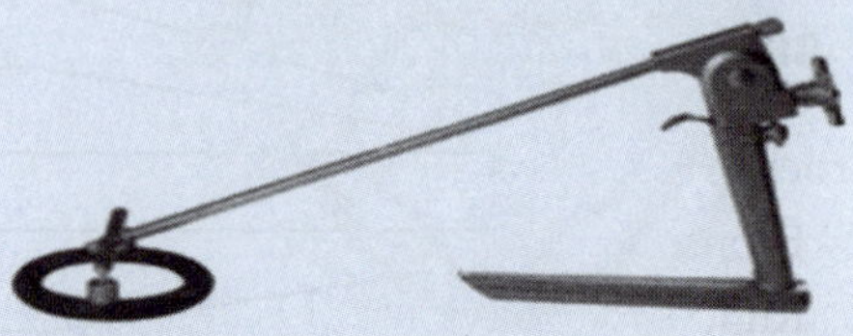 **Fig. 9:** Laryngoscope fitted onto the stand

FIBEROPTIC LARYNGOSCOPE

Fiberoptic laryngoscope is a flexible laryngoscope.

It is only used for diagnostic purpose.

The picture is given below.

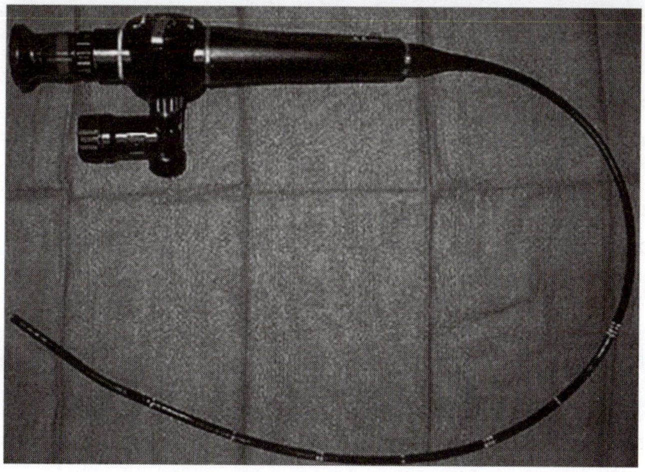

Fig. 10: Fiberoptic laryngoscope

Hidden areas of larynx are

These are areas that are seen only in direct laryngoscopy and not in indirect laryngoscopy:
- Anterior commissure
- Apex of the pyriform fossa
- Ventricle or saccule of larynx
- Laryngeal surface of infrahyoid epiglottis
- Subglottis

LARYNGOSTROBOSCOPY/VIDEOLARYNGOSTROBOSCOPY

We know that larynx vibrates at a very fast pace. The speed of vibration of larynx is approximately 100/sec.

Therefore the mucosal movement cannot be properly seen on laryngoscopy.

Laryngostroboscope is an instrument which has flashes of light. The pulse of the lightflash can be adjusted as per ones requirement.

This makes the mucosal movement appear very slow.

This therefore helps in proper examination.

It is mainly useful for examination/diagnosis of:
- ***Vocal fold mucosal movement and vocal waves***
- ***Voice disorders and***
- ***Lesions of the vocal cord.***

BRONCHOSCOPY

Brochoscopy is examination of the inside of airway.

Bronchoscopes are of two types:
1. Rigid bronchoscope
2. Flexible bronchoscope

1. Rigid bronchoscopes are being used traditionally.

   Chevalier Jackson bronchoscope is one of the earliest rigid bronchoscope.

   Note: Chevalier Jackson sign is pooling of saliva in pyriform fossa. This is seen in esophageal growths.

   One of the most common uses of rigid bronchoscopy is **removal of foreign body/debris from the bronchus.**

   In infants, rigid brochoscopy is "gold standard" for airway examination.

   During rigid bronchoscopy, patient has to lie in ***Boyce-Jackson position.***

The different options of anesthesia during rigid bronchoscopy are:

- Apneic oxygenation
- ***Jet ventilation using Sander's injection***
- ***Via side port (Racine adaptor).***

2. Flexible bronchoscopy

   Flexible bronchoscopes are very similar to flexible laryngoscope.

   They are easier to use and are very comfortable for diagnostic purposes.

   However, for foreign body removal the rigid bronchoscope is better.

Last minute revision

- Areas of larynx that cannot be seen on indirect laryngoscopy are called hidden areas of larynx
- Important hidden areas are:
  - Anterior commissure
  - Saccule
  - Apex of pyriform fossa
  - Subglottis (this is controversial)
- Kleinsasser is the father of microlaryngoscopy
- Laryngeal stroboscopy is the best investigation to see vocal fold movement and waves
- Jet ventilation is required during bronchoscopy.

QUESTIONS

1. **Flexible bronchoscopy is better than rigid in all, *except*:**
   a. Foreign body removal
   b. Bleeding
   c. Aspiration of saliva
   d. Bronchoalveolar lavage
2. **In indirect laryngoscopy, which of these is difficult to visualize:**
   a. Base of the tongue b. Pyriform fossa
   c. Glottis d. Subglottis
3. **Laryngeal mirror is warmed by placing:**
   a. Glass surface over flame
   b. Back of mirror on flame
   c. Whole mirror in boiling water
   d. Hot water on mirror
4. **Which is the best method of visualizing vocal fold movement?**
   a. Indirect laryngoscopy
   b. Direct laryngoscopy
   c. Fiberoptic laryngoscopy
   d. Video laryngostroboscopy
5. **Which of these is used during microlaryngeal surgery (MLS) of vocal cord?**
   a. Direct laryngoscope
   b. Fiberoptic laryngoscope
   c. Kleinsasser self-retaining laryngoscope
   d. Only microscope
6. **Jet ventilation is used during which of these procedures:**
   a. Flexible bronchoscopy
   b. Rigid bronchoscopy
   c. Esophagoscopy
   d. All of the above
7. **Functions of videostroboscopy include all except:**
   a. Examination of vocal fold mucosa
   b. Vocal fold anatomical defect
   c. Differentiate vocal cord cyst from vocal nodule
   d. Vocal fold biochemical disturbances
8. **In right handed person, direct laryngoscope is held in which hand.**
   a. Right hand b. Left hand
   c. Both d. either
9. **Function of videostroboscopy includes all except:**
   a. Examine vocal cord mucosa for general health
   b. Vocal fold anatomical defects
   c. Differentiate vocal cord cyst from vocal cord nodule
   d. Vocal cord biochemical disturbances
10. **The instrument shown below is used for:**

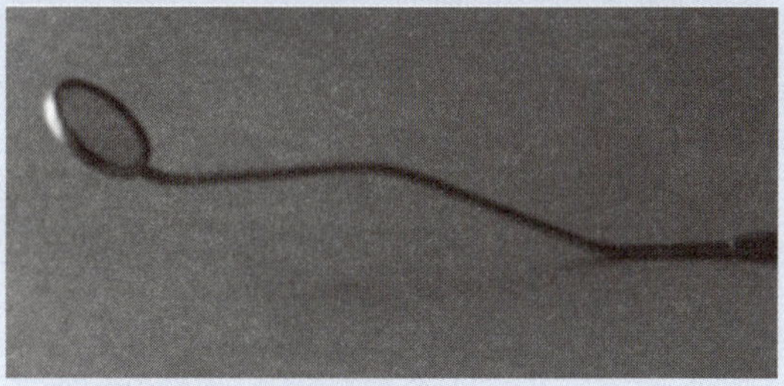

   a. Indirect laryngoscopy
   b. Direct laryngoscopy
   c. Posterior rhinoscopy
   d. Anterior rhinoscopy

ANSWERS AND EXPLANATIONS

1. **a. Foreign body removal**
   Flexible bronchoscope is a fiberoptic bronchoscope which can be easily negotiated through various brochioles and provides better magnification and illumination. It is a very handy instrument for diagnosis and treatment of chest pathologies but is mainly used for diagnosis.
   One of a very big advantage of flexible bronchoscope is that it can be passed through the endotracheal tube. However, foreign bodies of chest cannot be removed by it. For removal of foreign bodies, rigid bronchoscopy is preferred.
2. **b. Pyriform fossa.**

Advantages of Indirect Laryngoscopy Are

- It is an OPD procedure
- No anesthesia required
- Vocal cord movement is assessed better

Disadvantages of Indirect Laryngoscopy

- Laryngeal procedures cannot be done
- ***Hidden areas cannot be seen***

PART 4: LARYNX

Important Hidden Areas Are

- **Anterior commissure**
- **Undersurface of vocal cord. However *subglottis can be seen.***
- **Ventricles/saccule**
- **Apex of pyriform fossa**

3. **a. Glass surface over flame**
Laryngeal mirror is used for indirect laryngoscopy. During this procedure, the mirror has to be inserted in the mouth and oropharynx so that reflected image of the larynx can be seen in this mirror.
When the mirror is inserted in the mouth, it may get fogged by the warm air of breathe, thus blurring the image.
To avoid this, the mirror should be warmed over the flame.
We should avoid the heating of the back of mirror which may cause burning of the uvula and soft palate.
4. **d. Video laryngostroboscopy**
All the above mentioned procedures are good to visualize the vocal folds. But video laryngostroboscopy is the best method for vocal fold movement.

Laryngostroboscope

Laryngostroboscope is an instrument which has flashes of light. The pulse of the lightflash can be adjusted as per ones requirement.
This makes the mucosal movement appear very slow.
This therefore helps in proper examination.
It is mainly useful for examination/diagnosis of:

- ***Vocal fold mucosal movement and vocal fold waves***
- ***Voice disorders and voice disorders***
- ***Lesions of the vocal cord like nodule, sulcus, polyp cyst, etc.***

5. **c. Kleinsasser self-retaining laryngoscope**

Kleinsasser's Self-Retaining Laryngoscope

This laryngoscope is fixed on the chest of the patient and the doctor does not need to hold it.
In this way, both the hands of the doctor are free to perform procedures.
The self retaining laryngoscope is usually used for procedures like microlaryngeal surgery (MLS).
This laryngoscope has two parts:

Self-retaining laryngoscope

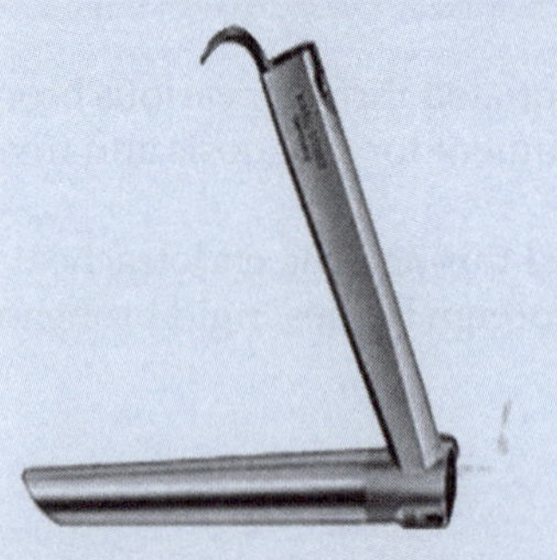
Kleinsasser laryngoscope

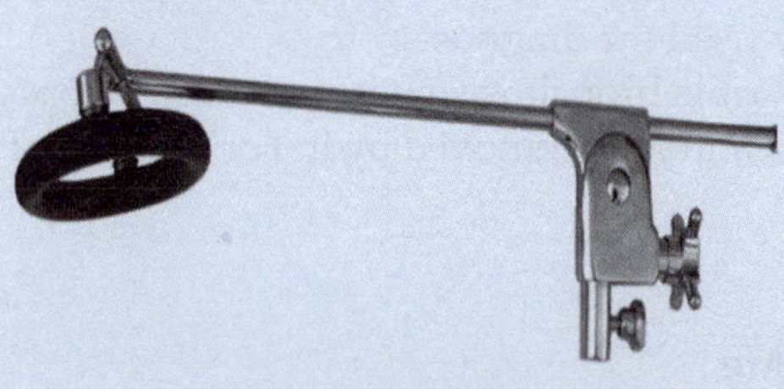
Self-retaining stand

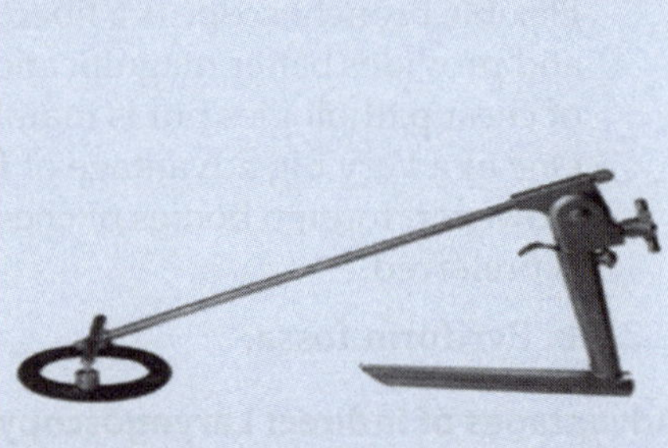
Laryngoscope fitted onto the stand

6. **b. Rigid bronchoscopy**
During rigid bronchoscopy, patient has to lie in ***Boyce-Jackson position.***
The different options of anesthesia during rigid bronchoscopy are:

- Apneic oxygenation
- ***Jet ventilation using Sander's injection***
- ***Via side port (Racine adaptor).***

7. **d. Vocal fold biochemical disturbances**
   Videostroboscopy is an investigation procedure mainly used for visualization of vocal fold wave and movement.
   Therefore it can visualize:
   - Vocal cord anatomy
   - Vocal cord anatomical defects
   - Differentiate between vocal cord lesions, etc.
     - It is not used for histopathological or biochemical examinations.
8. **b. Left hand.**
   The dominant hand has to be free so as to carry out any procedure, if required.
9. **d. Vocal cord biochemical disturbances**
   Videostroboscopy is a type of 'scopy' of the vocal cord where we just look at the cord with the help of a stroboscope.
   It is not a biochemical test.
10. **c. Posterior rhinoscopy**
    This is a picture of posterior rhinoscopic mirror. This is used to examine nasopharynx, choana and posterior part of nose.

CHAPTER 32

Inflammatory Diseases of Larynx

Inflammatory diseases of larynx can be of many types. We can classify the various laryngeal inflammatory conditions into the following types:

Flowchart 1: Inflammatory diseases of larynx

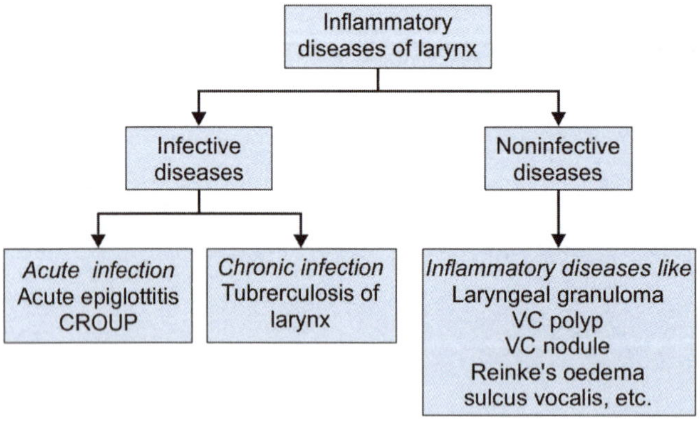

ACUTE EPIGLOTTITIS

- Acute epiglottitis also called ***supraglottic laryngitis***
- Acute epiglottitis is a sudden onset *rapidly progressive disease*
- It is more common in children between 2-7 years old
- In adults, it behaves differently.

Differences between Acute Epiglottitis of Children and Adult

Adult type	Child type
It is caused by H. influenzae type b	It is caused by Streptococcus
It is less common	It is more common
Gradually progressive	Sudden onset and rapidly progressive
Severe	Not severe
Never life threatening	May be life threatening

PRESENTATION

The main presenting features are:

- High grade fever
- Dysphagia and odynophagia with drooling of saliva
- Dyspnea/stridor.
  Stridor worsens when the patient is in supine position and relieves when the patient is sitting in **tripod position.**

Positions of patient affects stridor in the following diseases	
Laryngomalacia	Stridor worsens in supine position Stridor relieves in prone position
Acute epiglottitis	Stridor worsens in supine position Stridor relieves in tripod position
Retropharyngeal abscess	Stridor worsens in prone/sitting position Stridor relieves in supine position

When to suspect acute epiglottitis

A 4-5 years old child with fever having a triad of Ds:
- Dyspnea
- Dysphasia and
- Drooling

FINDINGS

- Laryngoscopy may show "**cherry red epiglottis**"
- X-ray may show **thumb sign.**

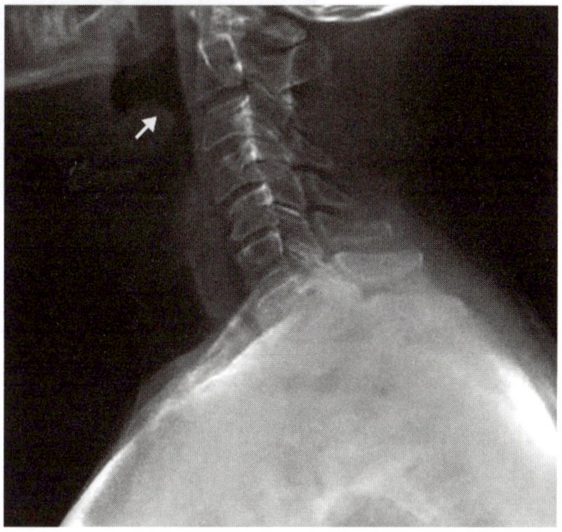

Fig. 1: X-ray showing **thumb sign** (arrow point)

Treatment

The main treatment option is medicinal:
- Higher generation cephalosporins
- Chloramphenicol and penicillin my be used.

Complication

Sudden enlargement of epiglottis may result in ***choking***.
This is the most common cause of death.
In such a situation; one of the following may be done:
- Steroids
- Intubation, in operation theater under special precautions
- Tracheostomy.

Prevention of Acute Epiglottitis

- Immunization against h. influenza type 1
- Rifampicin in non-immunizes child.

Croup

- Croup is also called **acute laryngotracheobronchitis**
- It is caused by parainfluenza virus type 1
- Croup is usually seen in children between 6 months to 3 years old.

It presents as:

- Mild fever
- Dyspnea and
- Hoarseness of voice.
  The voice of this child is described as **barking of seal**

X-ray may show **steeple sign which is also called pencil tip sign.**

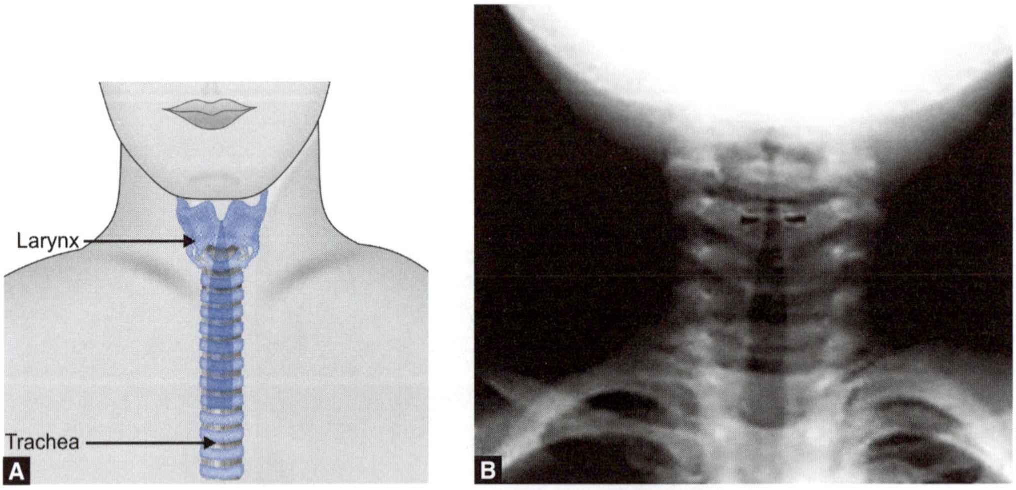

Figs 2A and B: Steeple sign

Treatment

Croup often has supra added bacterial infection, hence the most important drug is

- Ampicillin

In life threatening situation, the following may be done:

- Steroids
- Nebulized epinephrine
- Humidified oxygen
- Intubation, in operation theater under special precautions
- Tracheostomy.

Differences between Acute Epiglottitis and Croup

	Acute epiglottitis	Croup
Organism	*H. influenza type 1*	*Parainfluenza virus type 1*
Age	2–7 years	6 months–3 years
Fever	High grade	Low grade
Presentation	Stridor and odynophagia with drooling of saliva. Epiglottis is described as: • ***Cheery red, or*** • ***Rising sun sign***	Stridor with voice change which is described as: • ***Barking of seal***

	Acute epiglottitis	Croup
X-ray	Thumb sign 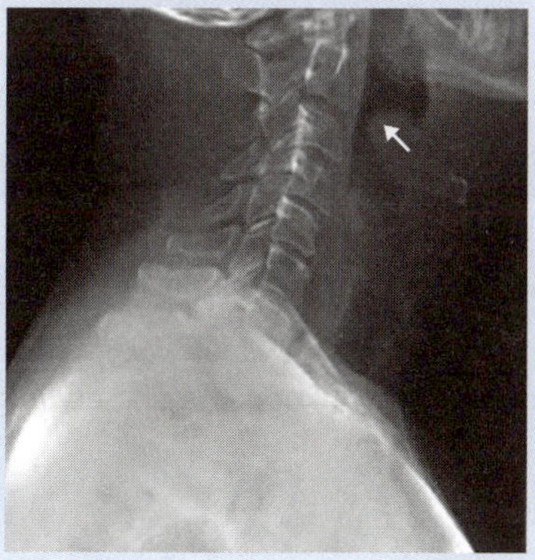	Steeple sign Pencil tip sign 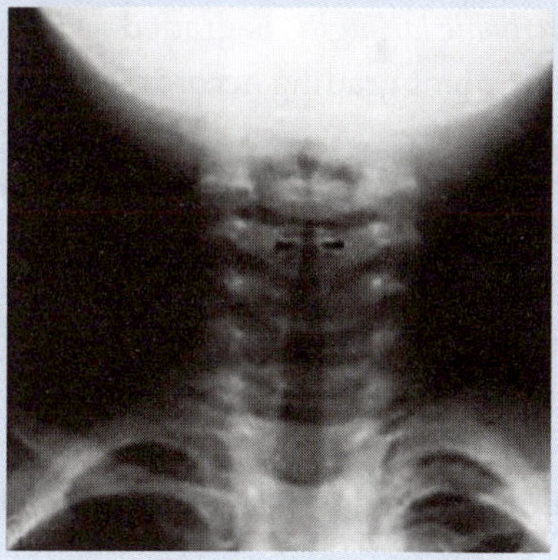

LARYNGOCELE

Laryngocele is ballooning or dilatation of saccule or ventricle which is filled by air or fluid or both.

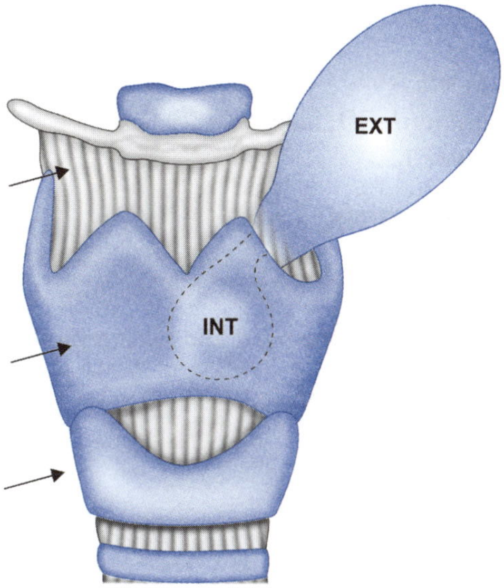

Fig. 3: X-ray showing **steeple sign**

It is commonly seen in *trumpet player, glass blower, etc.*
It may be of three types:

1. ***Internal laryngocele-*** is confined within the thyroid cartilage
2. ***External laryngocele-*** bulges out of the ***thyrohyoid membrane***
3. ***Mixed laryngocele-*** is partly inside and partly outside.

Bryce sign- on moving the laryngocele, it produces gurgling sound.
It is more commonly seen in external laryngocele.
X-ray- in this case X-ray is taken while performing **valsalvae maneuver.**
Ultra sound is the most useful investigation.

Treatment

- Surgical excision
- Marsupialisation.

CHRONIC LARYNGITIS

Chronic laryngitis can be divided into two main types:

- Hyperaemic laryngitis
- Hypertrophic laryngitis.

Hypertrophic laryngitis is graded as shown below:

1. Four point grading according to gross examination.

Four point grading on laryngoscopy	
Grade I	Mild erythema and piling of inter-arytenoid mucosa
Grade II	Diffuse oedema and mucosal thickening, with little erythema
Grade III	Diffuse erythema, with granular friable mucosa or ulceration
Grade IV	Discrete granuloma with/without oedema and erythema

Histological Grades of Hypertrophic Laryngitis

Grade I	Thickened epithelium and hyperkeratosis
Grade II	Limited disorganization of maturation process, cellular atypia, abnormal mitoses
Grade III	Severe dysplasia, also called Ca in situ

Treatment

Treatment of *keratosis of larynx and Ca in situ is*

- ***Decortication/stripping of vocal cord with CO_2 laser***

This surgery is also called ***cordectomy type 1.***

IMPORTANT TYPES OF CHRONIC LARYNGITIS

Tuberculosis of Larynx

Tuberculosis of larynx is the most common site in the head and neck region.

It is usually secondary to the tuberculosis of lungs.

The most commonly affected part is:

- ***Posterior part of glottis or***
- ***Posterior commissure or***
- ***Interarytenoids area.***

Presentation

Patient has pain in the throat with dysphonia.

Note: ***Please recall that tuberculosis of ear is painless whereas tuberculosis of larynx is painful.***

On examination, there is red granulation in the inter arytenoid area with oedema and ulceration.

There are three important features of tuberculosis of larynx. These are:

- ***Turban epiglottis.*** This is ***Pseudoedema of epiglottis***
- ***Mouse nibbled appearance***
- ***Cobble stone appearance.***

Sometimes ***adduction movement of vocal cord is compromised.***

Biopsy may be done for confirmation.

Treatment is anti tubercular therapy.

LARYNGOPHARYNGEAL REFLEX DISEASE (LPR)

Laryngopharyngeal reflex disease is similar to GERD.

In this condition, the oesophageal contents reflex into the larynx.

This juice contains acid and activated pepsin, a proteolytic enzyme needed to digest food in the stomach.
If the reflex of this juice into the larynx is long term, it may lead to a number of chronic inflammatory diseases like:

- Reinke's oedema
- Vocal cord nodule
- Vocal cord polyp
- ***Pseudosulcus laryngitis***
- ***Sulcus glottidis, etc.***

Treatment

- Treatment is similar to GERD. Patient is given proton pump inhibitors'
- Patient has to quit smoking
- Surgery may be required in some cases.

REINKE'S OEDEMA

It is also called ***polypoid degeneration of vocal folds.***
As the name suggests, there is oedema of the Reinke's space.
It is caused due to:

- Smoking and
- Talkative females
- Voice abuse
- Hypothyroidism.

Presentation

- Dysphonia is the main complaint
- On examination there is ***uniform and diffuse swelling of the membranous vocal cord***
- This looks of the vocal cord is described as "***Water balloon cords***".

Treatment

- Stop smoking and vocal abuse
- Surgical aspiration of fluid and excision of mucosa
- This procedure is called ***reduction glottoplasty.***

CONTACT ULCERS/ PACHYDERMA LARYNGITIS

Contact ulcer has many names. Some of the common names are:

- ***Intubation granuloma***
- ***Pachyderma laryngitis***

The main contributing factors are:

- Chronic irritation of larynx
- Smoking
- GERD.

It is formed mainly due to *misuse of voice* in which to two vocal cords hammer each other during speech.
The other contributing factors is *GERD.*
It involves the arytenoids (post. 1/3 of glottis), which has ***ulcer and granulation (heaping of epithelium)***.
Hoarseness of voice is the main complaint.
Microscopy may show *hyperkeratotic lesion in the posterior commissure.*

Biopsy

- From the ulcerative area may be *normal (there are* ***no*** *ulcerative changes)*
- From the pachyderma area may show hyperkeratosis.

Hence contact ulcer is **not a true ulcer;** it is a **false ulcer.**

Treatment

- *Speech therapy*
- *Treatment of GERD*
- *Stop smoking*
- ***Botulinum toxoid in thyroarytenoid muscles***
- ***Laser vaporization.***

VOCAL CORD NODULE

It is also called ***singer's nodule/teacher's nodule/screemer's nodule***

Vocal cord has two parts:

1. ***Membranous part. It is the anterior 2/3 of the vocal cord, and***
2. ***Cartilaginous part. It is posterior 1/3 of the vocal cord.***

The cartilaginous is part is formed by ***vocal process of arytenoids.***

During speech, the maximum vibration is seen in the *centre of membranous vocal cord*. This is also the junction of ***anterior 1/3 and posterior 2/3 of vocal cord.***

Hence, this is the most common site of vocal cord nodule.

During chronic misuse of voice, this point vibrates with maximum amplitude.

Hence, this point has traumatic edema and bleed.

This then gets re-organized and fibrosed and hyalinized.

Therefore, vocal cord nodule is ***re-organized fibrotic/hyalinized tissue.***

Sequence that leads to vocal cord formation
Chronic misuse of voice ↓
Trauma and oedema of superior lamina propria ↓
Reorganization ↓
Hyalinization of superior lamina propria ↓
Nodule formation

Presentation

- Hoarseness of voice
- It is bilateral
- This gives ***hour glass appearance.***

Treatment

- ***Voice rest is the treatment of choice***
- Microlaryngeal surgery is second line of treatment
- Steroids may be added
- Botox injections are an alternative.

MICROLARYNGEAL SURGERY

- It is the surgery of larynx under microscopic vision
- The microscope used is the same as used during microscopic ear surgeries
- The difference between the two is the difference in focal length of the lens used in the microscope
- During microlaryngeal surgery (MLS), patient is placed in ***Boyce-Jackson position.***

Note: During tonsillectomy patient is placed in ***Rose position.***

The focal length of the microscope used during MLS is ***400 mm.***

Focal lengths of lens used are	
• *Ear surgery*	*200-250 mm*
• *Nose surgery*	*300 mm*
• *Throat surgery*	*400 mm*

VOCAL CORD POLYP

- Vocal cord polyp is hypertrophic tissue which can be seen anywhere on the ***membranous part of vocal cord***
- But most commonly it is seen at the junction of ***anterior 1/3 and posterior 2/3 of vocal cord***
- They usually have:
  - Hemorrhagic polyp, and
  - Non-hemorrhagic polyp.

Sequence that leads to formation of vocal cord polyp
Voice abuse and shearing forces ↓
Rapture of capillaries in the submucosal region ↓ Accumulation of blood (hematoma formation) ↓
Inflammatory cell infiltration ↓
New matrix formation ↓
Vocal cord polyp formation

Presentation

- Voice change
- Breathing problems
- It is unilateral.

Treatment

- Voice rest
- Treat LPR (proton pump inhibitors are given)
- Stop **anticoagulants**
- **MLS (microlaryngeal surgery) is the treatment of choice**
- Pulse dye laser is used for small polyps.

Differences between Vocal Cord Nodule and Vocal Cord Polyp

Vocal cord nodule	Vocal cord polyp
Caused due to **chronic misuse of voice**	This is caused by smoking and phonotrauma
Is reorganized and hyalinized fibrotic tissue	Is hypertrophic and haemorrhagic tissue
At junction of anterior 1/3 and posterior 2/3 of cord	Anywhere on membranous cord
Is bilateral	Usually is unilateral
Main presentation: • *Voice change* • *Finding is "**hour glass glottis**"*	Main complaint: • *Voice change* • *Respiratory difficulty* • *Diplophonia, etc.*
Treatment is: ***Voice rest followed by speech therapy.*** ***Microlaryngeal surgery (MLS)*** may be required	The main treatment is: ***Microlaryngeal surgery (MLS.) and quit smoking and stop anticoagulant***

SULCUS VOCALIS

In this condition there is ***invagination of the mucosa of vocal cord causing a groove or sulcus on the edge of the vocal fold along with degeneration of the superficial layer of lamina propria.***
Sulcus vocalis can be divided into three types:

Type I (superficial type)
Type IIa (sulcus vergeture)
Type IIb (true sulcus)

Sulcus vocalis should not be confused with ***pseudosulcus laryngitis.***

Pseudosulcus laryngitis is oedema of the subglottis caused by laryngopharyngeal reflex (LPR).

The Parts of Larynx Involved in Different Diseases

Disease	Parts involved
Tuberculosis	Posterior commissure
Contact ulcers	Posterior commissure
Intubation granuloma or pachyderma laryngitis	Posterior commissure and posterior 1/3 of vocal cord
Vocal nodules	Junction of anterior 1/3 and posterior 2/3
Vocal polyp	Anywhere on the membranous part of cord. But more commonly at the junction of ant. 1/3 and post. 2/3

Last minute revision

- *In India, epiglottis is caused by H. influenzae*
- *X-ray of epiglottitis showns thumb sign and patient sits in tripod position*
- *Croup is called laryngotracheobronchitis and is caused by Parainfluenza virus*
- *X-ray of croup has steeple sign/pencil tip sign*
- *Tuberculosis of larynx is painful and affects posterior part of larynx*
- *Reinke's oedema is seen in talkative and smoking females. It has water balloon cords*
- *Pachyderma laryngitis affects posterior part. It can be caused by intubation and laryngopharyngeal reflex*
- *Vocal cord nodule is called singer's nodule and affect the junction of anterior 1/3 and posterior 2/3*
- *Voice rest is the initial treatment of vocal nodule*
- *Vocal cord polyps best treated by microlaryngeal surgery (MLS)*
- *The focal length of microscope during MLS is 400 mm*
- *Laryngocele can be internal, external or mixed type and Bryce sign is positive.*

QUESTIONS

1. **Reinke's edema is:**
   a. Oedema of the uvula
   b. Oedema of the free margin of the vocal cord
   c. Oedema of the ventricular band
   d. Cyst of the ventricle of the larynx
2 **Laryngocele arises as a herniation of laryngeal mucosa through the following membrane:**
   a. Thyrohyoid b. Cricothyroid
   c. Cricotracheal d. Cricosternal
3. **A laryngocele arises from the:**
   a. True vocal cord
   b. Subglottis
   c. Saccule for the ventricle
   d. Anterior commissure
4. **A woman singer with singer's nodes and with h/o reflux. The best treatment is:**
   a. Voice therapy and PPI
   b. Laryngomicroscopic excision
   c. Laser excision
   d. Vocal cord stripping
5. **Most common site of vocal nodule is:**
   a. Anterior l/3rd
   b. Middle l/3rd
   c. Posterior 1/3rd
   d. Junction of anterior and middle 1/3 rd
6. **Most common cause of acute epiglottitis:**
   a. H. Influenzae b. Pneumococcus
   c. Pseudomonas d. Staphylococcus
7. **'Steeple sign' on AP radiograph is seen in:**
   a. Laryngotracheobronchitis
   b. Epiglottitis
   c. Retrobulbar abscess
   d. Laryngeal diphtheria
8. **Most common site involved in tuberculosis of larynx is:**
   a. Anterior commissure
   b. Posterior commissure
   c. Ventricular bands
   d. Vocal cords
9. **Most common age involved in tuberculosis of larynx:**
   a. 1-10 years b. 10-20 years
   c. 20-40 years d. > 40 years
10. **The antibiotic of choice in acute epiglottitis pending culture sensitivity report is:**
    a. Erythromycin b. Rolitetracycline
    c. Doxycycline d. Ampicillin
11. **Fatality in acute epiglottitis is due to:**
    a. Respiratory obstruction due to oedema
    b. Septicemia
    c. Severe haemorrhage
    d. Laryngeal paralysis
12. **Statement not true about acute epiglottitis in children is:**
    a. Rising sun sign positive
    b. Usually caused by pseudomonas
    c. Presents as dyspnoea
    d. May need tracheostomy, if there is respiratory distress
13. **Which is the preferred method of securing airway in a patient with laryngotracheobronchitis?**
    a. Nasal intubation
    b. Endotracheal intubation
    c. Tracheostomy d. Any of the above
14. **A female Mamta 26 years old presented with gradually increasing respiratory distress since 4 days. She gives h/o hospitalisation and mechanical ventilation with orotracheal intubation for 2 weeks. Now she is diagnosed of having severe tracheal stenosis. What would be the next line of management?**
    a. Laser excision and stent insertion
    b. Steroids
    c. Tracheal dilation
    d. Tracheal resection and end to end anastomosis
15. **The cause for contact ulcer in vocal cords is:**
    a. Voice abuse b. TB
    c. Smoking d. Malignancy
16. **All of the following conditions affect posterior part of Larynx *except:***
    a. Tuberculosis larynx b. Pachydermia laryngis
    c. Intubation granuloma
    d. Lupus larynx
17. **Patient following peanut consumption presented with laryngeal oedema, stridor, hoarseness of voice and swelling of tongue. Most likely diagnosis is:**
    a. Angioneurotic oedema
    b. Pharyngeal abscess
    c. Foreign body of larynx
    d. Foreign body of bronchus
18. **True of laryngitis sicca:**
    a. Caused by klebsiella ozaenae
    b. Caused by klebsiella rhinoscleromatis
    c. Antifungal is effective
    d. Microlaryngeal surgery (MLS) is the main treatment
19. **Site of involvement in pachyderma laryngitis:**
    a. Junction of anterior and middle 1/3 of the vocal cord
    b. Posterior commissure
    c. Anterior commissure
    d. Vestibular fold
20. **A child presents with biphasic stridor, barking cough and difficulty in swelling for 2-3 days. He has fever and elevated leukocyte count. All are true, *except:***
    a. Subglottic stenosis and hypopharyngeal dilation may be seen on X-ray
    b. Boys are more commonly involved than girls
    c. Symptoms are predominantly caused by involvement of supraglottis
    d. Antibiotics do not have any role in treatment

21. **A patient of hoarseness was found to be having pachyderma laryngitis. All are true, *except:***
    a. It is hyperkeratotic lesion present within anterior 2/3 of the vocal cord
    b. It is not a premalignant condition
    c. Diagnosis is made by biopsy
    d. On microscopy, it shows hyperkeratosis
22. **A middle aged male comes to the OPD with complaint of hoarseness of voice for the past 2 months. He has been a chronic smoker for 30 years. On examination, a reddish area of mucosal irregularity overlying a portion of both vocal cord seen. Management would include all *except:***
    a. Cessation of smoking
    b. Radiotherapy
    c. Biopsy
    d. Regular follow-up
23. **A 3.5 years old fully immunized child develops sore throat, dysphagia, fever and stridor in quick succession. Within 2 hours of onset of symptoms the child was sick, pale and looked terrified. An hour later the child became quite and floppy and then expired after one hour. The most likely diagnosis was:**
    a. Croup
    b. Acute epiglottitis
    c. Laryngeal diphtheria
    d. Foreign body aspiration
24. **Which of the following conditions is considered to be definitely precancerous in larynx?**
    a. Pachyderma laryngitis
    b. Laryngitis sicca
    c. Scleroma of larynx
    d. Laryngeal leukoplakia
25. **Pseudosulcus of larynx is due to:**
    a. Vocal abuse
    b. Tuberculosis of larynx
    c. Laryngopharyngeal reflex (LPR)
    d. Chronic steroid use
26. **Treatment of early vocal cord nodule is:**
    a. Radical excision
    b. Microlaryngeal surgery (MLS)
    c. Cryotherapy
    d. Voice rest and speech therapy
27. **A shopkeeper had a verbal quarrel with one of his customer a month ago. Following which the shopkeeper has hoarseness of voice. The latyngoscopic finding is shown in the picture. Which of the following is true:**

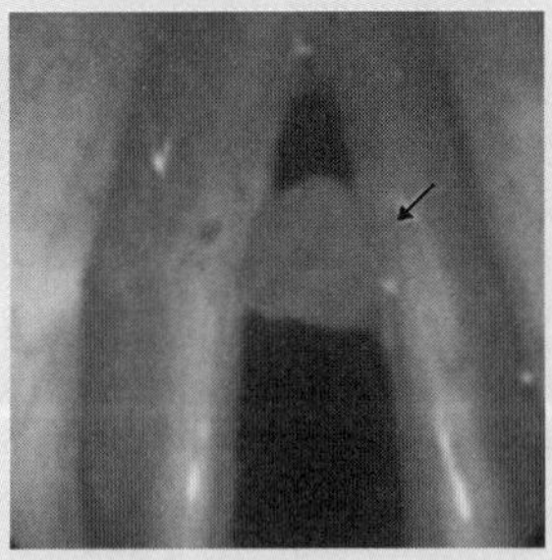

    a. This is a case of vocal cord nodule
    b. Voice rest is the first line of treatment
    c. Microlaryngeal surgery (MLS) is the treatment of choice
    d. This is a pre malignant condition of the larynx
28. **A patient presented with hoarseness of voice for the past few weeks. There is no history of smoking. Laryngoscopy finding is shown in the picture. Which of the following is true?**

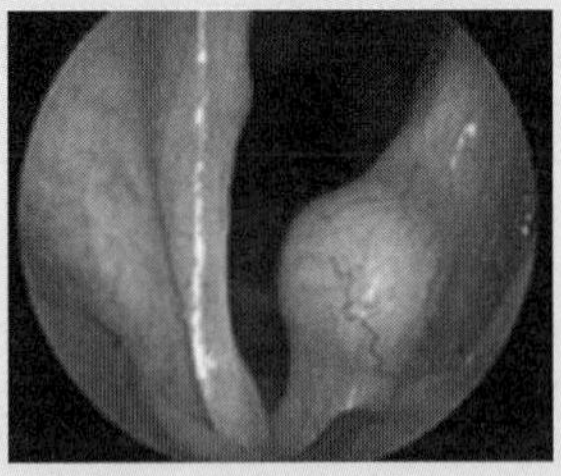

    a. This could be a case of carcinoma larynx
    b. This is a case of vocal polyp
    c. This is a case of vocal cyst
    d. This a case of laryngocele
29. **In this X-ray of lateral view of soft tissue neck (STN), the arrow shows ?**

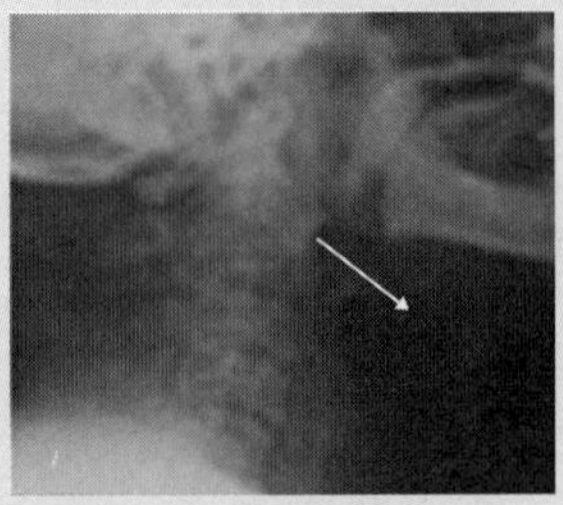

    a. Thumb sign of epiglottitis
    b. Thumb sign of croup
    c. Steeple sign of epiglottitis
    d. Steeple sign of croup

ANSWERS AND EXPLANATIONS

1. **b. Oedema of the free margin of the vocal cord**
   It is also called ***polypoid degeneration of vocal folds.***
   If cross-section of vocal cord is seen, it consists of four layers. They are:
   1. The deepest layer or skeleton of vocal cord is formed by the vocalis muscle which are the fibres of thyroarytenoid muscles.
   2. Around the muscles is the vocal ligaments formed by intermediate and deep layers of lamina propria.
   3. Superficial to this is the Reinke's space which is formed by superficial layer of lamina propria and is filled with loose fibrous substance and finally.
   4. Epithelial covering of stratified squamous epithelium.

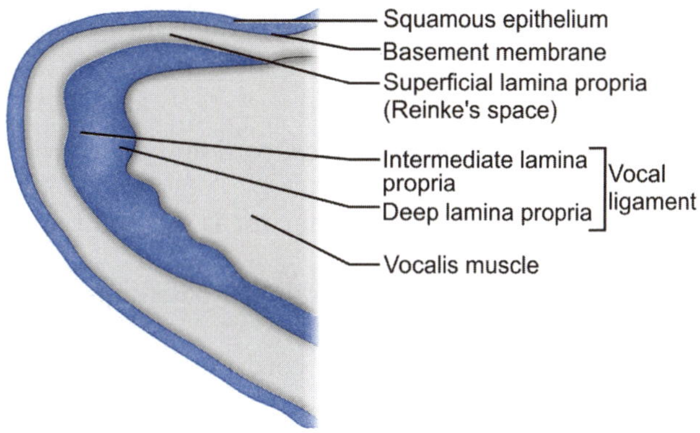

Layers of vocal cord

Reinke's edema is the edema of the Reinke's space just below the squamous epithelium of vocal cord.

PRESENTATION OF REINKE'S OEDEMA

- Dysphonia is the main complaint
- On examination there is ***uniform and diffuse swelling of the membranous vocal cord***
- This look of the vocal cord is described as ***water balloon cords:***
  - Oedema of uvula may be seen in ***Quincke's disease***
  - ***Cyst of the ventricle may be seen in laryngocoele.***

2. **a. Thyrohyoid**
3. **c. Saccule for the ventricle**
   Laryngocele is ***herniation of laryngeal saccule or ventricle of morgagni.***
   Laryngocele is herniation of saccule of larynx seen in people who has increased intraglottic pressure for long time (Like glassblower, wind instrument players, etc.).

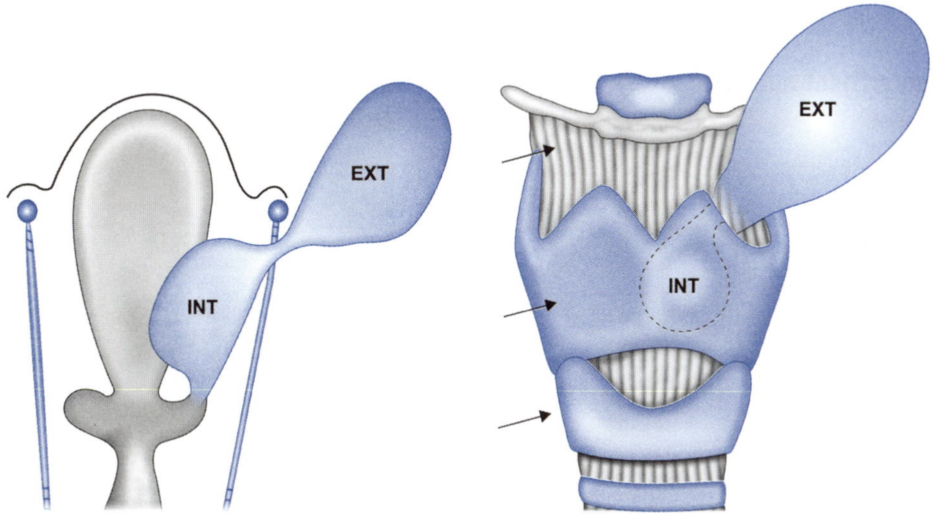

Diagrams showing laryngocele

PART 4: LARYNX

They are divided into three types:
1. Internal
2. External and
3. Combined or mixed.

External laryngocele is the one which herniates through the thyrohyoid membrane.
Bryce sign is a feature of external laryngocele.

4. **a. Voice therapy and PPI.**
Singer's nodule also called vocal cord nodule and is usually due to chronic misuse of voice which is compounded by gastric reflex (LPR).
Therefore the treatment is mainly voice therapy. If the patient has reflex then PPI should be added:
- Microscopic laryngeal excision is the second line of management, if the primary treatment fails.
- Laser excision is usually done for tumorous growths. Even if it is done, it is NOT the first line of treatment.
- Vocal cord stripping also called Type I cordectomy is done for ***carcinoma in situ of the vocal cord or T1 tumour of vocal cord.***

5. **d. Junction of anterior and middle 1/3rd**
Vocal cord nodules are formed due to misuse of vocal cord and hence will be seen at the point of maximum vibration of the vocal cords.
The junction of anterior 1/3 and middle 1//3 of vocal cord is the point of maximum vibration and hence the commonest site of vocal cord nodules.
It is also called singer's nodule and is usually bilateral. The patient presents as hoarseness of voice and voice rest is the treatment of choice.
Voice rest always succeeds in cases of early vocal cord nodules, but in cases of late V.C nodules, microlaryngoscopic surgery (MLS) may be required.
After the treatment, some patients may require speech therapy.

6. **a. H. Influenzae**
Some of the books claim that pneumococcus (streptococcus pneumonia) is the most common organism. Since H. influenza infections has decreased due to increased vaccination against this.
This may be true for western countries, but in India vaccination against H. influenza is still not in the national programs. Hence H. influenza Type B is still the most common organism causing acute epiglottitis.

> Traditionally, acute epiglottitis has been a manifestation of invasive Hib infection. This can be confirmed as the cause in partially treated patients by Hib antigen detection in concentrated urine specimens.
>
> *Scott-Brown's, ENT and HNS, pg 1131*

However in adults, streptococcus is the most common pathogens.

Haemophilus influenzae is the causative organism of three important ENT infections
1. Acute suppurative otitis media (ASOM) 2. Acute epiglottitis especially in children 3. Acute sinusitis

7. **a. Laryngotracheobronchitis**

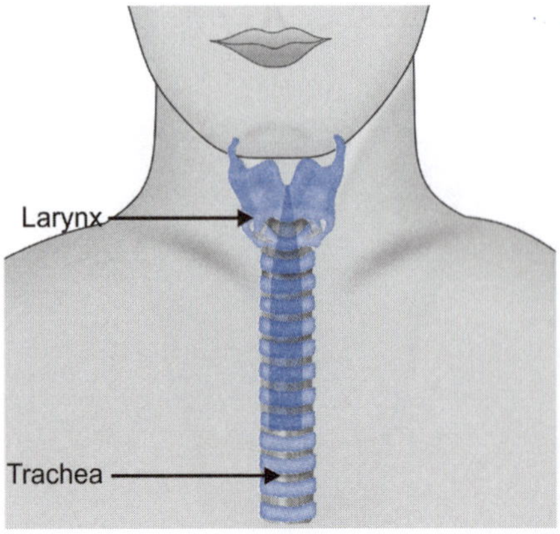

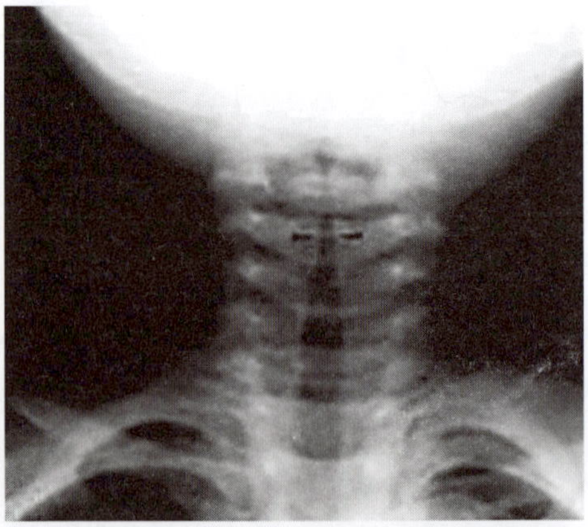

Steeple sign

Laryngotracheobronchitis also called **croup** is viral infection of trachea, larynx and bronchus.
It is caused by parainfluenza virus.
It is seen mainly in males between 6 months to 3 years old.
X-ray is diagnostic in which steeple sign is seen.
Note: the X-ray finding in epiglottitis is thumb/sore thumb sign.

8. **b. Posterior commissure**
Tuberculosis of larynx is usually secondary to the tuberculosis of lungs.
It usually involves the posterior part of larynx which is called posterior commissure in glottis.
Important features of tuberculosis of larynx are:
   - ***Turban epiglottis which is pseudoedema of epiglottis***
   - ***Cobble stone appearance***
   - ***Mouse nibbled appearance***
   - ***Adduction movement of vocal cord is compromised.***

9. **c. 20-40 years**
Most common age group involved in tuberculosis of larynx is 20-40 years. It is now increasingly seen in higher age group. It is more common in males.
Tuberculosis of larynx is usually secondary to the tuberculosis of lungs. It usually involves the posterior part of larynx which is called posterior commissure in glottis.

10. **d. Ampicillin**
The most common organism causing acute epiglottitis is haemophilus influenza. Hence the drug of choice is either ampicillin or cephalosporins.
    - ***1st line of drug is cephalosporin***
    - 2nd line of drug is ampicillin
    - Chloramphenicol is used in patients who are allergic to the above mentioned drugs
    - Immunization against Hib should be done to prevent this infection.

This disease can cause respiratory obstruction and hence the primary aim should be to maintain airway either by giving steroid, by intubation and in severe cases even tracheostomy.

11. **a. Respiratory obstruction due to oedema**
In acute epiglottitis the epiglottis gets swollen up and looks like rising sun and this is called the ***rising sun sign also called Cherry Red Epiglottis.***

Rising sun sign is seen in two diseases of ENT

- Glomus tumour in ear
- Acute epiglottitis

Due to oedema and swelling of epiglottis, the patient presents with high grade fever, dyspnea and change of voice.
Sudden edema of epiglottis may cause respiratory obstruction and may lead to death hence death is due to respiratory obstruction.
Tracheostomy may be required in some patients to save life of the patient.

12. **b. Usually caused by pseudomonas**
Acute epiglottitis is common in children between the age group of 2-7 years. It is most commonly caused by ***Hemophilus influenza type B***.
In western countries, this has been replaced by streptococcal infection due to aggressive immunization against *H. influenza:*
    - The epiglottis gets swollen up and looks like rising sun
    - Patient presents with high grade fever, dyspnea and change of voice
    - Tracheostomy may be required in some patients to save life of the patient because death is due to respiratory obstruction
    - The drug of choice is either ampicillin or cephalosporin.

Note: Rising sun sign is also a feature of glomus tumour.

13. **b. Endotracheal intubation**

Laryngotracheobronchitis is also called croup.

They are of two types:

- Viral croup. This is more common and is caused by parainfluenza virus.
- Bacterial croup. This is caused by ***staphylococcus.*** The bacterial croup is more dangerous and there is repeated sloughing of mucosa in the airway.

Therefore the airway needs to be secured in these patients:

- Nasal intubation is done only when oral intubation is not possible
- Tracheostomy is NOT a good option because trachea is also inflamed in croup
- Therefore endotracheal intubation is the preferred method for securing the airway
- The endotracheal tube has to be cleaned regularly otherwise it will get blocked.

14. **a. Laser excision and stent insertion**

Tracheal stenosis can be divided in the following ways:

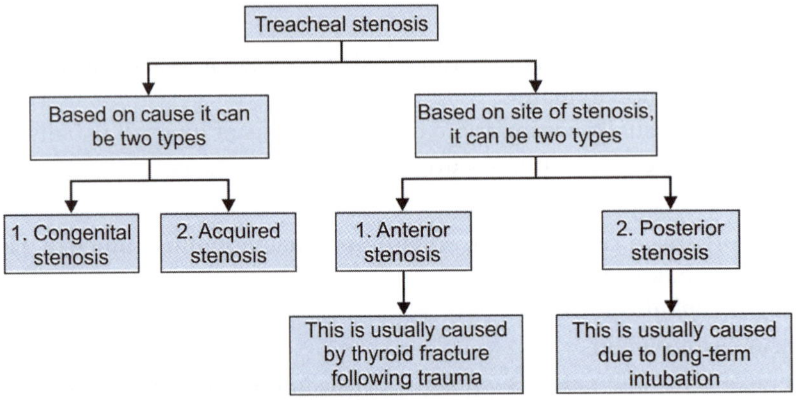

This is a case of acquired posterior stenosis.

Treatment Options for Tracheal Stenosis

- **Endoscopic laser excision** is the best option. Usually CO_2 laser is used. KTP can also be used.
- In case of anterior web a ***keel*** will have to be place for few weeks. However, NO keel needed in posterior stenosis.
- For large anterior web, repair through ***laryngofissure*** can be done
- In severe stenosis of less than 2 cm, there is an option of ***excision followed by end to end anastomosis***
- For long stenosis, tracheoplasty can be done
- Steroid alone is NOT an option. Steroid along with surgery may be useful.

15. **a. Voice abuse**

Contact ulcer has many names. Few of these names are:

- Arytenoids granuloma
- Intubation granuloma
- Contact pachyderma.

It is usually caused by mechanical trauma on the arytenoids part of the vocal cord. The common forms of trauma are:

- ***Intubation and***
- ***Voice abuse.***

This condition is aggravated in:

- Smoker and
- Laryngopharyngeal reflex (LPR).

Important Diseases Caused by Vocal Abuse

- Contact ulcers
- Vocal cord nodule
- Vocal cord polyp.

Treatment of Contact Ulcer

- Voice therapy and voice hygiene
- Stop smoking and treat LPR
- Laser vaporization of the granuloma
- Botulinum injection into the thyroarytenoid muscles, etc.

16. **d. Lupus larynx**
- Tuberculosis affects the interarytenoid area in the posterior part of larynx. The most commonly affected movement is adduction
- Pachyderma laryngitis and intubation granuloma are different names for the same disease. this affects the arytenoids part of vocal cord which is in the posterior end
- Lupus laryngitis is an indolent tuberculosis of the anterior part of larynx. It involves epiglottis and then spreads to rest of he larynx.

Diseases and the Part of Larynx Involved

Anterior part	Middle part	Posterior part
Lupus laryngitis Amyloidosis of larynx Vocal cord polyp Sarcoidosis of larynx	Vocal nodule Carcinoma larynx Vocal cyst and sulcus Vocal cord polyp	Tuberculosis Intubation granuloma or pachyderma laryngitis or contact ulcer

Note:
- Wegener's granulomatosis of larynx is most commonly seen in the ***subglottic region.*** This usually presents as subglottic stenosis
- Leprosy of larynx most commonly involves supraglottis and epiglottis
- Syphilis of larynx most commonly involves epiglottis and aryepiglottic fold.

- Wegener's granulomatosis of the gingival presents as *strawberry gingival*
- Wegener's granulomatosis of larynx presents as subglottic stenosis
- Rhinosporidiosis of nose, oral cavity, eye present as *strawberry polyp*

17. **a. Angioneurotic oedema**
- Angioneurotic oedema is rapid oedema with swelling of the deep layers of skin (dermis), subcutaneous tissue, mucosa and submucosa
- When it involves the uvula, it is called ***Quincke's disease.***

Causes or Types of Angioneurotic Oedema

- Idiopathic
- Allergic. This is most common type
- Drug induced and
- Hereditary due to deficiency of C-1 esterase inhibitor enzyme.

The above mentioned type is allergic type caused by consumption of peanut.
Rest of the conditions mentioned in the choices cannot involve such a wide area ranging from larynx to tongue.

18. **a. Caused by Klebsiella ozaenae**
- Laryngitis sicca is a condition where the laryngeal tissues become vary dry with crust formation over the surface of larynx
- It is sometime continuation of *rhinitis sicca/atrophic rhinitis*
- For this reason, this condition is also called *atrophic laryngitis.*

Causes of Laryngitis Sicca

- Klebsiella ozaenae
- Excessive dryness

- Dehydration
- Radiotherapy, etc.

Management

- The primary cause has to be treatment. In some case, antibiotic may be required
- To prevent loss of moisture, *glycerine with glucose* may be used.

19. **b. Posterior commissure**

The Parts of Larynx Involved in Different Diseases

Disease	Parts involved
Tuberculosis	Posterior commissure
Contact ulcers	Posterior commissure
Intubation granuloma or Pachyderma laryngitis	Posterior commissure and posterior 1/3 of vocal cord
Vocal nodules	Junction of anterior 1/3 and posterior 2/3
Vocal polyp	Anywhere on the membranous part of cord. But more commonly at the junction of ant. 1/3 and post. 2/3

20. **c. Symptoms are predominantly caused by involvement of supraglottis**
    - This is a classical case of **croup**
    - The alternate name of croup is *laryngotracheobronchitis*, suggesting that the sub glottis, trachea and bronchi are involved and NOT the supraglottis
    - Croup gives steeple sign on X-ray because the subglottis and trachea is involved.
21. **a. It is hyperkeratotic lesion present within anterior 2/3 of the vocal cord**
    Pachyderma laryngitis involves posterior part of larynx.

Biopsy

- From the ulcerative area may be *normal (there are **no** ulcerative changes)*
- From the pachyderma area may show hyperkeratosis
- Hence contact ulcer is **not a true ulcer;** it is a **false ulcer.**

Treatment

- *Speech therapy*
- *Treatment of GERD*
- *Stop smoking*
- ***Botulinum toxoid in thyroarytenoid muscles***
- Laser vaporization.

22. **b. Radiotherapy**
    - Since a portion of both the vocal cords are involved it is unlikely to be a malignancy
    - In malignancy, the lesion has to be continuous and NOT in portions
    - Therefore, it is likely to be a chronic laryngitis caused by smoking
    - Radiotherapy is indicated in malignancies and NOT in chronic inflammatory conditions.
23. **b. Acute epiglottis**

Croup	Has fever, stridor and voice change (barking) and NO dysphagia
Diphtheria	Unlikely in a fully immunized child
Foreign body aspiration	Will not have fever, sore throat and dysphagia

24. **d. Laryngeal leukoplakia**

Premalignant (definite) condition of throat	Risk factors for throat
• *Leukoplakia* • *Erythroplakia* • *Chronic hyperplastic candidiasis* • *Keratosis of larynx* • *Laryngeal papillomatosis, etc.*	• *Submucosal fibrosis* • *Lichen planus* • *Xeroderma pigmentosa* • *Dyskeratosis congenita*

25. **c. Laryngopharyngeal reflex (LPR)**
Laryngopharyngeal reflex (LPR) may lead to a number of chronic inflammatory diseases like:
- Reinke's oedema
- Vocal cord nodule
- Vocal cord polyp
- ***Pseudosulcus laryngitis***
- ***Sulcus glottitis, etc.***

26. **d. Voice rest and speech therapy**

Treatment of Vocal Cord Nodule

- *Voice rest and speech therapy are the treatment of choice*
- Microlaryngeal surgery is second line of treatment
- Steroids may be added
- Botox injections are an alternative.

27. **c. Microlaryngeal surgery (MLS) is the treatment of choice**
The picture is that of vocal cord polyp where MLS is the treatment of choice.
- Vocal cord nodules are very small growths and are bilateral.

Vocal cord nodule, vocal cord polyp, vocal cyst etc are NOT premalignant.

28. **c. This is a case of vocal cyst**
Laryngeal carcinoma and vocal polyp are growths on the vocal cord whereas the swelling seen in this picture is a bulge on vocal cord due to a growth in the subepithelial area. This is probably a vocal cyst.
Laryngocele is NOT a swelling in the vocal cord but is bulging of saccule of larynx.

29. **a. thumb sign of epiglottitis**
This is an X-ray showing thumb sign, which is a feature of acute epiglottitis.

CHAPTER

33 Voice and Speech Disorders

Although, the main function of larynx is protection of airway; phonation is also an important function.

Therefore, any abnormality of larynx will cause some voice problems. We are going to discuss few of these problems.

In the previous chapter, we have already discussed few of these conditions that is:

- Reinke's oedema
- Intubation granuloma
- Vocal cord nodule
- Vocal cord polyp
- Sulcus vocalis
- Pseudosulcus laryngitis etc.

In this chapter we are going to discuss the remaining conditions.

DYSPHONIA PLICA VENTRICULARIS

Dysphonia plica ventricularis is a condition where voice is produced by ***false cords/ventricular bands instead of true cord.***

Diagnostic Finding

Adduction of false cord takes before true cords.

Treatment is *speech therapy*

FUNCTIONAL APHONIA/HYSTERICAL APHONIA

It is a functional disease seen in young to middle age female

Presentation

It presents as sudden and complete loss of voice.

Laryngoscopic Finding

Vocal cords are seen in ***complete abduction.***

They do not adduct during speech, but adduct during *coughing*

Treatment

Counsel the family.

PUBERPHONIA AND ANDROPHONIA

It is also called ***mutational falsetto voice.***

Puberphonia is adult male having *high pitch or female like voice.*

Androphonia is female having male like voice

Treatment

- Puberphonia treatment:
  - Counseling
  - ***Isshiki's Thyroplasty Type III.***
  - Before the surgery, a procedure is done to know if the surgery is going to be effective. The procedure is called ***Gutzmann's technique***
- Androphonia treatment
  - ***Isshiki's Thyroplasty Type IV***

PHONASTHENIA

Phonasthenia is a condition where the laryngeal muscles are weak and get fatigued or tired very fast.

Mainly affected muscles are:

1. ***Inter arytenoid***
2. ***Thyroarytenoid***
3. ***Both the muscles involved together***

Laryngoscopic findings	
• *Elliptical glottis/spindle-shaped glottis*	• When ***thyroarytenoid muscle*** is involved
• *Triangular posterior glottis*	• When ***interarytenoid muscle*** is involved
• *Key hole glottis*	• When ***both muscles*** are involved.

Note:

- **Diamond shaped posterior glottis is seen in Cri- Du- Chat Syndrome**
- **Hour glass glottis is seen in vocal cord nodule.**
- **Water balloon vocal cords are seen in Reinke's oedema**

Treatment

- Voice rest

RHINOLALIA APERTA

Also called ***hypernasality***

Causes of hypernasality are:

1. ***Cleft palate***
2. ***Oroantral fistula***
3. ***Softpalate palsy***
4. ***Postadenoidectomy***
5. ***After UPPP***
6. ***Velopharyngeal insufficiency***

RHINOLALIA CLAUSA

It is also called ***hyponasality***

Causes of hyponasality are

1. *Nasal blockade*
2. *Nasopharyngeal blockade.*

MUSCLE TENSION DYSPHONIA (MTD)

Muscle tension dysphonia (MTD) is a condition where patient has voice disturbance without any structural or neurological pathology.

In this condition, the tension of intrinsic and extrinsic muscles is high as a result of compensation to some laryngeal pathology.

Muscle tension dysphonia has many synonymous.

- Hyperfunctional dysphonia
- Muscle misuse dysphonia
- Hyperkinetic dysphonia
- Laryngeal tension-fatigue syndrome
- Laryngeal isometric dysphonia.

SPASMODIC DYSPHONIA

Spasmodic dysphonia is also called ***laryngeal dystonia.***

This is a type of focal muscle dystonia of larynx (discussed above).

Causes

Cause is not known. But one of these may be possible cause.

- ***Idiopathic***
- ***Neurological***
- ***Psychogenic***

It can be divided into three types depending on the muscles that go into spasm.

1. Adductor spasm
2. Abductor spasm, and
3. Both spasms together.

The ***most common type is the adductor spasm.***

Treatment

Many treatment options are available for spasmodic dysphonia. Some of these are:

- Psychotherapy
- ***Injections of Botox (botulinum toxoid).***
  - In adductor spasm it is injected in vocalis muscle and thyroarytenoid muscle
  - In abductor spasm it is injected in posterior cricoarytenoid muscle.
- ***Isshiki's thyroplasty type I for abductor spasm***
- ***Isshiki's thyroplasty type II for adductor spasm***
- ***In severe cases, resection of recurrent laryngeal may benefit.***

Note: In palsy of vocal cord; type I thyroplasty is done in adductor palsy and Type II thyroplasty is done in abductor palsy (opposite of spasm).

BOGART-BACALL SYNDROME

This is a syndrome where the patient has dysphonia due to professional overuse/misuse of voice without any positive finding in larynx.

Voice rest followed by speech therapy is useful:

Last minute revision

- *Dysphonia plica ventricularis is voice production by the false cords*
- *Puberphonia is also called falsetto mutational voice*
- *Puberphonia can be treated by counselling, gutzman's technique, thyroplasty type III, etc*
- *Phonasthenia has key hole shaped glottis*
- *Rhinolalia aperta is caused by cleft palate, adenoidectomy, uvulopalatopharyngoplasty, palate palsy*
- *Rhinolalia clausa is caused by adenoid hypertrophy, nasal polyp, angiofibroma, nasal carcinoma*
- *Most common type of spasmodic dysphonia is the adductor type which has strangulated voice*
- *Spasmodic dysphonia is treated by botox injection, thyroplasty, recurrent nerve resection, etc*

QUESTIONS

1. **Androphonia can be corrected by doing:**
   a. Type 1 Thyroplasty
   b. Type 2 Thyroplasty
   c. Type 3 Thyroplasty
   d. Type 4 Thyroplasty
2. **Rhinolalia clausa is associated with all of the following *except:***
   a. Allergic rhinitis b. Palatal paralysis
   c. Adenoids d. Nasal polyps
3. **The quality of voice in a patient with gross adenoid hypertrophy is described as:**
   a. Hoarse b. Rhinolalia clausa
   c. Rhinolalia aperta d. Hot potato voice
4. **All are true of spasmodic dysphonia *except:***
   a. Local laryngeal disorder
   b. May be associated with other focal dystonias
   c. Adductor groups are having the strangulated voice while abductor type are having breathy voice
   d. Botulinum toxin is used in treatment
5. **Feature of functional aphonia:**
   a. More common in males
   b. Caused by vocal cord palsy
   c. Patient can cough
   d. Speech therapy is the treatment
6. **A 26-year-old lady comes complaining of scratchy croaky voice. Which of the following is true?**
   a. The best treatment is botulinum in cricoarytenoid
   b. Type I thyroplasty can be an option
   c. Adductor dysphonia is the cause
   d. Abductor dysphonia is the cause
7. **Key knob appearance is seen in:**
   a. Functional aphonia b. Puberphonia
   c. Phonasthenia d. V C Palsy
8. **Habitual dysphonia is characterized by A/E:**
   a. Seen in females
   b. Related to stressful event
   c. Treatment is vocal exercise and reassurance
   d. Quality of voice is constant

ANSWERS AND EXPLANATIONS

1. **d. Type 4 Thyroplasty.**
   Androphonia is a condition where females have male like or low pitch voice.
   Therefore, the pitch of voice needs to be raised.
   The pitch of voice is a function of mass and tension of the vocal cord.
   Increase in tension increases the pitch and for this the length of vocal cord has to be increased.
   Increasing the length of vocal cord is thyroplasty type IV.
2. **b. Palatal paralysis**
3. **b. Rhinolalia clausa**
   Rhinolalia clausa also called hyponasality is caused by conditions that cause blockade of nose.
   Palatal paralysis will cause velopharyngeal insufficiency and this will cause rhinolalia aperta ie hypernasality and will not cause rhinolalia clausa.
   Rest of the given choices will cause rhinolalia clausa.

Causes of hypernasality are	Causes of hyponasality are
• *Cleft palate* • *Oroantral fistula* • *Soft palate palsy* • *Post adenoidectomy* • *After UPPP* • *Velopharyngeal insufficiency*	• *Nasal blockade like:* – Nasal polyp – Rhinosinusitis – Turbinate hypertrophy – Tumours and growths • *Nasopharyngeal blockade.* – Adenoid hypertrophy – Nasopharyngeal angiofibroma – Nasopharyngeal carcinoma, etc.

4. **a. Local laryngeal disorders**
   Muscle dystonias are disease of muscles.

Dystonias can be:

Types	Examples
Focal	Spasmodic dysphonia Writer's cramp Blepharospasm Oromandibular dystonia, etc
Segmental	Cranial Axial, etc
Multifocal	More than one focal types at the same type, i.e Spasmodic dysphonia + blepharospasm
Generalized	Ambulatory Non ambulatory

Spasmodic dysphonia is a type of *focal muscle dystonia of laryngeal muscle*

Causes

- Idiopathic
- *Neurological or*
- *Psychogenic*

Therefore it is NOT a Local Problem

Important Presentation

- *In adductor type both the arytenoids are against each other causing strangulated voice*
- *In abductor type the arytenoids are far apart and the air escapes through the gap causing breathy voice*
- *In the multifocal type it may be associated with other focal problems*

Treatment

- *First line of management is injection of botulinum toxoid*
- *Second line of management is thyroplasty of larynx.*
- *Resection of recurrent laryngeal may be required.*

Note: It is a focal disease but is NOT a local disease.

5. **c. Patient can cough**
Fuctional aphonia is a psychological problem in which the patient has complete loss of voice.
It is more common in females and psychotherapy is the treatment.
Patient can cough. In fact the diagnosis is made when the patient is made to cough.
The vocal cords in this condition are in abduction position. When the patient is made to cough, the vocal cord adducts and this is diagnostic of this condition.

6. **c. Adductor dysphonia is the cause**
A lady with scratchy croaky voice is having high pitch voice due to adductor dysphonia.

Treatment of Spasmodic Dysphonia

Many treatment options are available for spasmodic dysphonia. Some of these are:

- Psychotherapy
- *Injections of Botox (botulinum toxoid).*
  - In adductor spasm it is injected in vocalis muscle and thyroarytenoid muscle
  - In abductor spasm it is injected in posterior cricoarytenoid muscle.
- *Isshiki's thyroplasty type I for abductor spasm*
- *Isshiki's thyroplasty type II for adductor spasm*
- *In severe cases, resection of recurrent laryngeal may benefit.*

7. **c. Phonasthenia**
Key knob appearance also called key-hole appearance is a feature of phonasthenia. .

8. **d. Quality of voice is constant**
Habitual dysphonia is also called functional aphonia
The voice quality is NOT constant. It changes and there is sometimes aphonia.

CHAPTER

34 Vocal Cord Palsy

Vocal cord palsy is the paralysis of the intrinsic muscles of the larynx.

We have already discussed the various intrinsic muscles of the larynx with their nerve supply and their functions. It will be helpful if you revise this before you start reading further.

NORMAL POSITIONS OF VOCAL CORD DURING VARIOUS SITUATIONS

Vocal cord position	Distance from midline	Distance between two cords	Action that causes this position
Median	Midline	0.0 mm	Phonation
Paramedian	1.5 mm	3.0 mm	Whisper
Cadaveric	3.5 mm	7.0 mm	Neutral position
Mild abduction	7.0 mm	13-14 mm	Respiration
Full abduction	9.5 mm	19 mm	Deep inspiration

POSITION OF VOCAL CORD DURING PALSY

Vocal cord positions	Diseases causing these positions
Median	Normal
Paramedian	Recurrent laryngeal nerve palsy
Cadaveric	Recurrent laryngeal nerve and superior laryngeal nerve palsy
Mild and full abduction	Adductors palsy

CAUSES OF VOCAL CORD PALSY

- *The most common cause of vocal cord palsy is* ***Idiopathic.***
- *The second most common cause is* ***Thyroidectomy surgery (Iatrogenic).***

Note: ***Usually idiopathic is not given in choices, hence thyroidectomy is the usual correct answer.***

ADDUCTOR PALSY

This is usually due to damage of the **vagus nerve** before it branches.

In this condition, both the nerves get paralyzed, i.e.

- ***Recurrent laryngeal nerve (RLN) and***
- ***Superior laryngeal nerve (SLN).***

Therefore, all the muscles of that side get paralyzed ***except interarytenoid muscle.***

This is because the interarytenoid has bilateral nerve supply so receives supply from RLN of the other side also.

Vocal Cord Position

- *Cadaveric/intermediate position or*
- *Paramedian position.*

Presentation

- *Hoarseness of voice.*
- *Aphonia in case of bilateral palsy*
- *Aspiration*

Treatment

- *Speech therapy*
- ***Medialization of vocal cord.*** Various methods of medialization are:
  - **Thyroplasty *type I.*** This is done by placing a silastic block lateral to vocal cord.
  - ***Injection of Teflon paste/collagen/fat, etc.***
- ***Arthrodesis of cricoarytenoid joint***
- ***Nerve or muscle pedicle grafting (Tucker's surgery)***
- ***Permanent Tracheostomy/Total Laryngectomy-*** for aspiration.

ABDUCTOR PALSY

This is due to **recurrent laryngeal nerve palsy (RLN Palsy).**

Left side recurrent laryngeal palsy is more common as compared the right side because the left recurrent laryngeal nerve is longer than the right nerve.

In this case, all the laryngeal muscles get paralyzed ***except cricothyroid.***

The most common cause of recurrent laryngeal nerve palsy is ***thyroidectomy.***

Uncommon cause like:

- ***Ortner's syndrome:*** In this syndrome recurrent laryngeal nerve is involved by cardiomegaly.

Position of Vocal Cord

- ***Initially paramedian position***
- ***Median or midline position may be seen later.***

Important points to remember

- *Semon's law:* ***states that, abductor fibres of vocal cord are phylogenetically newer fibres and hence gets paralysed first.*** *This causes paramedian/median* ***position due to unopposed action of adductors. Ultimately, the adductors also gets paralysed and therefore the*** *cadaveric position.*
- *Wagner and Grossman hypothesis:* ***States that recurrent laryngeal nerve does not supply the*** *cricothyroid muscles,* ***which are spared during RLN palsy. This causes*** *paramedian/median position* ***of the vocal cord.***
- ***Partial/incomplete damage of RLN causes paramedian/median position, whereas, complete damage causes cadaveric position.***
- ***Hence, bilateral partial/incomplete palsy of RLN is more dangerous than bilateral complete palsy of RLN.***
- ***The position of the vocal may also be decided by the*** *level/site of damage on the RLN.*

Presentation

- ***Voice change or hoarseness of voice.*** This may **not** be significant as **compensation** takes place by the other side vocal cord.
- Voice change is more severe in case of bilateral palsy.

- ***Stridor/dyspnoea:*** Seen only in case of ***bilateral palsy*** when both the cords are in median position. This can sometimes be life threatening.
- Therefore, it is believed that ***partial palsy of RLN is more dangerous than complete palsy.*** Partial palsy causes paramedian / median position causing dyspnoea, whereas, complete palsy causes cadaveric position.
- ***Aspiration*** *may be seen in case of* ***bilateral RLN palsy.*** However, this is not common.

Treatment

The problem with RLN palsy is that median/paramedian position may cause stridor/dyspnoea, and paramedian/ cadaveric position may cause hoarseness of voice.

Therefore

- To improve the voice, the cord has to be pulled medially.
- Whereas to relieve stridor, the cord has to be pulled laterally.
- Hence, when we try to improve one, the other gets compromised.

Voice Improvement

- ***Thyroplasty Type I***

Relieve Stridor

- ***Tracheostomy***
- ***Thyroplasty Type II***
- ***Arytenoidectomy(woodman's surgery)***
- ***Cordectomy-*** *usually by* ***CO_2 laser excision***
- ***Dennis and Kashima's procedure***
- ***Nerve grafting***
- ***Muscle pedicle grafting (Tucker's). Omohyoid or Stylohyoid muscles*** are used.

Relieve Aspiration (usually not required)

- ***Tracheostomy*** *- is a temporary method*
- ***Permanent Tracheostomy/Total Laryngectomy*** *- this is the* **gold standard treatment** *for aspiration.*
- ***Epiglottopexy***
- *Vocal cord plication.*

Superior Laryngeal Nerve Palsy (SLN Palsy)

The most common cause of SLN palsy is ***thyroidectomy.***

It is usually damaged along with RLN.

The most commonly damaged during **thyroidectomy** is the ***external laryngeal branch of superior laryngeal nerve.***

Presentation

- ***Weak voice/patient is unable to raise the pitch of voice.***
- ***Aspiration-*** in case of bilateral palsy.
  This is because the supraglottic sensory supply is by the *internal laryngeal nerve, a branch of SLN.*

Laryngoscopic Finding

- ***Askew position of glottis***
- ***Loose or flaccid cords***
- ***Flapping of cords during breathing.***

Treatment

- ***Wait for 6 months to 2 years for spontaneous recovery***
- ***Aspiration-*** same as in case of RLN Palsy.

Isshiki's Thyroplasty

Thyroplasty	What is done	Indication
Thyroplasty Type I	Medialisation	Adductor palsy (improve voice) and abductor spasm
Thyroplasty Type II	Lateralization	Abductor palsy (relieve dyspnoea) and adductor spasm
Thyroplasty Type III	Shorten/loosen	Puberphonia
Thyroplasty Type IV	Lengthen/tense	Androphonia

Last minute revision

- *Commonest causes of vocal palsy are idiopathic and thyroidectomy*
- *Adductor palsy is caused when vagus is damaged and it causes voice change and aspiration*
- *Adductor palsy is treated by medialization with injections of Teflon, collagen or thyroplasty type I*
- *Abductor palsy is caused by recurrent laryngeal nerve damage. Bilateral palsy can be life threatening*
- *It can be treated by thyroplasty type II, Woodman's surgery, Kashima's surgery, etc.*
- *Superior laryngeal nerve palsy may show askew vocal cord which is loose and hanging downward*
- *Thyroplasty are of four types*
- *Kashima's procedure (Dennis and Kashima) is useful for B/L abductor palsy.*

QUESTIONS

1. **Most common cause of vocal cord palsy is:**
   a. Bronchogenic carcinoma
   b. Tuberculosis lymph nodes
   c. Thyroidectomy
   d. Aneurysm of aorta
2. **Quality of the voice is nearly normal in:**
   a. Unilateral abductor paralysis of the vocal cord
   b. Bilateral incomplete paralysis of the vocal cords
   c. Unilateral adductor paralysis of vocal cords
   d. Bilateral abductor paralysis of the vocal cords
3. **Type I thyroplasty is for:**
   a. Vocal cord medialization
   b. Vocal cord lateralization
   c. Vocal cord shortening
   d. Vocal cord lengthening
4. **A 10-year-old boy developed hoarseness of voice following an attack of diphtheria. On examination, his Rt vocal was paralysed. The treatment of choice for paralysed vocal cord will be:**
   a. Gel foam injection of right vocal cord
   b. Fat injection of right vocal cord
   c. Thyroplasty - Type -I
   d. Wait for spontaneous recovery of vocal cord
5. **Kashima operation is done for which of these conditions?**
   a. B/L abductor vocal cord palsy
   b. B/L adductor palsy of vocal cord
   c. Cholesteatoma
   d. laryngocele
6. **Effect of bilateral recurrent laryngeal nerve damage is:**
   a. Aphonia with stridor
   b. Aphonia without stridor
   c. Stridor
   d. Depends upon level of injury
7. **Right side vocal cord palsy seen in:**
   a. Larynx-carcinoma
   b. Aortic aneurysm
   c. Mediastinal lymphadenopathy
   d. Right apical lung carcinoma
8. **Most common nerve injured during ligation of superior thyroid artery:**
   a. Recurrent laryngeal nerve
   b. Facial nerve
   c. Mandibular nerve
   d. External laryngeal nerve
9. **Most common nerve pressed by enlargement of left atrium is:**
   a. Phrenic nerve
   b. External laryngeal nerve
   c. Recurrent laryngeal nerve
   d. Sympathetic nerve
10. **On laryngoscopy, vocal cords are described in cadaveric position. This means they are:**
    a. Paralysed and abducted
    b. Paralysed and bowed
    c. Fixed
    d. None
11. **Following total thyroidectomy, the patient develops respiratory stridor. The cause is:**
    a. B/L recurrent laryngeal nerve palsy
    b. U/L recurrent laryngeal nerve palsy
    c. B/L complete palsy
    d. U/L complete palsy
12. **Maximum stridor is seen in:**
    a. U/L incomplete palsy
    b. B/L incomplete palsy
    c. U/L complete palsy
    d. B/L complete palsy
13. **Anastomosis of branches of superior laryngeal and recurrent laryngeal nerves is:**
    a. Pure sensory
    b. Motor
    c. Secretomotor
    d. Sympathetic
14. **A 30 years old female presents with stridor following URTI. Indirect laryngoscopy shows glottis gap of 3 mm. This can be managed by all except:**
    a. Tracheostomy
    b. Type II thyroplasty
    c. Type I thyroplasty
    d. Cordectomy
15. **Gold standard surgical procedure for prevention of chronic aspiration is:**
    a. Thyroplasty
    b. Tracheostomy
    c. Tracheal diversion and permanent tracheostomy
    d. Feeding gastrostomy
16. **A patient with Pancoast's tumour develops hoarseness after radiation. It is due to:**
    a. Vocal cord infiltration with secondaries
    b. Involvement of recurrent laryngeal nerve
    c. Irradiation of vocal cord
    d. Radiation stenosis of larynx
17. **A 10 years old child develops hoarseness of voice following an attack of diphtheria. There is no other significant history. On examination the right vocal cord is paralysed. The treatment for paralysed vocal cord will be:**
    a. Gel form injection in the right vocal cord
    b. Fat injection in the right vocal cord
    c. Type I thyroplasty
    d. Wait for spontaneous recovery

ANSWERS AND EXPLANATIONS

1. **c. Thyroidectomy**

   The common case of vocal cord palsy are:

   1. ***Idiopathic and***
   2. ***Thyroid surgery***

   Both the above mentioned causes are considered and accepted as the commonest cause of vocal cord palsy. However, if one of the two is to be selected, then idiopathic is a better choice in comparison to thyroid surgery.

2. **a. Unilateral abductor paralysis of the vocal cord**

   The four important movement of vocal cords are adduction, abduction, tension and relaxation.

   Out of these, adduction of vocal cord is most important for the production of voice.

   In case of unilateral abductor paralysis of the vocal cord, this vocal cord will be adducted to lie in the median position. As mentioned above, adduction of vocal is most important for production of voice and in this condition where the vocal cord is already in adduction, the voice will be nearly normal. Even if there is some change of voice, it will soon be compensated by the other vocal cord.

   In some cases of unilateral abductor paralysis, the voice is normal in the morning but by the end of the day it gets tried.

   Bilateral incomplete paralysis of the vocal cord leads to same condition as bilateral abductor paralysis. In both these conditions, the vocal cord will be in adduction position and the voice of the patient will be very good. In this case the patient mainly has respiratory difficulty and hence may have stridor.

   In case of unilateral adductor paralysis of vocal cord, the vocal cord comes to lie in abducted position and the patient has significant change of voice.

   Some important points about vocal cord paralysis:

   - The most common cause of vocal cord paralysis is **thyroidectomy** (*idiopathic* is also acceptable).
   - Incomplete paralysis of recurrent laryngeal nerve is more dangerous as compared to complete paralysis of recurrent laryngeal nerve
   - The position of vocal cord after nerve palsy may depend on the level of lesion. Lesions at higher level will cause cadaveric position of vocal cords where as lesions at lower level will lead to adduction of vocal cords.
   - Ortner's syndrome, is vocal cord paralysis due to compression of recurrent laryngeal nerve due to cardiomegaly.
   - In bilateral abductor paralysis, tracheostomy may be required to maintain airway.
   - In bilateral adductor paralysis, the larynx may have to be excised from the trachea or total laryngectomy may be required to prevent aspiration.

3. **a. Vocal cord medialization**

Isshiki's Thyroplasty

Thyroplasty	What is done	Indication
Thyroplasty Type I	Medialisation	Adductor palsy (improve voice) and abductor spasm
Thyroplasty Type II	Lateralization	Abductor palsy (relieve dyspnoea) and adductor spasm
Thyroplasty Type III	Shorten/loosen	Puberphonia
Thyroplasty Type IV	Lengthen/tense	Androphonia

4. **d. Wait for spontaneous recovery of vocal cord**

   In cases of Diphtheria laryngitis, paralysis is caused by toxins of the organism affecting the laryngeal nerve. Neuritis of laryngeal nerve has a tendency to recover spontaneously. Hence we wait for spontaneous recovery of vocal cord for at least 6 months.

5. **a. B/L abductor palsy of vocal cord, palsy**

   In bilateral abductor palsy both the vocal cords assume median or midline position. This may lead to serious laryngeal blockade.

   Sometimes this condition is life threatening.

To relieve stridor, the following procedures can be done:
- *Thyroplasty Type II*
- *Arytenoidectomy(Woodman's surgery)*
- *Cordectomy- usually by CO_2 laser excision*
- *Dennis and Kashima's procedure*
- *Nerve grafting*
- ***Muscle pedicle grafting (Tucker's). Omohyoid or Stylohyoid muscles*** are used.
  - ***In Dennis and Kashima's procedure, a small wedge is excised from the posterior of one vocal cord so that the patient can breathe through that small opening without compromising the voice.***
  - In adductor palsy, medialization of the vocal cord is required.
  - In patients of cholesteatoma, mastoidectomy is done.
  - In laryngocele, surgical excision or marsupialization is done.

6. **a. Aphonia with stridor**
Bilateral abductor palsy is seen in palsy of both the recurrent laryngeal nerves.
This condition most commonly happens due to trauma during thyroidectomy.
When recurrent laryngeal nerve is damaged, all the muscles of the larynx stop functioning except cricothyroid.
Cricothyroid has adductor function and so ***vocal cord will assume a median or midline position.*** This is called abductor palsy.
In unilateral palsy, there is enough space for breathing and voice is satisfactory due to ***compensation by the other (normal) vocal cord.***
In bilateral abductor palsy, both the vocal cords assume midline position and there can be no compensation.
This leads to aphonia with stridor. Sometimes this condition can be life threatening.
Immediate tracheostomy may be required in such a situation.

Other Surgical Options in this Patient

- *Thyroplasty Type II*
- *Arytenoidectomy(Woodman's surgery)*
- *Cordectomy- usually by CO_2 laser excision*
- *Dennis and Kashima's procedure*
- *Nerve grafting*

7. **d. Right apical lung carcinoma**
Vocal cord palsy is most commonly caused due to palsy of the recurrent laryngeal nerve.
Left recurrent nerve is longer than the right recurrent laryngeal nerve. Therefore left side nerve damage is almost times more common than the right nerve.
Left side nerve being longer; travel deep into the neck and therefore is more easily damaged by mediastinal diseases like mediastinal lymphadenopathy.
Arch of aorta and aortic artery are present on the left side and so will involve the left recurrent nerve.
Laryngeal carcinoma does not often cause vocal cord palsy. It may cause fixation of the vocal cord by:
- *Involving the cricoarytenoid joint*
- *Mass effect*
- *Involvement of laryngeal muscle*
- *Recurrent laryngeal nerve involvement (rarely)*

Therefore right apical lung carcinoma will cause right nerve palsy.

8. **d. External laryngeal nerve**
Ligation of superior thyroid artery damages the external laryngeal nerve and ligation of inferior thyroid artery damages the recurrent laryngeal nerve.
Facial nerve and mandibular nerve are no where close to the thyroid gland.

9. **c. Recurrent laryngeal nerve**
As we know that the left recurrent laryngeal nerve winds around the arch of aorta. This anatomy brings this nerve very close to the left atrium. Hence the enlargement of left atrium (Cardiomegaly), may press this nerve causing vocal cord palsy.
Cardiomegaly pressing the recurrent laryngeal nerve causing vocal cord palsy is also called **Ortner's syndrome.**

10. **b. Paralysed and bowed**
Cadaveric position of the vocal cord is also called the intermediate position. This is also the resting position of the vocal cord.
However, this position is also attained during adductor palsy of the vocal cord. Adductor palsy is due to palsy of both the nerves, i.e. *recurrent laryngeal nerve and superior laryngeal nerve.*
This leads to paralysis of all the laryngeal muscles and hence the cadaveric position.
Since external laryngeal branch of superior laryngeal nerve is also paralysed, there will be loss of tension and hence ***bowing*** of the vocal cords.
Vocal cord is abducted only during respiration. Palsies of vocal cord does not give rise to abducted position.
Fixed vocal cord is the term which is usually NOT used for palsies. This term is used when the joints are affected and causes fixation of the cords.

Conditions that Causes Fixed VC

- Laryngeal carcinoma involving joints
- Hypopharyngeal carcinoma spreading into the larynx
- Fibrosis/sclerosis of joints, etc.

11. **a. B/L recurrent laryngeal nerve palsy**
As already discussed, in recurrent laryngeal palsy/abductor palsy, the vocal cord will be either in median or paramedian positions.
When the vocal cord assume median positions on both the sides in case of B/L recurrent laryngeal nerve palsies, there will be difficulty in breathing and lead to stridor.
In complete paralysis of vocal cord and all other conditions of vocal cord paralysis, stridor is NOT seen.

12. **b. B/L incomplete palsy**
Partial/incomplete damage of RLN causes paramedian/median position, whereas, complete damage causes cadaveric position.
Hence bilateral partial/incomplete palsy of RLN is more dangerous (because it will cause stridor) than bilateral complete palsy of RLN.

13. **a. Pure sensory**
Anastomosis of internal laryngeal nerve a branch of superior laryngeal and recurrent laryngeal nerve is called ***Galen's anastomosis.***
This is the pure sensory supply of the glottis in the larynx.
- We know that supraglottis develops from 4th branchial arch and it's nerve is superior laryngeal nerve
- Subglottis develops from 6th branchial arch and it's nerve is recurrent laryngeal nerve
- Glottis is neither from the 4th arch nor from the 6th arch and is therefore is *watershed area of larynx.*
- Hence glottis does NOT have it's own nerve and it receives sensory from *Galen's anastomosis* (formed by superior laryngeal nerve and recurrent laryngeal nerve).

14. **c. Type I thyroplasty**
The lady with **stridor** and 3 mm glottis gap is a case of abductor palsy with paramedian position of vocal cords.

Treatment of Abductor Palsy

The problem with RLN palsy is that median/paramedian position may cause stridor/dyspnoea, and paramedian/cadaveric position may cause hoarseness of voice.
Therefore
- To improve the voice, the cord has to be pulled medially.
- Whereas to relieve stridor, the cord has to be pulled laterally.
- Hence, when we try to improve one, the other gets compromised.

Voice Improvement

- ***Thyroplasty Type I***

Relieve Stridor

- ***Tracheostomy***
- ***Thyroplasty Type II***

- ***Arytenoidectomy(Woodman's surgery)***
- ***Cordectomy-*** *usually by* ***CO_2 laser excision***
- ***Dennis and Kashima's procedure***
- ***Nerve grafting***
- ***Muscle pedicle grafting (Tucker's). Omohyoid or Stylohyoid muscles*** are used.

Relieve Aspiration (Usually Not Required)

- ***Tracheostomy -*** *is a temporary method*
- ***Permanent Tracheostomy/Total Laryngectomy -*** *this is the* ***gold standard treatment*** *for aspiration.*
- ***Epiglottopexy***
- *Vocal cord plication*

15. **c. Tracheal diversion and permanent tracheostomy**
    Treatment options for aspiration are:
    - Tracheostomy
    - Epiglottopexy
    - Tracheal diversion and permanent tracheostomy/total laryngectomy (Gold standard).

16. **c. Irradiation of vocal cord**
    Pancoast's tumour is also called *pulmonary sulcus tumour* and is present near the apical area of lungs.
    Hoarseness of voice is NOT a very common symptom in this tumour. However, if hoarseness does happen, it is most commonly due to *compression of the recurrent laryngeal nerve.*
    Infiltration of vocal cord with secondaries is uncommon.
    In this case, the hoarseness appears after radiation which suggests that hoarseness is due to radiation of vocal cord and not by the tumour.

17. **d. Wait for spontaneous recovery**
    All the treatment options given are used for treatment of hoarseness in vocal cord palsies.
    But here, the hoarseness and vocal cord palsy is caused by the toxins of diphtheria.
    Once the diphtheria gets treated and the effect of toxin goes off, the vocal cord may recover.
    Hence, we should wait for spontaneous recovery.

CHAPTER

35 Tumours of Larynx

Larynx is in the upper airway and therefore everything that effect the lung can also affect the larynx. It is not suprising that carcinomas of both these areas are very common.

Laryngeal tumours are the most common tumours in the head and neck region.

All types of tumours are possible in the larynx. We are going to discuss the important ones.

RECURRENT RESPIRATORY PAPILLOMATOSIS (RRP)

Recurrent respiratory papillomatosis (RRP) has many other names like:

- **Laryngeal papilloma**
- ***Juvenile onset recurrent respiratory papillomatosis (JORRP)***
- ***Multiple papilloma of larynx***

Recurrent respiratory papillomatosis (RRP) is the **most common** benign tumour of larynx in adult.

Juvenile onset recurrent respiratory papillomatosis (JORRP) is the **most common laryngeal tumour (including benign and malignant) in children.**

Aetiology

Recurrent respiratory papillomatosis (RRP) is caused by **HPV 6c-f and HPV 11**

Viruses causes head and cancinomas	
Nasopharyngeal carcinoma	*Epstein-Barr virus (EBV)*
Oropharyngeal carcinoma	*Human papilloma virus (HPV) 16 and 18*
Recurrent respiratory papillomatosis (RRP)	*Human papilloma virus (HPV) 6 and 11*
Laryngeal carcinoma	*No virus implicated*

Presentation

The most common symptom is ***hoarseness of voice and breathing difficulty.***

On examination it is a ***warty papilloma usually at the junction of squamous epithelium and columnar epithelium. It involves only the superficial layer of lamina propria of glottis.***

Differences between Adult Onset RRP and Juvenile Onset RRP

Adult onset RRP	Juvenile onset RRP
• It is less common	• It is more common
• Single in number	• Multiple in number
• Present near true cords	• May be seen in entire respiratory tract
• Is less severe	• Is more severe
• No recurrent after treatment	• Usually recurrent after treatment
• Is not premalignant	• Is premalignant

Investigation

The following investigations are done

- Fiberoptic laryngoscopy
- ***Microscopic examination***
- ***Bronchoscopic examination.***

Treatment

Treatment of RRP must have two aims:

1. Excision of tumour/growth, and
2. Treat the virus HPV 6 and 11.

For tumour excision	For treating virus infection
• **Microdebridement- This is the gold standard treatment**	• Systemic **interferons**
• CO_2 laser vaporization	• Indole-3-carbinol
• Photodynamic therapy • Tracheostomy to relieve obstruction	• ***Intralesional*** – Cidofovir (preferred) – Acyclovir

LARYNGEAL CARCINOMA

Laryngeal carcinoma is the most common head and neck tumour in adult.

Aetiology

- **Smoking. Tobacco act through its chemical benzopyrene**
- **Alcohol**
- **Asbestos**

Site of Laryngeal Carcinoma

- **Glottis**—It is the ***most common site*** of laryngeal carcinoma
- **Supraglottis**—It is second most common site
- **Subglottis**—It is least common site

Presentation

It is more commonly seen in ***males*** above the age of 55–60 years

The earliest presentation depends on the site involved

- Glottic carcinoma- ***hoarseness of voice***. This is also the most common presentation of laryngeal carcinoma.
- **Supraglottic carcinoma- *pain in the throat or lymphadenopathy***
- **Subglottic carcinoma-** voice change and stridor

Investigations

Important investigations are:

- Direct laryngoscopy and biopsy
- CT Scan and MRI are equally useful
- Positron emission tomography (PET) is useful when metastasis is suspected.
- ***Toluidine blue dye*** is used to differentiate carcinoma from leukoplakia.

TNM Staging and Classification

Tumour

T1	Tumor limited to *one subsite* with normal vocal cord mobility.
T1a	In case of glottic Ca, there is:
T1b	Tumor involves *one* vocal cord
	Tumor involves *both* vocal cords

T2	Tumor invades ***adjacent subsites*** without fixation of the larynx. In case of supraglottic ca, the following may be involved • Mucosa of base of tongue • Vallecula • Medial wall of pyriform sinus
T3	Tumor limited to larynx with ***vocal cord fixation*** and/or invades any of the following: • Postcricoid area • Preepiglottic tissues • Paraglottic space
T4a	Tumor invades through the thyroid cartilage and/or invades extra-laryngeal tissues like • Trachea • Soft tissues of neck including deep extrinsic muscle of the tongue, strap muscles • Thyroid • Esophagus
T4b	Tumor invades • Prevertebral space • Encases carotid artery • Mediastinal structures

NODES

N0	No neck nodes
N1	Single, ipsilateral lymph node less than 3 cm
N2 N2a N2b N2c	Lymph nodes more than 3 cm but less than 6 cm Single ipsilateral lymph node between 3 cm to 6 cm Multilateral lymph nodes less than 6 cm Bilateral or contralateral lymph nodes less than 6 cm
N3	Lymph nodes more than 6 cm

Treatment

Carcinoma in situ	• *Endoscopic excision with laser with regular follow-up* • *In case of glottis tumour this surgery is called "Cordectomy/Stripping of cord"*
T1 andT2 glottic CA	• Transoral laser microsurgery with regular follow-up • Radiotherapy is the 2nd option
T1 andT2 supraglottic CA	• Horizontal partial laryngectomy is the best option • Transoral laser microsurgery with regular follow-up • Radiotherapy is the 2nd option
T3 CA of larynx (glottis+supraglottis)	• Radiotherapy plus chemotherapy (chemoradiation) • Conservative or total laryngectomy followed by radiotherapy • Bilateral neck dissection is combined to the above mentioned therapy
T4 CA of larynx (glottis+supraglottis)	• Radiotherapy plus chemotherapy (chemoradiation) • Total laryngectomy followed by radiotherapy is 2nd option • Salvage surgery and combined chemoradiotherapy • Bilateral neck dissection done wherever possible – Chemotherapeutic agents are: ♦ Cisplatinum ♦ 5-Fluorouracil (5-FU)

SURGERIES FOR LARYNGEAL CARCINOMA

1. **Total laryngectomy**
2. **Conservative laryngectomy.** This may be of many types
3. **Transoral laser microsurgery (TLM)**

Voice Rehabilitation

- Oesophageal speech
- Tracheoesophageal speech

These are used to produce speech. This speech is amplified by using

- *Electrolarynx*
- *Transoral pneumatic device*

For tracheoesophageal speech, prosthetic valves are used. Few types of valves are:

- ***Blom-singer prosthesis***
- ***Panje prosthesis***

VERRUCOUS CARCINOMA OF LARYNX

Verrucous carcinoma is a variant of squamous cell carcinoma.

Presentation

It presents as slow growing exophytic mass with pushing (NOT infiltrating) margins.

Histopathology

It has thick papillary projections and bulbous invaginations of well differentiated keratinizing squamous epithelium around fibrovascular core.

Treatment

Total laryngectomy or conservative laryngectomy is the only option.

Role of radiotherapy is controversial.

Last minute revision

Respiratory recurrent papillomatosis (RRP) is the most common laryngeal tumour in children
RRP is caused by HPV type 6 and 11. It is diagnosed by bronchoscopy
RRP is treated by microdebridement + interferon + intralesional cidofovir
Laryngeal carcinoma is caused in males who smoke and glottis is the most common site
Voice change is the most common presentation with lymphadenopathy in supraglottic carcinoma
Laryngeal carcinoma stage I and II is treated by excision with laser or radiotherapy
Stage III and IV are treated by concomitant chemoradiation or surgery + radiotherapy.
Verroucous carcinoma is a variant of squamous carcinoma which looks like papillated and warty
Verrucous carcinoma is treated by surgical excision

QUESTIONS

1. **A 70-year-old chronic smoker male comes with complain of hoarseness of voice. Which of these could be the likely diagnosis?**
   a. Epiglottitis
   b. Carcinoma of larynx
   c. Reinke's oedema
   d. Vocal cord nodule
2. **A 7-month-old child, presents with failure of gaining weight and noisy breathing which becomes worse when the child cries. Laryngoscopy shows a reddish mass in subglottis. Treatment modality may include all, except:**
   a. Radiation
   b. Steroids
   c. Tracheostomy
   d. Carbon dioxide laser treatment
3. **True about juvenile laryngeal papillomas is all, *except:***
   a. Usually single
   b. Disappear spontaneously after puberty
   c. Viral in origin
   d. Cause hoarseness of voice
4. **Treatment of choice in juvenile papillomas of larynx is:**
   a. Repeated local excision
   b. Vocal cord stripping
   c. Radiotherapy
   d. Chemotherapy
5. **The most common and earliest manifestation of carcinoma of the glottis is:**
   a. Hoarseness
   b. Haemoptysis
   c. Cervical lymph nodes
   d. Stridor
6. **First symptom of glottic cancer is:**
   a. Swelling in neck b. Dysphagia
   c. Cough d. Hoarseness
7. **A middle aged male comes to the outer patient department (OPD) with the only complaint of hoarseness of voice for the past 2 years.**
   He has been a chronic smoker for 30 years. On examination, a red dish area of mucosal irregularity overlying a portion of both cords was seen. Management would include all *except:*
   a. Cessation of smoking
   b. Bilateral cordectomy
   c. Microlaryngeal surgery for biopsy
   d. Regular follow-up
8. **A-50-year old male chronic smoker complains of hoarseness for the past 4 months. Microlaryngoscopic biopsy shows it to be keratosis of the larynx. All are suggested treatment modalities for this condition, *except:***
   a. Laser vaporizer b. Stop smoking
   c. Stripping of vocal cord
   d. Partial laryngectomy
9. **The treatment of choice of a T1N0M0 glottic carcinoma is:**
   a. External beam radiography
   b. Brachytherapy
   c. Surgery
   d. Chemotherapy
10. **Treatment of Ca larynx in stage. T1 M0 N0 is:**
    a. Radiotherapy b. Surgery
    c. Chemotherapy
    d. Radiotherapy + Chemotherapy
11. **A patient with Pancoast's tumour, develops loss of voice after radiation. It is due to:**
    a. Vocal cord infiltration with secondaries
    b. Involvement of recurrent laryngeal nerve
    c. Irradiation to vocal cords
    d. Radiation stenosis of larynx.
12. **Which of the following is NOT an indication for near total laryngectomy?**
    a. Stage T3
    b. Anterior commissure involvement
    c. Free lateral arytenoids cartilage
    d. Interarytenoid plane involvement
13. **Treatment of choice in stage III carcinoma larynx is:**
    a. Chemotherapy b. Surgery + radiation
    c. Surgery + chemotherapy
    d. Only radiotherapy
14. **An elderly male presents with T3N0 laryngeal carcinoma. What would be the management:**
    a. Neoadjuvant chemotherapy followed by radiotherapy
    b. Concurrent chemoradiation
    c. Radiotherapy followed by chemotherapy
    d. Radical radiotherapy without chemotherapy
15. **A patient with carcinoma of larynx involving the left false cord, left arytenoids and left aryepiglottic fold with bilateral mobile true cords. Treatment of choice is:**
    a. Vertical hemilaryngectomy
    b. Horizontal hemilaryngectomy
    c. Radiotherapy followed by chemotherapy
    d. Total laryngectomy
16. **The preferred treatment of verrucous carcinoma of the larynx is:**
    a. Pulmonary surgery
    b. Electron beam therapy
    c. Total laryngectomy
    d. Endoscopic removal
17. **Involvement of pre-epiglottic space is seen in:**
    a. Carcinoma larynx
    b. Ludwig's angina
    c. Submandibular gland infection
    d. Vincent's angina
18. **Which of the following carcinoma presents with neck nodes commonly?**
    a. Hypopharynx b. Glottic area
    c. Epiglottis d. Hard palate

19. A 4-year-old child presents with hoarseness for 4 months and stridor for 4 days. The most likely diagnosis is:
a. Laryngomalacia
b. Foreign body aspiration
c. Epiglottitis
d. Laryngeal papillomatosis

20. Topical treatment for recurrent respiratory papillomatosis includes:
a. Acyclovir b. Cidofovir
c. Ranitidine d. Zinc

21. Contraindication of supraglottic laryngectomy are all *except:*
a. Poor pulmonary reserve
b. Tumour involving pryriform fossa
c. Tumour involving pre-epiglottic space
d. Vocal cord fixation

22. Juvenile papillomatosis is caused by:
a. HSV b. EBV
c. CMV d. HPV

23. Ridhi 4-year-old presented in emergency with mild respiratory distress. On laryngoscopy she was diagnosed to have multiple juvenile papillomatosis. Next line of management is:
a. Tracheostomy
b. Microlaryngoscopic excision
c. Steroids
d. Antibiotics

24. True of papilloma are all *except:*
a. Solitary is more common in adults and most common presentation is voice change
b. Solitary type is more aggressive, has bad prognosis and malignant transformation is common
c. Multiple type is more common in children and hoarse cry is the most common presentation
d. Early treatment gives better results in multiple type

25. Lymph node metastasis in the neck is almost NOT seen in:
a. Carcinoma vocal cord
b. Supraglottic carcinoma
c. Carcinoma tonsils
d. Papillary carcinoma of thyroid

26. True statement about infraglottic carcinoma of larynx:
a. Commonly spread to mediastinal lymph nodes
b. Second most common carcinoma
c. More common in females
d. Spreads to sub mental lymph nodes

27. The most common cause of laryngeal stridor in 60 years old male is:
a. Nasopharyngeal carcinoma
b. Laryngeal carcinoma
c. Reinke's oedema
d. Acute asthma

28. In a case of glottic carcinoma with fully mobile cords, the treatment of choice is:
a. Total laryngectomy b. Hemilaryngectomy
c. Radiotherapy d. Chemotherapy

29. A 50-year-old male presents with 4 cm hard and immobile node in the middle deep cervical region. FNAC shows metastatic squamous cell carcinoma. O/E no lesion was found in the head and neck. Further management will be:
a. Oesophagoscopy
b. Triple endoscopy
c. Laryngoscopy
d. Supravital staining

30. Which of the following is inappropriate indication for concomitant chemotherapy in case of head and neck cancer?
a. Primary treatment in a patient with unresectable disease
b. As an organ safeguarding method
c. Postoperative case of intermediate stage resectable tumour
d. Metastatic advanced head and neck tumour

31. An 8-year-old child presents with hoarseness of voice for the past few years. During fiberoptic laryngoscopy examination the following is seen:

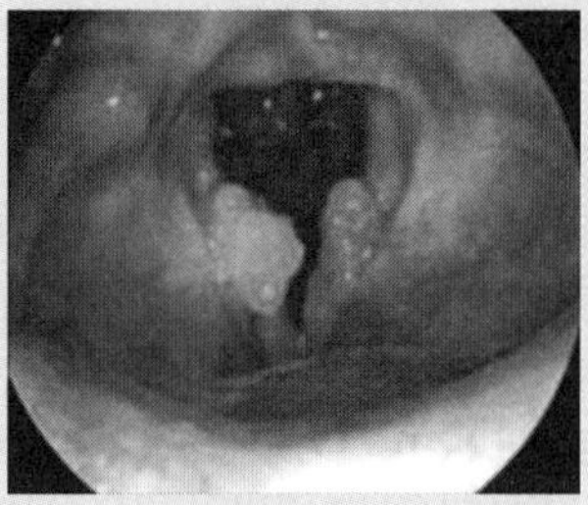

This child is most probably suffering from which of these
a. Laryngeal carcinoma
b. Vocal cord nodule
c. Vocal cord polyp
d. Recurrent respiratory papillomatosis (RRP)

ANSWERS AND EXPLANATIONS

1. **b. Carcinoma of larynx.**
   - Epiglottitis is usually seen in children between 2-7 years of age. The child is toxic with fever and drooling of saliva. X-ray may show ***thumb sign.***
   - Reinke's oedema is seen is ***smoker and talkative females.*** Vocal cord may look like ***water balloon.***
   - Vocal cord nodule is usually present in chronic misuser of voice like singer and teachers. It is also called ***singer's nodule and teacher's nodule.*** Vocal cord may look like ***hour glass.***
   - Laryngeal carcinoma is commonly seen in elderly (more than 55 years) chronic smoker males. Glottis is the most common site and therefore hoarseness of voice is the most common presentation. The above mentioned patient fits this description and therefore this is the correct answer.

2. **a. Radiation**
   The commonest subglottic reddish mass in infants is benign vascular tumour. It is usually a ***subglottic haemangioma***.
   Subglottic haemangioma can be a congenital disease of the subglottis which presents as ***stridor between 6 months to 1 year of age.***

TREATMENT OF SUBGLOTTIC HAEMANGIOMA

- ***Tracheostomy*** may be required in most patients.
- Systemic steroid is given to relieve acute respiratory obstruction and regression of tumour.
- Intralesional steroids may be useful
- CO_2 laser vaporization is done for small lesions.
- Radiotherapy may induce thyroid malignancy.

3. **a. Usually single**
   Juvenile laryngeal papilloma is the most common laryngeal tumour in children.
   It is also called multiple papilloma because they are multiple in number and can be seen any where in the respiratory tract. For this reason, microlaryngoscopy or bronchoscopy is usually done in these patients.
   It is caused by human papilloma virus and presents as hoarseness of voice and stridor. They tend to disappear after puberty.
   Three very important features of these tumours are:
   1. They are recurrent
   2. They are premalignant
   3. They are best treated by microdebridement or CO_2 laser excision.

   The adult laryngeal papillomas are single, NOT recurrent and NOT pre-malignant.

4. **a. Repeated local excision**
   Juvenile papilloma of larynx also called multiple papilloma is a squamous papilloma of larynx. In adults, it presents and behaves differently. The treatment in both adult and juvenile is *microdebridement or CO_2 laser excision.*
   Juvenile papilloma is a recurrent disease and is also pre-malignant. In the past, when laser was not used, multiple local excision was done due to recurrent nature of the disease.
   Microlaryngoscopy or bronchoscopy is usually done before treating juvenile papilloma, this is not required for adult papilloma.

TREATMENT OF LARYNGEAL PAPILLOMA MUST HAVE TWO AIMS:

- Excision of tumour/growth, and
- Treat the virus HPV 6 and 8.

For tumour excision	For treating virus infection
• **Microdebridement- This is the gold standard treatment**	• Systemic **interferons**
• CO_2 laser vaporization	• Indole-3-carbinol
• Photodynamic therapy • Tracheostomy to relieve obstruction	• ***Intralesional*** – *Cidofovir* – *Acyclovir*

5. **a. Hoarseness**
6. **d. Hoarseness**
   Vocal cords are primarily used for production of speech although the main function of larynx is protection of airways. Hence, when VC are involved, the earliest symptom is change of voice.

PRESENTATION LARYNGEAL CARCINOMA

It is more commonly seen in ***males*** above the age of 55-60 years
The earliest presentation depends on the site involved
- Glottic carcinoma- ***hoarseness of voice.*** This is also the most common presentation of laryngeal carcinoma.
- **Supraglottic carcinoma-** ***pain in the throat or lymphadenopathy***
- **Subglottic carcinoma-** voice change and stridor

7. **b. Bilateral cordectomy**
   In such a patient, the diagnosis has to be made. However the history is very long ie 2 years, hence possibility of benign disease is high.
   Hence, patient should be advised to stop smoking and put on regular follow-up.
   Bilateral cordectomy is usually is done in any glottic carcinoma stage Ib.
   Bilateral Vocal Cord stripping is done in carcinoma in situ.
8. **d. Partial laryngectomy**
   The biopsy clearly mentions keratosis of larynx which is a premalignant condition and is not a malignancy hence laryngectomy is not required in this patient.
   When patient has such premalignant conditions as keratosis, two modalities are to be achieved:
   1. Remove all risk factors like
      a. Smoking
   2. Treat the existing disease.
   - ***Smoking has to stop and hence remove risk factor.***
   - ***Keratosis has to be removed by:***
     1. ***Laser vaporizer***
     2. ***Stripping of vocal cord.***

   Partial laryngectomy is done for confirmed malignancy. Therefore it is NOT required in this condition.
9. **c. Surgery**
10. **b. Surgery (Transoral laser microsurgery-TLM)**
    T1N0M0 glottic carcinoma is Stage 1 Carcinoma of glottis.
    There are two treatment options for T1N0M0:
    - ***Transoral laser microsurgery (TLM) of tumour with follow-up and***
    - ***External beam radiation.***

    The prognosis with either is very good. Five year survival rate is more than 85–100%.
    - ***Transoral laser microsurgery (surgery) of tumour with follow-up is the preferred option***
    - External beam radiotherapy is the second best option
    - Brachytherapy is local radiotherapy. It is only possible in easily accessible area like:
      - Oral cavity and
      - Oropharynx
    - Chemotherapy is used for ***Stage IV tumours.***
    - Open surgery (laryngectomy) is indicated in one of the following situations:
      - ***Fixed vocal cord***
      - ***Involvement of laryngeal cartilage***
      - ***Palpable lymph nodes.***
11. **c. Irradiation to vocal cords**
    Pancoast's tumour is a tumour of apex of lung and recurrent laryngeal nerve passes close to this area. Hence in such a tumour, recurrent laryngeal nerve may be involved leading to vocal cord palsy and loss of voice.
    Radiotherapy of vocal cords is also known to cause loss of voice.
    Hence, if the loss of voice takes place after radiation then the most probable cause could be irradiation to vocal cords

12. **d. Interarytenoid plane involvement**
Near total laryngectomy is a surgical procedure in which the entire larynx is remove with preservation of ***one arytenoids along with its joint with cricoids cartilage (one cricoarytenoid joint is preserved).***
This is done because this joint can be used for reconstruction of speech.

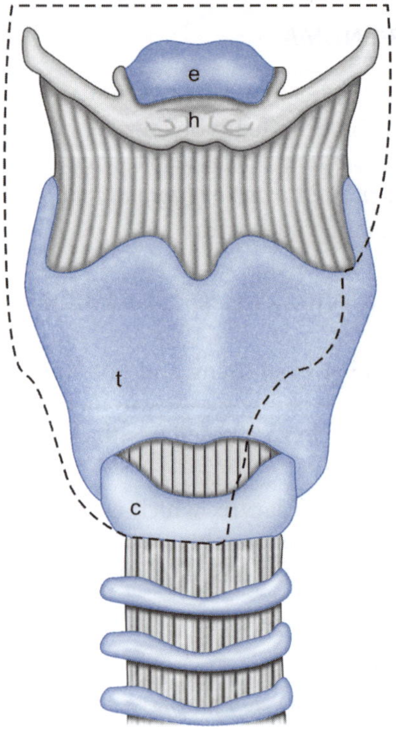

Dotted line shows the removed part in near total laryngectomy

INDICATION OF NEAR TOTAL LARYNGECTOMY

The only important indication is wherever total laryngectomy is contemplated but one cricoarytenoid joint is free of disease. This free join can be saved for voice restoration.

- Hence, it is done for stage T3 and T4 carcinoma of larynx
- Whether the anterior commissure is involved or not, has nothing to do with this surgery. Which means that the decision; to DO OR NOT DO near total laryngectomy; does not depend on anterior commissure.
- One arytenoid has to be free of disease. This arytenoid will be preserved/saved.
- In patients where interarytenoid plane is involved, the chances of free arytenoid/joint is bleak. Interarytenoid plane is the space between the two arytenoids cartilages. There might be micrometastasis of both the arytenoids. Therefore, near total laryngetomy should NOT be done in these patients.

13. **b. Surgery + radiation**

14. **b. Concurrent chemoradiation**
In stage III carcinoma of larynx, there are two treatment options:
- ***Combined radiotherapy and chemotherapy (concurrent).***
- ***Laryngectomy followed by radiotherapy.***

OTHER IMPORTANT POINTS

- Only chemotherapy is NOT used in laryngeal carcinoma.
- Surgery + chemptherapy is used for stage IV carcinoma
- Only radiotherapy is used for stage I and stage II carcinoma.

15. **b. Horizontal hemilaryngectomy**
The carcinoma involves one side false cord, arytenoids and aryepiglottic fold means the carcinoma is confined to supraglottic area.

Bilateral vocal folds are mobile mean that glottis is free of disease.
This makes it stage T2 carcinoma of supraglottis.

Treatment Options for Stage T2 Supraglottic Carcinoma

- ***Transoral laser microsurgery (TLM).*** This is the best option
- ***Open supraglottic hemilaryngectomy (horizontal hemilaryngectomy)***
- ***Radiotherapy.***

From the option gives, the best answer is horizontal hemilaryngectomy.

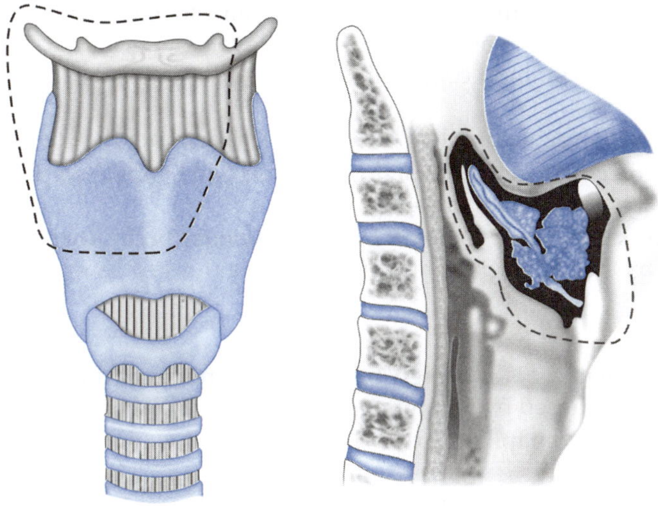

Showing supraglottic hemilaryngectomy

16. **c. Total laryngectomy**
Verrucous carcinoma is well- differentiated keratinizing squamous epithelial carcinoma.
It is a very rare carcinoma of larynx.
It presents as warty papillary tumour of glottis and does not have deep infiltration.
Treatment of choice for verrucous carcinoma is either partial laryngectomy or total laryngectomy.
Radiotherapy is contraindicated in this case as radiotherapy may convert verrucous carcinoma from relatively benign into malignant tumour.

17. **a. Carcinoma larynx**
Pre-epiglottic space called the ***space of boyer.*** It is in front of the larynx.
It is bounded:
- Anteriorly by the ***thyroid cartilage and thyrohyoid membrane.***
- Posteriorly by the ***epiglottis.***
- Superiorly ***hyoepiglottic ligaments***
- On either side it opens into the paraglottic spaces.

Petiole of epiglottis has number of microscopic holes in it.
Carcinoma of larynx (supra-glottic carcinoma) can spread into this pre-epiglottic space through these holes.
From here it may spread through the thyroid cartilage involving extra laryngeal tissue.

18. **c. Epiglottis**
Head and neck has very rich and extensive lymphatic supply. Tumours of head and neck area involve lymph nodes very commonly.
- In some of these tumours, cervical lymphadenopathy is the ***most common presentation (nasopharyngeal carcinoma).***
- In some tumours, lymphadenopathy is very uncommon. This is true for ***glottis carcinoma.*** It is well known that glottis has NO lymphatic supply.
- Hard palate has ***salivary gland tumours.*** Lymph node involvement is uncommon.
- In India, squamous cell carcinoma may be seen in hard palate due to practice of ***reverse smoking.*** They present as ulcer on the palate.

PART 4: LARYNX

- Hypopharynx has three areas;
  - Pyriform fossa. This is most common site of carcinoma.
  - Post cricoids area. This is second common site of tumour.
  - Posterior pharyngeal wall
- Hypopharyngeal carcinomas commonly involve lymph nodes. But they usually involve ***Mediastinal nodes (group VII nodes).*** These nodes do not present clinically. They can only be diagnosed radiographically.
- Supraglottic carcinoma including carcinoma of epiglottis may present with cervical lymphadenopathy

19. d. Laryngeal papillomatosis

From the history we understand that the child is suffering from a long duration disease of larynx (hoarseness for 4 months), which is progressive in nature (stridor for 4 days).

- Laryngomalacia is the most common congenital disease of larynx and does NOT cause voice change or hoarseness.
- Foreign body aspiration is an acute problem. It will NOT have 4 months old history of hoarseness.
- Epiglottitis is an acute infective disease of epiglottis caused by H. influenza. The child is around 5-year-old and has fever, stridor, dysphagia with drooling.
- Laryngeal papillomatosis is the ***most common laryngeal tumour in children.*** They are multiple in numbers and can cause symptoms like hoarseness and stridor. Since this is a benign tumour, the history can be of long duration.

20. b. Cidofovir

Recurrent laryngeal papillomatosis is a benign tumour of respiratory tract. They are usually multiple in numbers and is believed to be caused by human papilloma virus (**HPV 6c-f and HPV 11**)

Treatment of recurrent respiratory papillomatosis should have following parts:

Aim of treatment	Treatment option
1. Relieve stridor	• Tracheostomy
2. Tumour excision	• Microdebridement • CO_2 laser excision • Photodynamic therapy
3. Intralesional injections of antivirals	• Cidofovir • Acyclovir
4. Systemic antiviral	• Interferons • Indole-3-carbinol

21. c. Tumour involving pre-epiglottic space

Supraglottic laryngectomy is a surgical procedure in which supraglottis is removed and glottis and subglottis are retained.

It should only be done for tumours confined to supraglottic area such as:

- False cords or ventricular folds
- Epiglottis
- AE fold
- **Pre-epiglottic space,** etc.
  - It should not be done when vocal cord is fixed because this involves glottis also.
  - Pyriform fossa is a part of hypopharynx, and supraglottic laryngectomy does not remove this area.
  - In supraglottic laryngectomy, the epiglottis is also removed, because this is a part of supraglottis. We know that epiglottis is the main protector of airway and if this is removed the patient may start having aspiration. Therefore this surgery should NOT be done in patients with poor pulmonary status.

22. d. HPV

Viruses causes head and cancinomas	
Nasopharyngeal carcinoma	*Epstein Barr virus (EBV)*
Oropharyngeal carcinoma	*Human papilloma virus (HPV) 16 and 18*
Recurrent respiratory papillomatosis (RRP)	*Human papilloma virus (HPV) 6 and 11*
Laryngeal carcinoma	*No virus implicated*

23. **b. Microlaryngoscopic excision**
This is a very old question. It was asked in 2001 in AIIMS. The best answer from among the choices given is microlaryngoscopic excision. However, the recent treatment options are as:

Treatment of Laryngeal Papilloma must have Two Aims

- Excision of tumour/growth, and
- Treat the virus HPV 6 and 8.

For tumour excision	For treating virus infection
• **Microdebridement- This is the gold standard treatment**	• Systemic **interferons**
• CO_2 laser vaporization	• Indole-3-carbinol
• Photodynamic therapy • Tracheostomy to relieve obstruction	• ***Intralesional*** – Cidofovir – Acyclovir

Tracheostomy is not required for three reasons:
1. Stridor is mild
2. Laryngeal papilloma may be present in the lower part of trachea and bronchi. Hence, tracheostomy is not useful.
3. If papilloma is present in the area where tracheostomy is done, this papilloma may get pushed more distally.

24 **b. Solitary type is more aggressive, has bad prognosis and malignant transformation is common**
Differences between adult onset RRP and juvenile onset RRP

Adult onset RRP	Juvenile onset RRP
• It is less common	• It is more common
• Single in number (solitary)	• Multiple in number
• Present near true cords	• May be seen in entire respiratory tract
• Is less severe	• Is more severe
• No recurrent after treatment	• Usually recurrent after treatment (bad prognosis)
• Is not premalignant	• Is premalignant

25. **a. Carcinoma vocal cord**
Glottis has almost no lymphatic supply and therefore carcinoma of this area does not have neck nodes.

26. **a. Commonly spread to mediastinal lymph nodes**
Infraglottic carcinomas are least common laryngeal carcinoma and are more common in males. They spread to mediastinal lymph nodes (group VII nodes).

27. **b. Laryngeal carcinoma**

28. **c. Radiotherapy**
Among the choices given, radiotherapy is the best option.
However, local excision (***transoral laser microsurgery)*** with cessation of smoking and regular follow up is best option in glottis carcinoma with mobile vocal cords (stage I or stage II).

29. **b. Triple endoscopy**
This is a case of ***unknown primary.***
Unknown primary where a metastatic lymph node is detected but the primary tumour is not found.
In such cases, now a days **PET Scan** has become extremely popular and is the best answer if given in choices.

Triple endoscopy includes
1. Nasopharyngoscopy 2. Oesophagoscopy 3. Laryngoscopy

30. c. Postoperative case of intermediate stage resectable tumour

- Concomitant chemotherapy is the preferred option in advanced unresectable tumour of head and neck (stage III and stage IV tumours)
- Organ conservation and organ safe guarding methods are both chemotherapy and radiotherapy.
- Metastatic advanced head and neck tumours that have spread to a wide area. In such a case surgery and radiotherapy alone or in combination are NOT useful. Hence, concomitant chemotherapy is used.
- Intermediate stage resectable tumours are best treated with surgery. In post-op case of such a tumour, radiotherapy may be combined if needed. Chemotherapy (if additional treatment is required) is usually used for advanced tumour and not intermediate tumours.

31. d. Recurrent respiratory papillomatosis (RRP)

The picture clearly shows two separate papillomatous growths on each vocal cord.

- Laryngeal carcinoma is continuous growth and is NOT papillomatous. However, verricous carcinoma may give a papillomatous appearance.
- Vocal cord nodule is a very small growth and is at the junction of anterior 1/3 and posterior 2/3 of the cord. It gives an appearance of an hour glass.

Vocal cord polyp is usually unilateral and is in the anterior 1/3 of the cord.

CHAPTER 36

Neck and Airway Surgeries

LARYNGECTOMY

Laryngectomy is usually done for carcinoma of larynx.

Laryngectomy can broadly be divided into three types:

1. Total laryngectomy
2. **Conservative laryngectomy.** This may be of many types
3. **Transoral laser microsurgery.**

Incision

A number of incisions are used during laryngectomy.

The most common incision is **Gluck Sorensen's incision.**

Gluck Sorensen's incision is a "**U**" shaped incision.

The main advantages of this incision are:

- Very good exposure of surgical field
- The skin has NO post surgery contraction.

Disadvantages of Total Laryngectomy

- Complete loss of voice
- Permanent tracheostomy
- Supplement of thyroid hormones, vitamin D3 and calcium will be required lifelong
- Carotid blowout, etc.

Conservative laryngectomy types:

Types	Subtypes	
Cordectomy According to European laryngological society (ELS) are of 5 types	Type I Subepithelial Type II Subligamental Type III Transmuscular Type IV Total Type V Extended	Subepithelial is also called stripping of vocal cord
Vertical partial laryngectomy	1. Type I Standard vertical	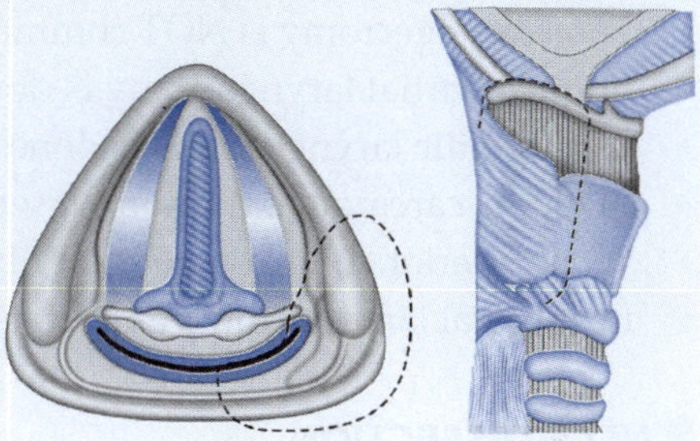

Contd...

Contd...

Types	Subtypes	
	2. Type II Frontolateral	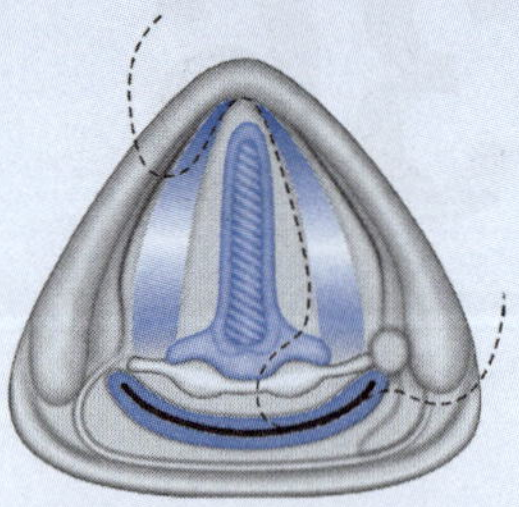
	3. Type III Anterofrontal 4. Type IV Extended	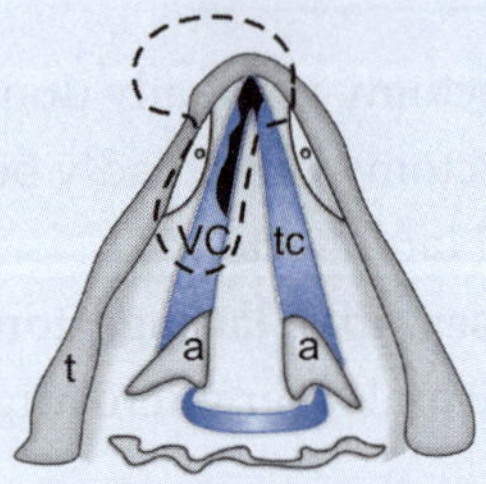
Horizontal partial laryngectomy	1. Supraglottic laryngectomy 2. Supracricoid laryngectomy	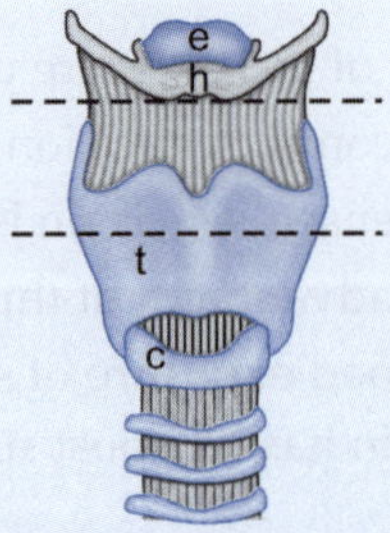
Subtotal laryngectomy		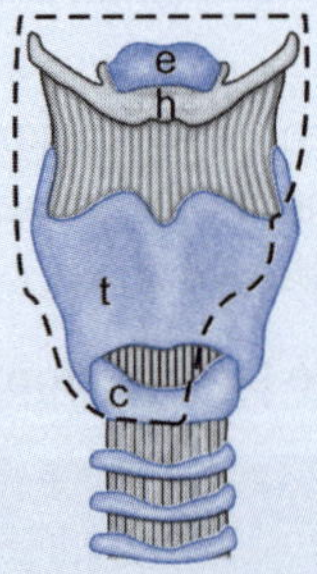
Near total laryngectomy		

IMPORTANT POINTS ABOUT LARYNGECTOMIES

- Total laryngectomy is NOT common now a days
- Vertical partial laryngectomy is done if tumour is confined to on side of the glottis
- Supraglottic laryngectomy is done when disease is confined to supraglottic area only.
- In glottis carcinoma, transoral laser microsurgery is preferred unless anterior commissure is also involved
- When anerior commissure is involved in glottis carcinoma, anterolateral hemilaryngectomy is done
- In subtotal laryngectomy and near total laryngectomy, one ***cricoarytenoid joint is preserved.***

NECK DISSECTION

The neck nodes are divided into six groups:

These are:

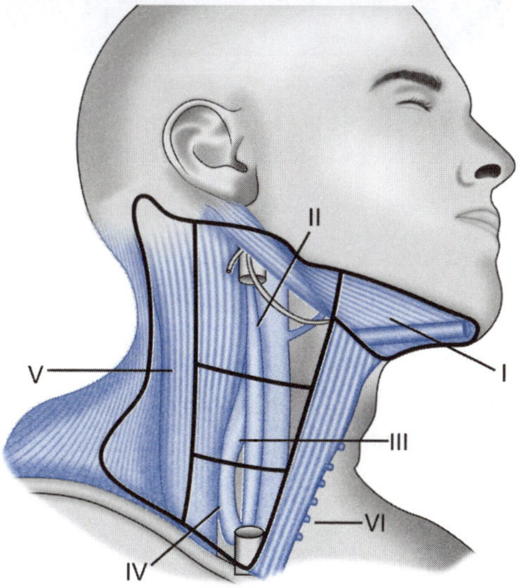

Level I	Is divided into two levels
	IA submental nodes
	IB submandibular nodes
Level II	located in the upper 1/3 of jugular vein above the hyoid bone.
Level III	located in the middle third of jugular vein or between the hyoid and upper border of cricoid cartilage
Level IV	located between the cricoid and clavicle
Level V	located in the posterior triangle, between the anterior border of sternomastoid and trapezius.
Level VI	Midline nodes. In between the two sternomastoid muscles.

Neck Dissections are Divided into Four Main Types

1. Radical neck dissection
2. Modified neck dissection
3. Selective neck dissection
4. Extended neck dissection

RADICAL NECK DISSECTION (RND)

This is enblock removal of lymph nodes between **level I to V**, along the following structures:
- Sternomastoid muscle
- Internal jugular vein
- Spinal accessory nerve

Many types of incisions are used for radical neck dissection. Few common ones are:
- ***Schobinger incision***. This is the ***most common incision*** used for (RND)
- Hetter incision
- McFee incision, etc.

MODIFIED NECK DISSECTION

Modified neck dissection is removal of groups I to V lymph nodes with preservation of one or more of the three structures:
- Sternomastoid muscle
- Internal jugular vein
- Spinal accessory nerve

Depending on the structures that are preserved, it is divided into types.

Types	Structures preserved
Type I	Structure preserved is • Spinal accessory nerve
Type II	Structures preserved are • Spinal accessory nerve and • Internal jugular vein
Type III	Structures preserved are • Spinal accessory nerve • Internal jugular vein and • Sternocleidomastoid muscle
Note: In type III modified neck dissection, the function of all the three structures are preserved. Therefore this is also called ***functional neck dissection.***	

SELECTIVE NECK DISSECTION

In selective neck dissection, one or more of the lymph nodes groups are preserved along with preservation of all the three structures.

In other words, it means that in selective neck dissection only few groups of lymph nodes are removed.

They are of the following types:

Supraomohyoid neck dissection	Lateral neck dissection	Posterolateral neck dissection	Anterior neck dissection
Groups I, II, III	Groups II, III, IV	Groups II, III, IV, V	Group VI
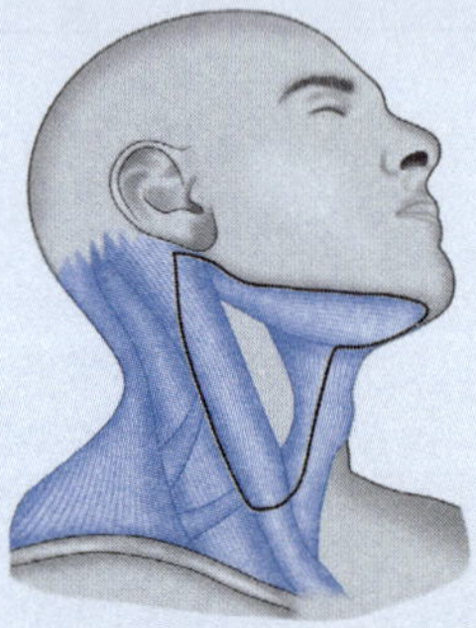	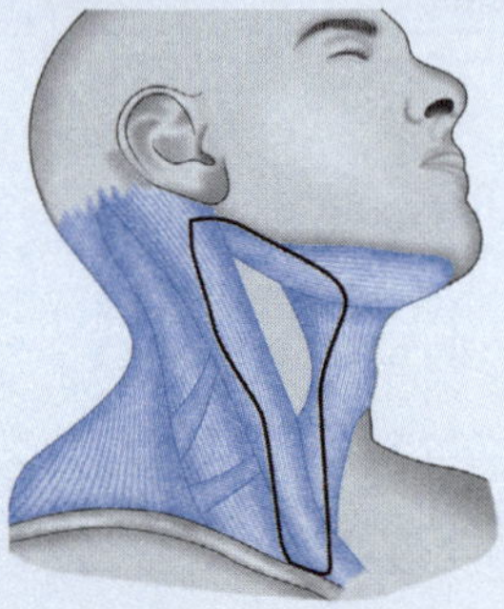	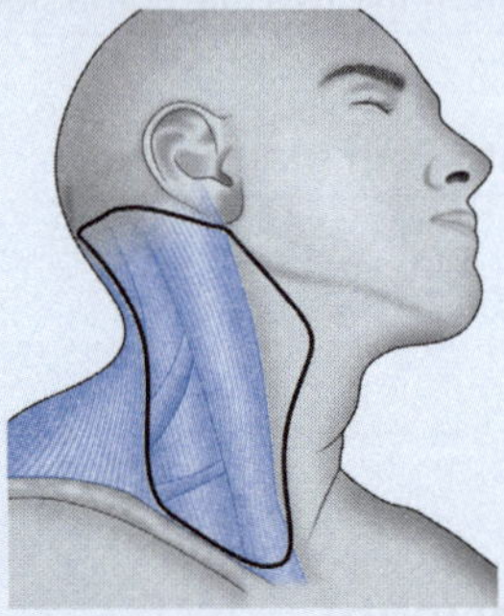	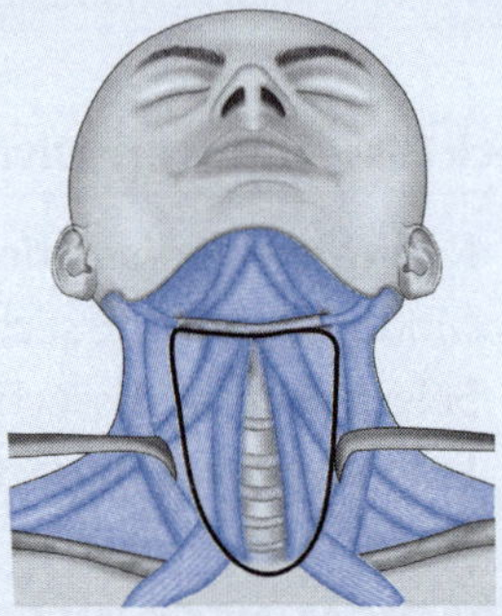

EXTENDED NECK DISSECTION

In this, additional structures are removed.

Tracheostomy

Tracheostomy is a surgical procedure where an opening is created in the tracheal ring so as to bypass the larynx.

Common indications of tracheostomy are:

- *Laryngeal obstruction. This is the most common indication. It is usually done for carcinoma.*
- *To decrease the dead space. To assist breathing*
- *For lung toilet. To suck out secretions*
- *To prevent secretion of pharynx from entering the trachea/lungs*
- *As an assistant for other procedures, etc.*

Tracheostomies can be of various types. Few common ones are:

1. Cricothyroidotomy/Minitracheostomy
2. Percutaneous tracheostomy
3. Conventional tracheostomy
4. Translaryngeal tracheostomy, etc.

CRICOTHYROIDOTOMY/MINITRACHEOSTOMY

Cricothyroidotomy is an emergency procedure in which a ***wide bore needle is passed through the cricothyroid membrane.***

PERCUTANEOUS TRACHEOSTOMY

In percutaneous tracheostomy a needle and cannula is passed through the skin and then below the ***first tracheal ring.***

Through this cannula; dilators of different sizes are passed and thus opening in the tracheal ring is dilated.

Finally a tracheostomy tube is passed through the cannula into the tracheal opening.

This procedure is very commonly used in ICUs.

CONVENTIONAL TRACHEOSTOMY

Conventional tracheostomy is the open surgical method and is most common type of tracheostomy.

Incision

- In adult a horizontal incision is made.
- In children a vertical incision is made

Tracheal Ring

- Incision is preferred in the ***2nd and 3rd tracheal rings (sometimes 3rd and 4th rings).***
- The second common site is ***3rd tracheal ring***

Complications

- ***Most common early complication is bleeding.***
- Subcutaneous emphysema is also common
- Late complication in *children* is ***difficult decannulation***
- Late complication in *adult* is ***tracheal stenosis and tracheomalacia***
- Tracheal stenosis are treated with **mitomycin C.**

Tracheostomy Tubes

Different types of tracheostomy tubes are used.

- The ***most common tracheostomy tube is the Portex tube.***
  Portex tube is non metallic and is made of polyurethane.
  It has a cuff around it.
  It is easy to clean, sterilize and change.
- Shiley tube is good for paediatric patients

Last minute revision

- *Cordectomy are of five types subepithelial, subligamental, transmascular, total cordectomy, extended*
- *Vertical partial laryngectomy is done when tumour involves only one side vocal cord*
- *Supraglottis hemilaryngectomy is done when tumour involves arytenoids, AE fold, epiglottis, pre-epiglottic space*
- *Radical neck dissection is removal of 5 groups of lymph nodes with sternomastoid, IJV, IX nerve*
- *Type III modified neck dissection is also called functional dissection where only lymph nodes are removed*
- *Selective neck dissection are of many types where all lymph nodes are not removed*
- *Tracheostomy is done on 2nd and 3rd ring.*
- *Most common indication for tracheostomy is carcinoma of larynx or laryngeal obstruction*
- *The most common complication is bleeding, emphysema, stenosis, difficult decannulation.*

QUESTIONS

1. **A case of carcinoma larynx with the involvement of anterior commissure and right vocal cord, develops perichondritis of thyroid cartilage. Which of the following statements is true for the management of this case?**
   a. He should be given radical radiotherapy as this can cure early tumours
   b. He should be treated with combination of chemotherapy and radiotherapy
   c. He should first receive radiotherapy and if residual tumour is present then should undergo laryngectomy
   d. He should first undergo laryngectomy and then postoperative radiotherapy.
2. **In esophageal speech, the dynamic component is:**
   a. Buccal segment
   b. Pharyngoesophageal segment
   c. Trachea
   d. Pharynx
3. **Which of the following structures are preserved in radical neck dissection?**
   a. Vagus nerve
   b. Accessory nerve
   c. Internal jugular vein
   d. Sternocleidomastoid muscle
4. **All are true about tracheostomy tube except:**
   a. Consist of 2 metallic tube
   b. Tubes are made of silver alloy and titanium oxide
   c. Metallic tubes are ideally changed every 2-3 days
   d. Cuffed tubes used for IPPV
5. **Montgomery tube used in ENT procedure is a:**
   a. Double barrel tube
   b. Lobster tail tube
   c. Airway tube
   d. Silicone T-tube
6. **The important complication of tracheostomy is:**
   a. Surgical emphysema
   b. Vocal cord trauma
   c. Recurrent laryngeal nerve palsy
   d. Haemorrhage"
7. **Advantage of tracheostomy are all except:**
   a. Bronchial toilet
   b. Decreased dead space
   c. Pharyngeal secretion toilet
   d. Increased dead space
8. **Early complications of Tracheostomy are all except:**
   a. Haemorrhage b. Apnoea
   c. Pneumothorax d. Stenosis
9. **A female mamta 26 years old presented with gradually increasing respiratory distress since 4 days. She gives h/o hospitalisation and mechanical ventilation with orotracheal intubation for 2 weeks. Now she is diagnosed of having severe tracheal stenosis. What would be the next line of management?**
   a. Laser excision and stent insertion
   b. Steroids
   c. Tracheal dilation
   d. Tracheal resection and end to end anastomosis
10. **Tracheostomy is done at which of these levels:**
    a. T_1 b. T_2
    c. T_3 d. None
11. **A construction worker met with an accident and presented to the trauma centre when a heavy concrete block fell over his face. He was found to have severe maxillofacial and laryngeal injury. He was not able to open his mouth and, on examination, he is found to have multiple fractures and obstruction in nasopharynx as well as oropharynx. In order to maintain a patent airway, the following procedure was done for him. Which of the following options correct define the procedure?**
    a. Submental endotracheal intubation
    b. Emergency tracheostomy
    c. Cricothyroidotomy
    d. Subcutaneous tracheostomy
12. **Laryngofissure is:**
    a. Opening the larynx in midline
    b. Making window in thyroid cartilage
    c. Removal of arytenoids
    d. Removal of epiglottis
13. **All of the following are true about tracheostomy tube except:**
    a. Consists of metallic tubes
    b. Consists of silicone and poly vinyl chloride (PVC) material
    c. Portex tube is ideally changed every 15 days
    d. Cuffed tube used for IPPV
14. **In emergency tracheostomy, the following structures are damaged except:**
    a. Isthmus of thyroid
    b. Inferior thyroid artery
    c. Thyroidea ima artery
    d. Inferior thyroid vein
15. **High tracheostomy is done in:**
    a. Laryngeal carcinoma
    b. Vocal cord palsy
    c. Laryngomalacia
    d. Subglottic stenosis

16. **Most common complication of high tracheostomy is:**
    a. Laryngeal stenosis
    b. Difficult decannulation
    c. Pneumothorax
    d. Subcutaneous emphysema
17. **Palpatory thud and audible slap seen in:**
    a. Tracheal foreign body
    b. Bronchial foreign body
    c. Laryngeal foreign body
    d. None
18. **Which of the following statement is false about tracheostomy:**
    a. Decrease dead space by 30–50%
    b. A frequent problem in infant is difficult decannulation
    c. In emergency tracheostomy, transvers incision is given 2 fingers above the sternal notch
    d. A complication of paediatric tracheostomy is pneumothorax
19. **Site of emergency needle cricothyroidotomy is:**
    a. Between 1st and 2nd tracheal rings
    b. Between 2nd and 3rd tracheal rings
    c. Thyrohyoid membrane
    d. Cricothyroid membrane
20. **Best treatment for lacerated and crush injury of larynx is:**
    a. Cricothyroidotomy
    b. Bag and mask ventilation
    c. Low tracheostomy
    d. None
21. **A 5 years old child having dinner suddenly becomes aphonic and develops respiratory distress. What should be the initial appropriate management?**
    a. Cricothyroidotomy
    b. Emergency tracheostomy
    c. Finger sweep manoeuvre
    d. Heimlich maneouvre
22. **A tracheostomised patient with portex tube in the ward develops sudden complete blockade of tube. Which is the best next step in the management?**
    a. Immediate removal of the tracheostomy tube
    b. Suction of the tube with sodium bicarbonate
    c. Suction of the tube with saline
    d. Transtracheal jet ventilation
23. **Tracheostomy is NOT indicated in:**
    a. Emphysema b. Bronchiectasis
    c. Atelectasis d. Pneumothorax
24. **We have done a supraomohyoid neck dissection thus we have removed:**
    a. Level I, II,III nodes
    b. Level II, III, IV nodes
    c. Level I, II,III, IV nodes
    d. Level I pretracheal and paratracheal nodes
25. **Which is the most common indication of tracheostomy in a child?**
    a. Carcinoma of larynx
    b. Laryngeal diphtheria
    c. Prolonged intubation
    d. Poliomyelitis
26. **$T_3N_1M_0$ carcinoma of larynx is treated by:**
    a. Radiotherapy
    b. Surgery
    c. Concomitant chemoradiation
    d. Surgery and radiotherapy

IMAGE BASED QUESTION

27. **Which of the following is true for the figures given:**
    a. Figs 1 and 4 are safe CSOM and Figs 2 and 3 are unsafe CSOM
    b. Figs 1, 2 and 4 are safe CSOM and Fig. 3 unsafe CSOM.
    c. Figs 1, 3 and 4 are safe CSOM and Fig. 2 unsafe CSOM.
    d. All are safe CSOM.

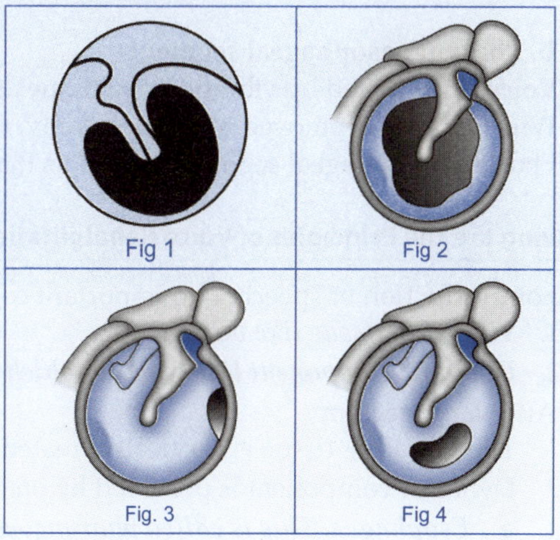

ANSWERS AND EXPLANATIONS

1. **d. He should first undergo laryngectomy and then postoperative radiotherapy.**
   A carcinoma of larynx involving anterior commissure and one sided vocal cord is stage I.
   - Development of perichondritis DOES NOT mean that the perichondrium or cartilage is involved by the tumour.

   Treatment of this is either frontolateral partial laryngectomy or radiotherapy.
   Since the growth is also causing pericondritis of the thyroid cartilage, RT cannot be given.
   This is because one of the complications of RT is perichondritis and RT in this patient might cause necrosis of the cartilage. Therefore, removal of the inflamed perichondrium and cartilage is done surgically.
   Therefore, among the choices given the best option is surgery followed by RT.
   - Even if we assume that perichondritis is due to cartilage involvement.

   This will make it stage IVa glottis carcinoma. The answer remains same because the treatment remains same.

Treatment Policy of Laryngeal Carcinoma

Carcinoma in situ	• *Endoscopic excision with laser with regular follow-up* • *In case of glottis tumour this surgery is called "Cordectomy/Stripping of cord"*
T1 and T2 glottic CA	• Transoral laser microsurgery (TLM) with regular follow-up • Radiotherapy is the 2nd option
T1 and T2 supraglottic CA	• Horizontal partial laryngectomy is the best option • Radiotherapy is the 2nd option
T3 CA of larynx	• Conservative or total laryngectomy followed by radiotherapy along with bilateral neck dissection
T4 CA of larynx	• Total laryngectomy followed by radiotherapy • Radiotherapy plus chemotherapy is 2nd option • Chemotherapeutic agents are: – Cisplatinum – 5-Fluorouracil (5-FU)

2. **b. Pharyngoesophageal segment**
   Voice is produced by vibration of a tissue. Normally it is the vibration of the vocal cords.
   When larynx is removed in laryngectomy, then esophagus is used for speech production.
   Pharyngoesophageal segment is used as the dynamic component.

Following are the Principles of Voice Rehabilitation

For production of speech, two important components are required:
1. ***Vibrating tissue like vocal cord***
2. ***Dynamic component like trachea which is source of air.***

After laryngectomy:
1. The vibrating tissue is surgically created in the remaining pharynx. This is called ***neolarynx.***
2. Dynamic component is provided by one of the two things.
   a. ***Esophagus. This is called pharyngoesophageal speech, or***
   b. ***Trachea and esophagus. This is called tracheoesophageal speech.***

In case of tracheoesophageal speech, a tracheoesophageal fistula is created. In this fistula a one way valve has to be inserted in the fistula.
- ***Blomsinger's valve***
- ***Panje's valve.***

3. **a. Vagus nerve**
   1. **Radical neck dissection**
      Radical neck dissection is a surgery in which ***enblock removal of the first five groups of neck***

lymph nodes (groups I to V) is done along with removal of three important structures. These three structures are:

1. ***Sternocleidomastoid muscle***
2. ***Internal jugular vein and***
3. ***Spinal accessory nerve.***

2. **Modified neck dissection**

   Modified neck dissection is removal of groups I to V lymph nodes with ***preservation of one or more*** of the three structures:
   - Sternomastoid muscle
   - Internal jugular vein
   - Spinal accessory nerve

3. **Selective neck dissection**

   In selective neck dissection, one or more of the lymph nodes groups are preserved along with preservation of all the three structures.

   In other words, it means that in selective neck dissection only few groups of lymph nodes are removed.

4. **c. Metallic tubes are ideally changed every 2–3 days**

   One of the advantages of metallic tracheostomy tubes is that it has two tubes and so it can be left in situ for a long time.

   In other words, frequently changing is not required.

Tracheostomy Tubes

Metallic tubes	Non metallic tubes
• **Made of silver alloy and titanium oxide** • **Has two tubes inner and outer** • **There is NO cuff around it** • **Positive pressure cannot be created** • **Need NOT be changed frequently** • **Is traumatic** • **NOT used commonly**	• Made of polyurethane (Portex tube) • Has only one tube • It has a cuff around it • Positive pressure can be created (IPPV) • Need frequent cleaning and changing • It is atraumatic • Is used more commonly

5. **d. Silicone-T-tube**

   Montgomery tracheostomy tube is a special type of tube which is made of silicon and is 'T' shaped.

   This is used in patients who need tracheostomy but have normal larynx and so can speak.

Advantages of Montgomery Tube

- It has to be left in the trachea for a long period of time
- Patient can speak if larynx is intact

Disadvantages

- It has to be surgically placed inside the trachea
- If it gets blocked, cleaning is very difficult
- Second surgery has to be done when removal of tube is required.

6. **a. Surgical emphysema**

   Surgical emphysema if happens may compress the trachea and cause respiratory distress.

   The most common complication of tracheostomy during surgery is **bleeding** due to trauma to ***anterior thyroid vein.***

   The common complication immediately after the surgery is surgical emphysema.

   Late complication in children is difficult decannulation and late complication in adults is tracheal stenosis.

7. **d. Increased dead space**

   Tracheostomy is a procedure of making an opening in the trachea.

Indications of Tracheostomy

- ***For respiratory obstruction which may be caused by infection, trauma, growths, etc.***
- ***To decrease dead space usually in cases of respiratory insufficiency***

- ***Protection of airway such as pharyngeal secretions, bleed from pharynx***
- ***Removal of excessive secretions from bronchus and lungs (bronchial toilet).***

8. **d. Stenosis**

Stenosis is a late complication of tracheostomy.
Rest of the mentioned conditions are early complications of tracheostomy.

- The most common complication of tracheostomy during surgery is *bleeding* due to trauma to anterior thyroid vein.
- The common complication immediately after the surgery is ***surgical emphysema.***
- Other early complications are ***apnoea, pneumothorax,*** etc.
- Late complication in children is ***difficult decannulation*** and
- Late complication in adults is ***tracheal stenosis and tracheomalacia.***

The gold standard treatment of stenosis is excision of stenosis trachea and end to end anastomosis

9. **c. Tracheal stenosis**

Tracheal stenosis can be divided in the following ways:

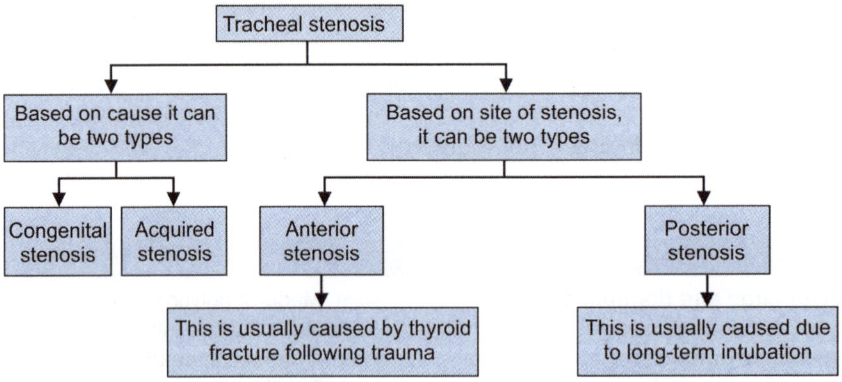

This is a case of acquired posterior stenosis.

Treatment Options for Tracheal Stenosis

- **Endoscopic laser excision** is the best option. Usually CO_2 laser is used. KTP can also be used.
- In case of anterior web a ***keel*** will have to be place for few weeks. However NO keel needed in posterior stenosis.
- For large anterior web, repair through ***laryngofissure*** can be done.
- In severe stenosis of less than 2 cm, there is an option of ***excision followed by end to end anastomosis.***
- For long stenosis, tracheoplasty can be done.
- Steroid alone is NOT an option. Steroid along with surgery may be useful.

10. **c. T_3**

Tracheal Ring

- Incision is preferred in the ***2nd and 3rd tracheal rings (sometimes 3rd and 4th rings).***
- The second common site is ***3rd tracheal ring.***

Note: The best answer is rings T_2 and T_3.
If this is not given in the choices, then T_3 is the accepted answer.

11. **c. Cricothyroidotomy**

A cricothyrotomy (or cricothyroidotomy) is an incision made through the skin and cricothyroid membrane to establish a patent airway during certain life-threatening situations.

Important Indications of Cricothyroidotomy

- Inability to intubate
- Inability to ventilate
- Severe facial or nasal injuries
- Massive midfacial trauma

- Possible cervical spine trauma
- Anaphylaxis
- Chemical inhalation injuries, etc.

12. **a. Opening the larynx in midline**
Laryngofissure is an approach usually used for thyroplasty in cases where endoscopic approach is NOT possible.

13. **c. Portex tube is ideally changed every 15 days**
Note: Also refer to answer no. 4.

14. **b. Inferior thyroid artery**
Isthmus is almost always damaged during emergency procedure.
The vessels that get damaged during emergency tracheostomy are:
- ***Inferior thyroid artery***
- ***Thyroidea ima artery***

Inferior thyroid artery is deep to thyroid gland and therefore is not damaged during this procedure.

15. **a. Laryngeal carcinoma**
Laryngeal carcinoma is the ***only indication for high tracheostomy where tracheostomy is done in 1st ring.***
Patients who require tracheostomy for laryngeal carcinoma may ultimately laryngectomy for carcinoma.
If high tracheostomy is done; than the tracheostomy can be easily removed during laryngectomy.
In these patients, if tracheostomy is in the usual area (ring 2nd and 3rd); then a large part of trachea will have to be removed.

16. **a. Laryngeal stenosis**

Complications

- ***Most common early complication is bleeding.***
- Subcutaneous emphysema is also common
- Late complication in *children* is ***difficult decannulation***
- Late complication in *adult* is ***tracheal stenosis and tracheomalacia***

17. **a. Tracheal foreign body**
- Most common site of foreign in the aerodigestive tract is ***right main bronchus.***
- Most common site of foreign body in the larynx is the glottis (narrowest part of larynx).

But in these two sites the foreign body is firmly stuck and does not move and therefore no sound is produced. Whereas in tracheal foreign body, the foreign body easily moves up and down with respiration producing sound (palpatory thud and auditory slap).

18. **c. In emergency tracheostomy, transvers incision is given 2 fingers above the sternal notch**
Transvers incision is given 2 fingers above the sternal notch is given during elective tracheostomy.
In emergency tracheostomy, vertical incision is given over the trachea.

19. **d. Cricothyroid membrane**
Cricothyroidotomy is an emergency procedure in which a ***wide bore needle is passed through the cricothyroid membrane (a membrane between thyroid cartilage and cricoids cartilage).***

20. **c. Low tracheostomy**
In lacerated and crush injury of larynx, the larynx is crushed and obstructed. In such a case air cannot pass through the larynx and so bag and mask ventilation is not possible.
If the lower part of larynx, i.e., cricoids is damaged, then cricothyroidotomy is not useful.
In such patients, low tracheostomy is preferred so as to avoid further damage to the larynx.

21. **d. Heimlich maneouvre**
This is most probably a care of foreign body in the larynx (aspiration of food).
In laryngeal foreign body, Heimlich maneouvre is the first line of management.

22. **a. Immediate removal of the tracheostomy tube**
Blockade of the tracheostomy tube is very common. To avoid respiratory obstruction in such patients, regular suction of the tube with sodium bicarbonate is done commonly.

But if the tube is completely and suddenly blocked, the better option is removal of the completely blocked tube.

23. **d. Pneumothorax**
Pneumothorax is one of the complications of tracheostomy.
Rest of the conditions may require prolonged ventilation. For prolonged ventilation, tracheostomy is the preferred.

24. **a. Level I, II, III nodes**
Supraomohyoid neck dissection is a type of selective neck dissection. In this surgery, the first three groups of lymph nodes (I,II,III nodes) are removed.
This surgery is done for oral cavity tumours and oropharyngeal tumours.
Neck dissections are divided into four main types
- ***Radical neck dissection***
- ***Modified neck dissection***
- ***Selective neck dissection***
- ***Extended neck dissection***

Radical Neck Dissection (RND)

This is enblock removal of lymph nodes between **levels I to V**, along the following structures
- **Sternomastoid muscle**
- **Internal jugular vein**
- **Spinal accessory nerve**

Many types of incisions are used for radical neck dissection. Few common ones are:
- ***Schobinger incision***. This is the ***most common incision*** used for (RND)
- Hetter incision
- McFee incision, etc.

Modified Neck Dissection

Modified neck dissection is removal of groups I to V lymph nodes with preservation of one or more of the three structures:
- Sternomastoid muscle
- Internal jugular vein
- Spinal accessory nerve

Depending on the structures that are preserved, it is divided into types.

Types	Structures preserved
Type I	Structure preserved is • Spinal accessory nerve
Type II	Structures preserved are • Spinal accessory nerve and • Internal jugular vein
Type III	Structures preserved are • Spinal accessory nerve • Internal jugular vein and • Sternocleidomastoid muscle
Note: In type III modified neck dissection, the function of all the three structures are preserved. Therefore this is also called ***functional neck dissection.***	

SELECTIVE NECK DISSECTION

In selective neck dissection, one or more of the lymph nodes groups are preserved along with preservation of all the three structures.
In other words, it means that in selective neck dissection only few groups of lymph nodes are removed.
They are of the following types:

Supraomohyoid neck dissection	Lateral neck dissection	Posterolateral neck dissection	Anterior neck dissection
Groups I, II, III	Groups II, III, IV	Groups II, III, IV, V	Group VI
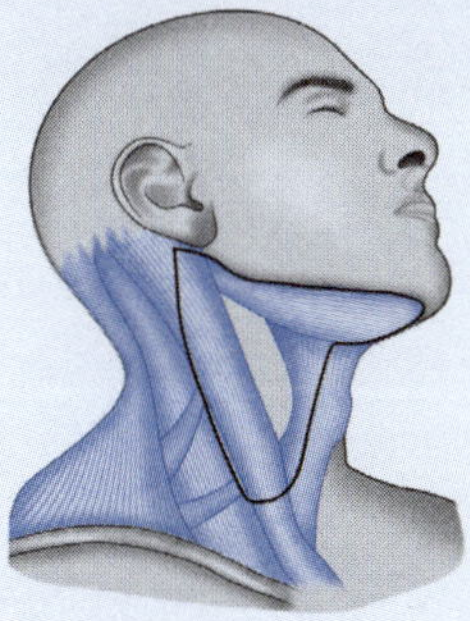	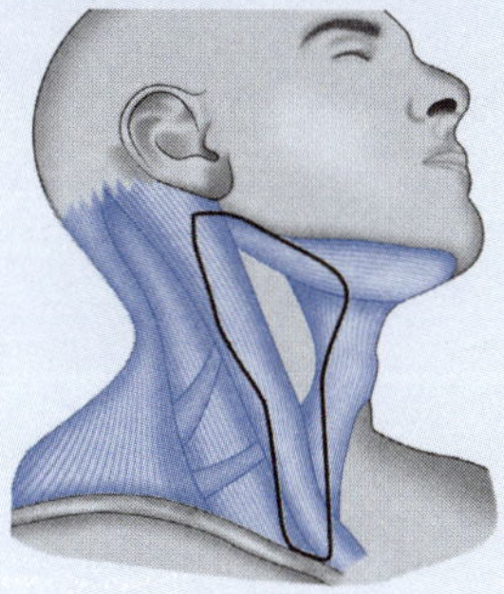	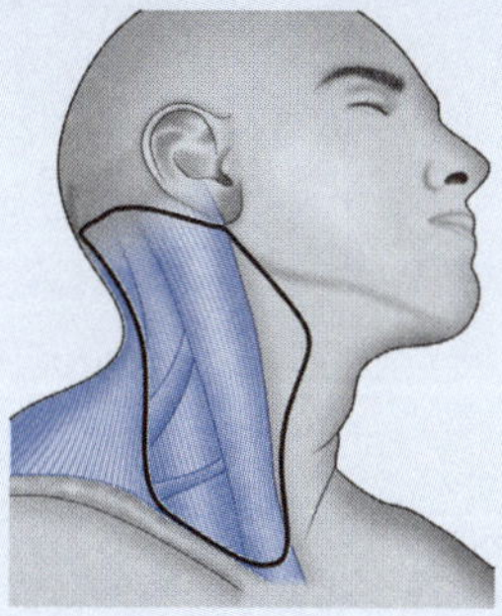	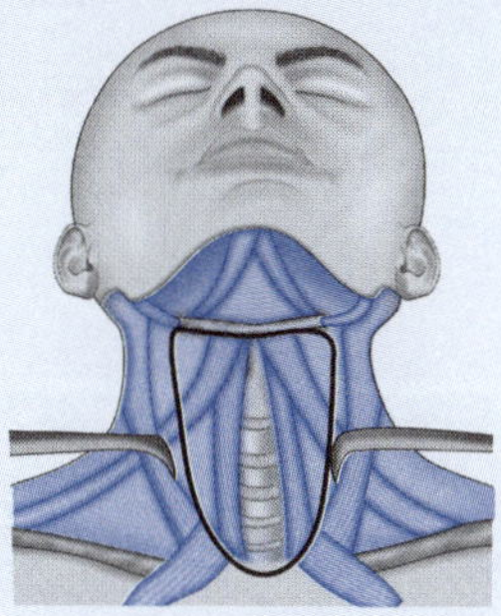

Extended Neck Dissection

In this, additional structures are also removed.

25. **c. Prolonged intubation**
There are a number of conditions where prolonged ventilation is required in children. As already discussed, for prolonged ventilation, tracheostomy is better than intubation.

26. **c. Concomitant chemoradiation**

IMAGE BASED ANSWER

27. **b. Fig 1, 2 and 4 are safe CSOM and fig 3 unsafe CSOM.**